Praise for *The Grain-Free, Sugar-Free, Dairy-Free Family Cookbook*

"As a busy mom and nutrition therapist, trying to strategize meals that everyone in my family will eat on a grain-, sugar-, and dairy-free diet can be exhausting. Leah Webb's book takes the work out of the daily 'what are we going to eat?' conundrum. The recipes are doable even on busy weekdays and have high kid-appeal. Her raw, relatable experiences with feeding and loving her children round this book into a parenting guide, nutrition primer, and cookbook. The best family focused cookbook I've ever come across."

—**Jess Higgins Kelley**, coauthor of *The Metabolic Approach to Cancer* and *Bioregulatory Medicine*

"Mothers are my heroes! And here another mother has had a steep learning curve in understanding how to heal her children. Having helped her own family, Leah Webb is now generously sharing what she learned on her journey. Parents will find this book very helpful! It is full of practical tips and good ideas on how to feed children from day to day and make the whole process happy and doable."

—**Natasha Campbell-McBride**, MD, author of *Gut and Psychology Syndrome*

"Leah Webb's *The Grain-Free, Sugar-Free, Dairy-Free Family Cookbook* should be in the hands of any family looking to manage multiple food allergies or simply eat healthfully in the face of chronic illness. If you are looking to learn the hows and whys of dietary change in an approachable way, as well as try some kid- and family-friendly recipes and meal plans, this book is for you!"

—**Mickey Trescott**, NTP, author of *The Autoimmune Paleo Cookbook* and *The Nutrient-Dense Kitchen*

"*The Grain-Free, Sugar-free, Dairy-free Family Cookbook* should not be seen as just part of an unusual dietary niche as more and more families are now faced with illnesses and will find important solutions in this comprehensive book. Leah Webb tells the compelling story of her own journey in a compassionate and informed manner. Inspired by her family's serious health conditions, she explored a grain-free, dairy-free, sugar-free diet due to its purported benefits on gut health and found it changed the way she cared for her two children. While filled with many time- and kid-friendly recipes, this book is more than just a cookbook. Practical strategies are offered to assist families transitioning to a healthful way of eating and in regaining health while on a budget. Sections on creating a kitchen, stocking the pantry, and meal planning offer practical advice for all readers and eaters, and the resources and thorough bibliography will help those desiring further inquiry. Make room for this book on your kitchen counter!"

—**Michelle Perro**, MD, author of *What's Making Our Children Sick?*

"Us mamas who walk the walk and have found the beautiful power of food as medicine want to shout from the rooftops to prevent others from enduring the pain of chronic illness. As we begin to understand the intricacies and differences of our microbiomes, we are realizing more and more that personalized medicine and intuitive eating are vital. Returning to a baseline with real food is where the magic unfolds. Yet for so many, with the swirling of life's busyness, this seems impossible. Leah not only inspires us with her own honest reflections, she sets us up for delicious success by teaching us the rudimentary and lost life skill of cooking. It does not have to be complicated, but you do have to be dedicated—a small price to pay for health. This is a must-read for anyone involved in the health and well-being of children! It's valuable information we all need to hear."

—**Hilary Boynton**, author of *The Heal Your Gut Cookbook*

THE
GRAIN-FREE
SUGAR-FREE
DAIRY-FREE
FAMILY COOKBOOK

Simple and Delicious Recipes for Cooking with Whole Foods on a Restrictive Diet

Leah Webb, MPH, CHC

Chelsea Green Publishing
White River Junction, Vermont
London, UK

Unless otherwise noted, all photographs by Thomas C. Webb.
Photographs on pages 87, 98, 111, 131, 159, 180, 196, 226, 232, and 259 from iStock.com.

Project Manager: Patricia Stone
Editor: Makenna Goodman
Copy Editor: Diane Durrett
Proofreader: Laura Jorstad
Indexer: Linda Hallinger
Designer: Melissa Jacobson

Printed in the United States of America.
First printing March, 2019.
10 9 8 7 6 5 4 3 2 1   19 20 21 22 23

Our Commitment to Green Publishing

Chelsea Green sees publishing as a tool for cultural change and ecological stewardship. We strive to align our book manufacturing practices with our editorial mission and to reduce the impact of our business enterprise in the environment. We print our books and catalogs on chlorine-free recycled paper, using vegetable-based inks whenever possible. This book may cost slightly more because it was printed on paper that contains recycled fiber, and we hope you'll agree that it's worth it. Chelsea Green is a member of the Green Press Initiative (greenpressinitiative.org), a nonprofit coalition of publishers, manufacturers, and authors working to protect the world's endangered forests and conserve natural resources. *The Grain-Free, Sugar-Free, Dairy-Free Family Cookbook* was printed on paper supplied by LSC Communications that contains at least 10% postconsumer recycled fiber.

Library of Congress Cataloging-in-Publication Data
Names: Webb, Leah M., 1983– author.
Title: The grain-free, sugar-free, dairy-free family cookbook : simple and delicious recipes for cooking with whole foods on a
   restrictive diet / Leah M. Webb, MPH, CHC.
Description: White River Junction, Vermont : Chelsea Green Publishing, [2019] | Includes bibliographical references and index.
Identifiers: LCCN 2018047428 | ISBN 9781603587594 (pbk.) | ISBN 9781603587600 (ebook)
Subjects: LCSH: Low-carbohydrate diet—Recipes. | Gluten-free diet—Recipes. | Sugar-free diet—Recipes.
Classification: LCC RM237.73 .W43 2019 | DDC 641.5/6383—dc23
LC record available at https://lccn.loc.gov/2018047428

Chelsea Green Publishing
85 North Main Street, Suite 120
White River Junction, VT 05001
(802) 295-6300
www.chelseagreen.com

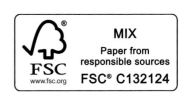

This book is dedicated to June and Owen,
the teachers I never knew I needed.
May they be a reminder to us all
that light comes from the darkness . . .
as long as you open the door to let it in.

contents

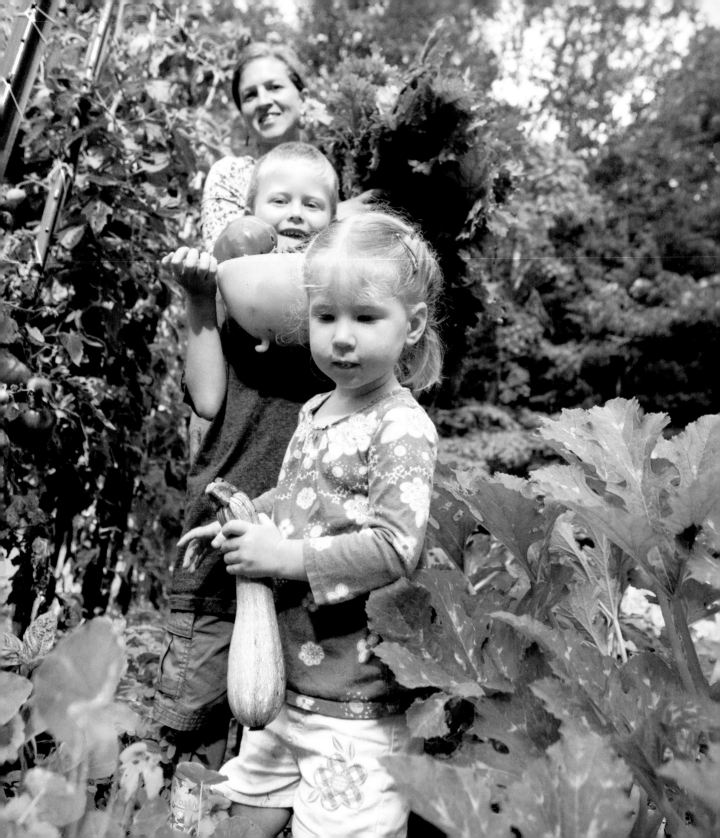

When Crisis Compels Transformation

I'm proud to say that I'm a fourth-generation gardener with a knack for cooking. As a child I was often required to help maintain our large vegetable garden, and it's a chore that has served me well in my adult life. I was also taught that home-cooked meals can be joyfully prepared on a daily basis and that healthy food takes priority. These traditions that were ingrained in me from a young age are now being passed along to my two kids, Owen and June.

I became a mother shortly after completing my master's degree in public health. While I was trained to work in environmental health sciences (think OSHA or the EPA), I knew that my education would propel me into a career of helping families follow healthier diets. After four years completing a bachelor's degree and three years of graduate work, the take-home message was that nutritional status affects most aspects of disease etiology (causes). While many exposures are out of our control—air pollution, water quality, indoor air pollution in public spaces—we all choose what to eat. So when it came to food, I knew that I wanted to make appropriate choices, especially once I became responsible for cultivating the early development of my own children.

I followed all of the rules while pregnant with my first child. I ate vegetables, walked daily, choked down my horse pill of a prenatal vitamin, read all the books, and did my best to nurture the growing human inside my womb. Owen, like the other babies born from small women in my family, was characteristically large—a healthy nine-pound, two-ounce baby who neared the 99th percentile for height and weight. But his weight suddenly plummeted, and at his four-month visit I learned that he had dropped to the 45th percentile over the course of just a few months. Something was wrong.

Owen's inability to gain weight was due to an underlying dairy allergy, the first of many food-related surprises from Owen. To say that he was sensitive is a gross understatement. We slowly learned that he had an anaphylactic (severe, potentially life-threatening) allergy to wheat, eggs, cashews, pistachios, almonds, and oddly enough, seaweed. Less easily discovered were his other food intolerances—coconut, beets, sesame, soy, melon, and cacao. Luckily, he has outgrown some of the allergies and many of the intolerances, but managing Owen's sensitive gut required creativity in the kitchen, persistence, and a whole lot of diaper cream. I had to adjust my boundaries surrounding food, which wasn't easy. In fact, it felt like one of the most challenging things I had ever done. My friends and family were sure I'd turned into a neurotic mother, fretting over the simplest foods as if they were kryptonite.

What these good-intentioned folks didn't understand was that trying to keep a constant watchful eye on an allergic toddler was exhausting. Dinner dates? Not fun. Potlucks? Even worse. Large parties? Stress city. What if Owen innocently grabbed a piece of bread or God forbid a cookie from the food table when someone wasn't watching? If you've ever seen someone in anaphylaxis (life-threatening allergic reaction) then you understand the severity of our situation. My husband and I would take shifts—one parent enjoyed the company of friends while the other watched over Owen like a hawk. We'd switch roles every 20 minutes or so, but sometimes the watchful effort wasn't worth the struggle and we'd skip social engagements altogether. Owen's issues have become less problematic, because he can now voice that he simply can't eat some of the foods that most people enjoy, but those first few years were difficult.

At some point during all of the stress of sorting through Owen's food allergies, he developed asthma. It started as a persistent dry cough at night, a symptom that someone inexperienced with asthma wouldn't recognize as being a threat, that soon developed into emergency room–worthy bouts of impaired breathing. We lived a mile from the closest hospital at the time, and proximity to 24-hour emergency care became an important criterion when looking for our next home. I remember one of the scariest nights when Owen coughed so hard and for so long that he simply couldn't catch his breath. He started vomiting from his inability to breathe and I silently hoped that he'd pass out, a last-chance mechanism that would prevent his situation from elevating past the point of no return. We rushed him to the ER where he quickly recovered after receiving inhaled and oral steroids, a routine that was all too familiar to his young little body. Over time, as we got to know Owen's symptoms, managing his condition became less frightening, but I spent a lot of time feeling like we were teetering on the edge of irreversible disaster.

My expectations of having two children shifted due to Owen's sensitive condition. What if we had another child with asthma and allergies? What if the allergies weren't the same and we had a whole additional set of restrictions? Some people tried to persuade me that the scenario would be much easier the second time, but I wasn't convinced. It's hard for someone to comprehend the anxiety that accompanies the protection of an allergic child in those early years. I didn't want to relive the stress of deciphering the unknowns. Despite my hesitations, my husband and I learned that I was pregnant again right around Owen's second birthday.

A girl this time. She was smaller, only eight pounds, four ounces, and she came bursting into this world as if she had a God-given purpose to fulfill. While Owen was the sensitive child, June appeared to be sturdier. I don't know how to explain it, but our acupuncturist confirmed my belief when she told me that June has particularly strong qi (in Chinese medicine this refers to one's life force). But June was just two weeks old when her pediatrician handed me a piece of paper and pointed to a series of letters and numbers that had been circled in the middle of the page, the results from June's routine newborn screening for common metabolic diseases. The results read "DF508," which meant that June had the most common genetic mutation for cystic fibrosis (CF). Alone, this mutation meant nothing, but the results warranted a visit to the CF clinic in Burlington, Vermont, to confirm the absence of a second CF-causing mutation. If June carried just the one gene, DF508, she would be deemed a carrier, but if a second gene was found, she would have the disease.

I was reassured that we had nothing to worry about. June didn't fit the description of a typical child with CF, but our doctor also believed that further testing was in her best interest. We made the hour-long journey to Burlington, strapped an archaic electrode machine on June's arm that stimulated the sweat glands, and waited as her sweat was meticulously collected. It would be analyzed later that day. People with CF have abnormally high concentrations of salt in their sweat, so the test was nothing more than an elegant method to measure salinity. Pretty simple.

We returned home and I didn't think much of it. After all, I had been convinced that June was likely a carrier and I had nothing to worry about. But then we got the call. I hadn't prepared myself for the worst. I assumed I was just going through the motions of pleasing the medical community while fully knowing that we'd get a positive outcome. I was wrong. I could say that I should've prepared myself, but how is a postpartum mother supposed to prepare herself for the worst news of her life? "Your daughter has cystic fibrosis. There is no cure."

While I wish that I could tell you that this day was difficult, but it eventually turned out to be a day full of motivational life lessons, I cannot. I will instead tell you that this was the worst day of my life. I lost a small piece of my inherent joy on that day. Never before had I felt so broken. The one-page CF Fact Sheet that I had been given earlier in the day shook every part of my soul. I couldn't stop reflecting on the bullet point stating that the life expectancy for someone with CF was around 27 years of age. I've since learned that this number is actually closer to 40 and that it's even higher in countries such as Canada that have better access to health care, but this number made me feel physically ill. My sweet baby, just two weeks old, was staring up at me and all I could think was that I would only get to enjoy her for the next 27 years. I didn't know anything else about CF except that it was going to break my heart in a way that nothing ever had.

The next few months were a crash course into a world that I denied being part of. Even when we got the results from June's genetic test that identified her second CF-causing mutation, 3272-26A>G, my husband and I often discussed a repeated sweat test. How could this possibly happen to *us*? Were *we* destined to care for a sick child? Would *our* child lead a life of suffering? Acceptance didn't come easily.

I don't know how else to describe the next eight months other than to say I was grieving. Part of this process involved numerous late nights spent frantically searching for an obscure cure. I don't always trust the advice of the medical community with their heavy reliance on pharmaceuticals and often complete neglect of preventive care, so I somehow hoped that independent research would reveal a solution to prevent the devastation of disease in a way unbeknownst to the professionals.

I never found the cure. I also found a complete lack of compelling evidence to show that pharmaceuticals wouldn't be necessary in June's life. Managing her disease was going to require that we approach preventive care from multiple angles—diet, lifestyle, antibiotics, herbs, drugs, and physical therapy. And then there was accepting the fact that much of her disease would be out of my control, an aspect of genetic disease management that has turned out to be the most heartbreaking and challenging part of the journey. There is no correcting her faulty genes; I cannot change that.

Now for the silver lining. CF, like many illnesses, is an inflammatory disease. Luckily, diet goes a long way toward controlling inflammation. I researched anti-inflammatory diets and came to the conclusion that a GAPS diet would be beneficial in establishing a healthy immune response early on. Dr. Natasha Campbell-McBride developed the GAPS—Gut and Psychology Syndrome—diet as a primary treatment for autism spectrum disorders and other conditions that she theorized to originate in the gut. Her belief is that repairing the gut using a specific combination of healing foods can result in a reversal of the child's condition. Establishing a healthy immune response for my daughter would mean developing a healthy gut, and the GAPS diet stood out as the most beneficial diet to achieve those results (see the *GAPS Diet and Early Foods for Baby* section on page 32 for more information regarding GAPS). My daughter was solely breastfed until six months of age, at which point I introduced homemade bone broths and healthy fats such as lard, organic coconut oil, organic olive oil, and avocado oil. I then introduced non-starchy vegetables including leeks, zucchinis, greens, and others that were boiled and blended in bone broth and fat to make simple soups. Around the same time I started to prepare simple egg preparations. Next came the well-cooked meats including beef, pork, chicken, and fish. Fruits and starchy vegetables weren't introduced until around ten months of age. Fermented vegetables, juice from ferments, and probiotics were added to foods throughout this entire process as a way to establish a healthy microbiota. Beans were introduced, but not until my daughter was around 18 months of age. I never introduced dairy, grains, sugar, or any type of processed oil, and with the rare exception, my daughter doesn't eat these foods to this day.

The diet I chose is slightly different from a complete GAPS diet since fermented raw dairy lies at the cornerstone of a true GAPS baby. I explain the depth of my reasons for avoiding dairy in chapter 1 (see *The Dairy Debacle* on page 20), but one of my primary reasons is because dairy is a mucus-producing food. The CF lungs suffer from abnormally thick and sticky mucus, so avoiding dairy is a choice that I continue to make for my daughter.

Here's what's amazing—while we started this diet for my daughter, our whole family has benefited from its implementation. My five-year-old son now requires limited medications to fully manage his asthma. (For those who are curious, his current dose of Qvar [beclomethasone dipropionate HFA] is at 40mcg/day. He takes just one puff every evening, but we're hoping to experiment with natural alternatives under the care of an integrative physician in order to completely ditch the medication. Regardless, this is an extremely low dose, especially for someone who has multiple environmental allergies. We've even had periods of time where he's been able to stop taking his daily dose of Qvar entirely, but this is challenging to maintain since some of his environmental allergies seem to be fairly persistent triggers for him.) Overall, I'd say his condition has improved since starting this diet and I believe that it will only continue to improve over the coming years.

Owen had his most severe anaphylactic reaction to date in November 2018 while I was halfway through writing this book. I questioned whether we were actually making headway with him, but the reaction prompted us to review some of his other allergies that had been diagnosed when he was a small child. Avoiding multiple foods can be challenging and stressful, so because Owen hadn't been tested since he was quite small our allergist felt it necessary to retest him so we could fully understand the extent and severity of his food allergies. The results from these tests revealed that Owen is now able to eat nuts, eggs, seaweed, and dairy without suffering from any type of noticeable reaction (he still doesn't eat dairy because I believe it's not in his best interest, but the potential for major reactions is gone). Owen is actually outgrowing some of his allergies! His wheat and barley allergies remain, but our list of avoided foods has gotten a whole heck of a lot smaller over the past four years. Did this result stem from our diet and my dedication to avoiding chemicals as much as possible? I'll never know for sure, but I know that he's not getting worse, which is always a possibility in kids with multiple food allergies.

My husband is also severely asthmatic, and exhibits many of the sensitive traits of my son (although to a lesser degree). Yet after a year of following this refined way of eating, he has completely stopped relying on daily meds. He has depended on varying medications since a very young age, so this transformation is quite impressive. Interestingly, the change for my son started only six months after we had been following the diet, which is perhaps a testament to the dynamic nature of a child's body.

A grain-free, sugar-free, dairy-free diet has been hugely beneficial for my family. We've experienced major improvements in medical conditions for my son and husband, I've drastically improved my mood by eliminating sugar, and my daughter has experienced limited digestive issues related to CF. My daughter's success is partially attributed to her genetic makeup (she has a class V mutation, meaning that she maintains residual function of CFTR proteins and is pancreas sufficient—does not require digestive enzymes with every meal—unlike the majority of people with CF; see the *Cystic Fibrosis and Our Journey with June* section, page 6, for more info regarding cystic fibrosis) and the luck of the draw, but I'm comforted by the fact that we've included diet as one part of a multifaceted preventive approach to health. How much of her success is due to diet? I'll likely never know, but why would I stop doing something if it seems to be working?

We're certainly not your typical family when it comes to health and medical needs, but it's not uncommon for families to seek a similar type of diet to help improve their own unique situation, whatever that may be. Our story is our own, but I know we're not alone. I want others to be inspired in knowing that a diagnosis doesn't mean the end. It means that you just have to work that much harder and with that much more passion to achieve the results you want. In fact, a diagnosis can sometimes mean the beginning of something you never thought possible. I'm not sure who said it originally, but I'll say it, too: *Not all storms come to disrupt your life; some come to clear your path.*

I also want people to remember that an ounce of prevention is worth a pound of cure. If you stumbled upon this book as a perfectly healthy individual, but you are interested in improving your diet, I say go for it! I'll be one of the first to tell you that managing disease is a path that's best avoided. And most of the foods available to us in grocery stores and restaurants will eventually make us sick. Changing your diet now can save you time, heartache, and money in the future. Don't settle for mediocrity when it comes to diet when the alternative is so much better.

I never imagined I'd be sharing my story and food wisdom in a book, especially a cookbook. Like most of us, I assumed my life would be different. Writing about food obstacles and solutions in the treatment of my children's unique medical issues never occurred to me as an imaginable future. As a young woman reflecting on my hopes of becoming a mother, I didn't even consider the possibility that life with children would mean having medical equipment piled in a corner of the living room, medications scattered throughout the house, frequent doctor visits with multiple specialists, an hour of daily treatments and therapies (more when sick), epinephrine and Benadryl, lists of restrictions and rules (each kid has their own), and living with stress of this magnitude. However, I can say with 100 percent certainty that I wouldn't appreciate life and health in the same way had I not been gifted these two special children who are a daily reminder that without health you have nothing. And for that reason, achieving optimal health is worth putting in a damn good effort.

The opportunity to write this book fell into my lap, which I've been told almost never happens. When I was in the early stages of grieving my daughter's disease, a friend wrote to me saying that she hoped I would someday find the gifts that come from the darkness. I believe this book is one such gift, and my hope is to offer parents like me a tool and platform to help improve their families' quality of life.

I chose a grain-free, sugar-free, dairy-free diet because of its benefits for gut health and its associated reduction in inflammation, an extremely desirable response in the treatment of any disease or condition. But as we began our journey, I quickly discovered that many of the recipes I found were attempts at mimicking traditional foods like mac 'n' cheese, a food that I'm sorry to say is impossible to re-create without grains and dairy. Store-bought Paleo Diet products proved equally disappointing for their inclusion of varying starches—potato, tapioca, arrowroot, and the like. Many grain-free recipes featured similar issues. The presence of sugar in recipes and packaged foods was in my opinion the worst of the issues. It was the number one food that I wanted to avoid. Marketers would have you believe that because their processed foods are gluten-free, all natural, heart healthy, low fat, or sugar-free, you're buying a healthy product. But this couldn't be further from the truth. When we learned that my son had a wheat allergy I remember being so disappointed to find that not only did store-bought gluten-free breads have the worst texture of any bread I had ever tasted, but this terrible texture was achieved using chemicals, fillers, starches, and other food-like substances that aren't worth eating. (Note that this microscopic loaf of a health hazard cost around $8.) Believe me when I say that many gluten-free products are some of the least healthy and least affordable options in the grocery store. And while I certainly have a handful of gluten-free products in my pantry that our family enjoys, the majority of them should be avoided. Attempts to re-create traditional grain-based foods without grains equates to a product full of chemicals and inscrutable ingredients. The bottom line is that we couldn't improve our diet simply by changing from grains to highly processed grain-free foods. We had to instead make some major upgrades and learn to cook more meals from real, whole ingredients—a skill that is mostly lost in today's busy world. I realized what we needed was more than just a new diet; we needed an entirely new way of looking at food and cooking.

As the fervently dedicated mother that I am, I started cooking more than I ever had. I was determined to supply my family with real, whole foods to support their health in the best way possible. Quality breakfasts, lunches, dinners, and snacks soon began flying out of the kitchen. But there was a downside: I was never leaving the kitchen. Our diet had turned me into the household cook and my other interests and responsibilities were being pushed to the wayside. I'm a firm believer that joy and happiness are two of the most important contributors to health. Although our diet was drastically helping us to reduce inflammation, it was also taking away precious time from other health-promoting activities such as spending quality time with family, exercise, and even sleep. If we were to continue life on this diet I knew I had to find a more sustainable, balanced approach to meal preparation.

So I started buying and cooking in bulk, meal planning, eating more leftovers, freezing leftovers, multitasking in the kitchen, asking for more help, and implementing numerous other tactics that slowly made this diet feel more sustainable. And now it's just a part of life! And although we stick with the diet for the most part, we occasionally cheat and eat convenience foods that aren't necessarily part of the diet. I occasionally buy a gluten- and dairy-free frozen pizza for my kids to share, and my husband and I share a grain-free version that's loaded with cheese. We always stay within the important boundaries necessary to maintain each individual's health, but a convenience food night allows us to enjoy a relaxing evening that requires little prep or cleanup. I've even cut the pizza boxes into "plates" so that I have zero dishes to clean. Everyone eats a salad while the pizzas bake and we enjoy our packaged Friday night dinner in front of the television. This book is not about turning you into a superhero, but about making it *work for you*. And making life enjoyable.

One of the takeaways I hope you get from reading through the following chapters is that life is about progress, not perfection. Sometimes that means letting go in one area so that you can gain some peace in another. Hopefully this book will help you achieve your own version of balance, one with less sugar, grains, and dairy, and more home-cooked meals.

I'll also say that this diet doesn't necessarily *feel* restrictive most of the time. I genuinely enjoy eating a grain-free, sugar-free, dairy-free diet and all of the nourishing foods that come along with it. I can't imagine going back to eating any other way now that we've grown accustomed to such a high standard of quality. Likewise, I'm quick to observe the negative way in which my body responds to unhealthy foods when we do break our own food "rules." There's a great deal of reward that comes with following a healthy diet, and my body clearly appreciates my efforts.

My hope is that you don't just treat this book like any other cookbook. This book is more about the process of food and how we can achieve healing when we commit to a better way of eating and living, and less about the perfect combination of herbs and spices. Tasty food doesn't have to be complicated. In fact, sometimes kids enjoy simple foods more than a complex mix of unfamiliar ingredients and flavors. Besides, this book is written to simplify the process of everyday food prep for a family. Why would I include a plethora of complicated recipes? I want someone to read this book, implement my strategies, use the menus, and prepare the recipes as everyday solutions to health and longevity. I want my readers (you!) to have success.

I hope you enjoy reading about my family, our tragedies, our solutions, and our celebrations. And most of all, I hope you enjoy the simple yet delicious and healthy recipes that I've shared with you and your family. A grain-free, sugar-free, dairy-free diet has been a true gift to my own family in more ways than I can explain, and I am certain that other families will experience similar benefits. This book is one of my gifts from the darkness that I have the joy and pleasure of sharing with you all.

How to Use This Book

In my health coaching practice I've noticed time and again that almost anyone can prepare a recipe, but cooking from scratch for nearly every single meal becomes a labor-intensive task that most aren't willing to take on. In this book I'll show you how to get organized, get cooking, and stay sane while keeping you and your family healthy. The only caveat is that you have to agree to be patient, commit to completing the recommendations in each chapter, and not give up when it's challenging, because it will be challenging at times.

Please don't immediately flip to the recipe section and ignore the rest of the contents like we so often do with other cookbooks. I suggest you instead start by reading chapter 1, *The Restrictive Diet for Optimal Health*. You're clearly interested in a grain-free, sugar-free, dairy-free family diet, but this chapter will help affirm your interest in this nutrient-dense, health-promoting way of eating. It's easy to lose interest or motivation with a change in diet if you don't understand the full reason behind its implementation. So do yourself a favor and start by soaking up some intellectual motivation!

You'll next want to gain a better understanding of how to get the whole family involved by reading chapter 2, *Feeding the Kids—Get Your Game Face On!* You simply will not have time to prepare multiple meals to cater to the desires of your kids if you're cooking from scratch every day, three to five times a day. Plus, your kids will need to start eating the same foods enjoyed by the entire family, which means you might need to brace yourself for some pushback. This chapter is designed to encourage and affirm your desire to abandon the picky eating trap and create healthier habits for the entire family. I've included tips on how to get your kids more involved, so that they're more likely to accept these new dietary changes. Incorporating kids in healthy eating habits is one of the central themes for this book, so please don't skip this chapter! If you're a grandparent, know that you're not off the hook. Grandparents are especially notorious for providing grandkids with foods that parents might not approve of. While this tradition may have been acceptable in the past, we're now in the midst of a major public health crisis due to drastic decline in food quality and extreme overconsumption of chemical-laden foods. Our children are being exposed to foods that weren't even thought possible 50 years ago, and these foods are resulting in severe negative health consequences. We all (grandparents, parents, teachers, educators, and anyone involved in the lives of children) need to start being part of the solution if we're ever going to get ahead of ourselves.

Chapters 3 and 4, *Get Prepared, You Can Do This!* and *The Importance of Meal Planning*, are the workhorses of this book. I simply wouldn't be able to cook so many meals from scratch if I wasn't prepared to do so. I've outlined every possible suggestion, from stocking your pantry to reducing your material possessions, so that you can get organized and ready to cook. If your freezer or pantry isn't stocked with the right foods, if you don't have the appropriate equipment, and if you have no clue how to organize your time, then you're going to fall short of your expectations. You need the information in these chapters to make this diet work!

Once you've implemented the organizational pieces from these preparatory chapters, you'll have the pleasure of perusing my absolute favorite grain-free, sugar-free, dairy-free family recipes, everything from Plantain Muffins for breakfast, to an Apple Spice Bundt Cake for dessert. I've included notes throughout the recipes with suggestions for batch cooking and meal planning to help you stay organized and find success in the kitchen.

There is an extensive appendices section where you'll find the following: four weeks of menus (including ingredients lists to help with managing grocery shopping); menus for kids' packed lunches; a list of recipes that freeze well; and menus for holiday meals and celebrations. Additionally supplementary resources are available on my website (deeprootedwellness.com) in which I outline daily prep recommendations for the menus and explain how to double and freeze meals to be used in later weeks. The menus can be reformulated to meet your family's specific needs, but you should follow a similar pattern in that you prep and cook in advance, and freeze leftovers whenever possible. Organizing your time in the kitchen is critical, and these menus are designed to help you become an efficient cook while investing as little time as possible.

My hope is that you're patient and persistent enough to keep working toward a healthier diet, and that this book is the catalyst for dramatic change. So let's get organized, get cooking, and keep sane while doing it!

chapter one

The Restrictive Diet for Optimal Health

Science repeatedly demonstrates that poor diet leads to chronic and acute illness, but I've observed that the consequences of such a diet don't always manifest in ways that science would predict. To truly understand the benefits of healthy eating you have to look beyond the textbook definition of disease and practice the lost art of listening to your body and observing the outcomes.

I haven't always been good at receiving cues from my own body, but my family's adoption of a restrictive diet free of grains, sugar, and dairy has helped me learn some positive listening skills. Although my kids may not consciously recognize the diet's benefits in the same way that my husband and I do, the results have been clear. So when I talk about a restrictive diet, I'm also talking about a choice to optimize your family's health. Families who are not in crisis mode might find my approach extreme and may instead favor a more moderate approach to their diet. These families can partially follow the included recommendations. But I've included details specific enough for those who may be in crisis so much that most available food choices, even in small quantities, can contribute to negative health outcomes in their families.

Processed flours, refined sugars, preservatives, fillers, refined oils, food dyes, and all of these other food-like substances are slowly making us sick, but even many of the restrictive diets encourage the use of highly processed foods. My approach is about *pure* food, such as flours made from seeds that are ground up right before you add it to a recipe. The bottom line is that I don't believe processed foods are worth eating, even if they may "technically" fit into a restrictive diet.

The hardest part of restrictive diets is that limiting your food choices can feel a lot like self-deprivation. What's a life without cheesy crackers or indulging in copious amounts of ice cream? Isn't this what makes a happy childhood? Even though these small "rewards" can be what get us through the day at times, the problem with this thinking is that we have created a false perception of reward. For example, we've all been trained to believe that food, especially sweets, makes an excellent reward for good behavior. I was at the playground recently when a mother told me the story of keeping M&M's on the back of her toilet as rewards for potty training. I was slightly put off by the idea of storing food on the toilet, but even more put off by teaching another human that good behavior equates to sweets, especially behavior that is so basic to the daily routine of being human. How have we gotten here? How many times in my life have I felt the need to reward myself with a brownie or ice cream when I'm feeling successful or when I've had a particularly bad day? Countless! If you're anything like me this is a habit you could happily live without.

At some point in my life I started to actually listen to my body. I came to realize that eating sugar made me feel fantastic for all of 30 minutes. But I noticed that the sugar crash left me irritable and feeling like I needed more. The cyclical deceit put my body at the mercy of variable blood sugar and hazed my brain. I was knee-deep in brain fog, addicted to sugar (God knows what it was doing to my microbiome), and feeling like my kids were the most annoying humans on the face of this planet. And I ate sweet treats as a reward? *This* was how I rewarded myself, by surrendering to legal substance abuse and living life on an emotional roller coaster. Shouldn't reward feel better than this?

When I talk about a restrictive diet, I'm talking about an act of self-love and respect. Next time you feel yourself craving a treat or another unhealthy food, first ask yourself whether you're making a loving, nourishing choice for your body. Will the crash that you experience later be worth the momentary pleasure? If the answer is no, then consider what would be a better choice. Is there a healthier food you could eat instead? Is your body really even hungry? Are you craving some other form of nourishment? Maybe what you really need is a break from your computer to take a step outside.

Using the principle of *primary vs. secondary foods* can help explain that nourishment comes from many sources. The idea is that our body is fueled by more than just the food we eat. Primary foods are things like career, social life, home environment, and exercise, which provide you with nonfood nourishment. Although it's beyond the scope of this book to discuss how these other elements factor into disease etiology, I will say that you can eat all the kale in the world, but you're not going to feel your best if you wake up every day to work a job that leaves you mentally drained. The same goes for secondary foods—the actual food that provides you with energy. You can feel satisfaction in most areas of life, but you're not going to feel your best if you have poor eating habits.

To demonstrate the principle of primary versus secondary foods imagine when you were a child, engaged in some type of incredibly fun activity, and your mother called you in for dinner. Were you hungry? Ravenous! But you were too busy playing to even notice that you needed to eat. You were fueling yourself with fun. Fast-forward to your adult self. If you're anything like me you count down the hours and minutes until you get the opportunity to snack again. At this point in my life I'm almost always willing to stop what I'm doing to eat, and I'm often eating when I'm not even really hungry. Sometimes I eat because I'm bored, sad, frustrated, hormonal, or tired. I'm fueling myself with secondary food when I should be thinking about primary food instead.

You can extend the idea of loving boundaries to almost every aspect of your life. We're not necessarily restricting just ourselves; we're making choices that create boundaries with ourselves and our loved ones. There are times when we unfortunately have to cut ties with people who we feel have repeatedly drained our emotional well-being. I once quit a job because I left work every single day feeling like I left my soul in my office. I had drawn a loving boundary to protect my emotional well-being.

You might be wondering how difficult it is to implement loving boundaries when it comes to food. The good news is that it's a lot easier to restrict your diet than it is to make many other life changes! Some of the difficult relationship issues that we often face are with our own family, and these issues can often be the most troublesome, time consuming, and energetically intensive. But in most cases we can't just walk away from family, nor should we. And not everyone has the luxury to quit their soul-destroying job, because they would lose important benefits, salary, and all of the financial security that comes along with being employed. But to lose a food that isn't supporting your body? What's the big deal? What do you have to lose? More important, what do you have to gain?

Slow Death by Sugar

Carbohydrates exist in one of three forms—fiber, starches, and sugar. Fiber is a structure unique to plants that is essential to the physical integrity of plant cells. Have you ever really thought about the fact that certain plants can stand hundreds of feet tall without any bones? Mammals would collapse into a pile of goop without their bones. Plants have fiber to thank for their rigid structures, while, among other things, we have fiber to thank for daily bowel movements. The recalcitrant structure of fiber makes it impossible for the human body to digest it. Fiber provides bulk to our stools and helps keep things moving along. Sugar and starches, on the other hand, are delivered to the bloodstream as glucose—readily available energy for our cells.

Muscles contain "storage units" in which excess glucose is stored as glycogen. This storage mechanism is helpful in times when food isn't immediately available, a phenomenon that rarely affects the modern Western human. When glucose blood levels remain high and glycogen stores are full, the body then converts the excess glucose to fat, another mechanism that has lost its purpose in a society of overeaters with access to an overabundance of food. Storing excess energy in the form of fat would have served us well in times of famine, but this conversion now leaves the majority of us with swollen waistlines and snug clothing.

Recommendations versus Actual Consumption

The American Heart Association (AHA) is particularly concerned with our sugar intake, because excess sugar intake leads to fat accumulation, which leads to metabolic syndrome, which leads to heart disease and other metabolic diseases. The AHA therefore recommends the following limits on sugar consumption: nine teaspoons (38 g) for men, six teaspoons (25 g) for women, and three to six teaspoons (12–25 g) for children 2 to 18 years of age. The World Health Organization (WHO) has set similar limits, stating that ideally no more than 5 percent of daily caloric intake comes from added sugars. While the WHO is as concerned with heart disease as the AHA, their interest is a bit more broad: Their objective is to prevent obesity, dental caries (cavities), and numerous noncommunicable diseases that are often avoided through positive

Table 1.1. Actual sugar intake vs. AHA- and WHO-recommended intake, age 2–18 years

Age	Actual daily intake		AHA-recommended daily limit		WHO-recommended daily limit*	
	Boys	Girls	Boys	Girls	Boys	Girls
2–5 years	13.5 tsp	12.25 tsp	3–6 tsp	3–6 tsp	5 tsp	4.7 tsp
6–11 years	21.5 tsp	18.3 tsp	3–6 tsp	3–6 tsp	6.5 tsp	5.8 tsp
12–19 years	28 tsp	19.6 tsp	3–6 tsp	3–6 tsp	7.8 tsp	5.9 tsp

* Data representing average caloric intake for different age groups was used to calculate the WHO-recommended daily limit in teaspoons of sugar. Five percent of the average number of calories consumed in a day was calculated and then converted to teaspoons of sugar.

lifestyle choices. The recommendations set by the AHA and WHO include any form of added sugar such as table sugar, high-fructose corn syrup, honey, syrups, fruit juices, and fruit juice concentrates.

It's no surprise that our intake of sugar far surpasses the recommendations of the AHA and WHO. In fact, Americans are eating two to three times the recommended limit. An average American is eating approximately 76 pounds of sugar every year, which works out to almost 1½ pounds of sugar every week or 22.4 teaspoons of sugar per day. This is an insane amount of sugar! Imagine cooking for your family in this way. A family of four would consume six pounds of sugar every week. Six! I'd have to put sugar in my water, eggs, fruit, all baked goods, salads, and pretty much every other meal that I prepared in order to use such a hefty load. Ah, now I'm starting to think like a processed food manufacturer.

I find it to be particularly problematic that youth, especially boys, are consuming even larger amounts of sugar when the effects are clearly negative. I'll discuss more about these effects later, but sugar consumption among children is staggering. Despite what you may believe, sugar intake does not correspond with income level. People often associate poverty with poorer eating habits, but that's simply not the case with sugar. Excess sugar consumption is a problem that transcends socioeconomic status.

Hidden Sugars Everywhere

Most added sugars (36 percent) appear in the food stream in the form of sodas, energy drinks, and sports drinks. Thirteen percent appear as grain-based desserts, 10 percent as fruit drinks, 6 percent as dairy-based desserts, 6 percent as candy, and the remaining percentage as miscellaneous foods. A quick look at the consumption patterns of children shows that 59 percent of added sugars come from foods while 41 percent come from beverages. A study of children's eating habits showed that 57 percent of children at the age of two are consuming cookies or candy in a given day and that 16 percent of toddlers are drinking carbonated beverages during lunch. This same study noted that the most commonly consumed food by toddlers was french fries. We're feeding our two-year-olds french fries, cookies, and soft drinks? There are certainly more nutritious options out there.

Sugar is found in 74 percent of packaged foods, from crackers and processed cheeses to canned and frozen meals. Some of the offenders contain minimal amounts while others give your body a toxic dose. For example, just one 12-ounce soda is 39 grams of sugar. Four grams of sugar is equal to 1 teaspoon, which means you're consuming nearly 10 teaspoons of sugar in just one soda—an amount that exceeds the AHA limits set for men, women, and children.

Identifying sugar in a food can be tricky because sugar is called by 61 different names. Some of the most common names for sugars include sucrose, fructose, high-fructose corn syrup, corn syrup, barley malt, maltose, dextrose, rice syrup, and concentrated fruit juice. Don't fool yourself, sugar is almost inescapable. As I discuss in the *A Note on Natural Sweeteners*, page 67, even natural sweeteners like honey, maple syrup, and agave are all forms of sugar (and even date paste is a sugar, though it's the least "sugar-y" of the lot because it has fiber). Reading labels is a good starting point when trying to reduce your sugar consumption, but labels often don't distinguish between naturally occurring sugars such as fructose in peaches or added sugars like simple syrup in canned fruits.

Many of the foods that are marketed as health foods are in fact as laden with sugar as their less healthy counterparts. You simply can't trust that because a food is marketed as healthy, you're buying a superior product. You can see in table 1.2 that sugar exists, often in incredible quantities, in foods that are commonly perceived as being healthy options.

Table 1.2. Sugar content in common foods

Food	Approximate sugar content in one serving (grams)
Granola bar (1 bar)	11
Organic fruit on the bottom yogurt (5 ounces)	21
Fat-free organic fruit on the bottom yogurt (5 ounces)	25
Apple juice (8 ounces)	26
Peanut butter (2 tablespoons)	3
Fat-free peanut butter (2 tablespoons)	4
Energy bar (1 bar)	24
Baked beans (½ cup)	16
Ketchup (1 tablespoon)	4
Whole wheat crackers (16 crackers)	4
Mint chocolate chip ice cream (½ cup)	20

Our accidental overconsumption of sugar is better understood when you're enlightened to the fact that some foods contain such large quantities of sugar. Not only that, but some of the serving sizes listed are incredibly small. Who eats just 16 crackers or a half cup of ice cream? And why do we have to add sugar to foods like peanut butter? The stuff is packed full of creamy, delicious fats for crying out loud! You can also see that the low-fat or fat-free versions of peanut butter and yogurt actually have more sugar (and more calories) than their fat-containing equivalents. When you remove the fats from a food you also remove the flavor, and removing the flavor requires a bit of a flavor boost—sugar. Upward

trends in the prevalence of obesity started at nearly the same time that low-fat foods were being marketed as health foods. Lo and behold, sugar turns out to be responsible for many of the negative health outcomes that were previously hypothesized to be associated with fat intake.

Glycation and Faulty Proteins

Experts unanimously agree that sugar consumption plays a role in diabetes, obesity, and fatty liver disease, yet we're only beginning to understand the extent of the damage. Traditional concerns over sugar consumption focused on sugar equating to empty calories, but we're now learning that sugar isn't just a caloric void. We're discovering that its biological effects on the body are actually toxic. Sugar can negatively impact your mood, effectively lower pH to disrupt the mineral balance in blood (which also leads to osteoporosis and osteopenia), lead to weight gain and obesity, cause insulin resistance, increase inflammation, and impair cognitive ability. I'll briefly describe each of these consequences momentarily, but I'd like to first discuss the process of glycation and how it's likely the culprit in these numerous and diverse outcomes.

Glycation is the process by which sugar effectively binds to other substrates in the body, such as proteins and fats. The end products are appropriately known as AGEs (advanced glycation end products). This discovery was noted in the early 1900s, but it wasn't until the mid-1980s that doctors tried to understand its link with diabetes and the aging process in general.

Proteins are largely responsible for completing most of the functions that occur between our cells, which keeps the body in balance. Cell membranes welcome uniquely shaped proteins, and these proteins then regulate the flow of varying substances in and out of the cell, and allow for cell-to-cell communication. Think of the toddler toys that include varying shapes that fit through corresponding holes. You can't very well fit a star through the rectangle hole. Proteins behave in much the same way. But when a sugar molecule effectively binds to a protein, a misshapen protein is formed via the process of glycation. After glycation, AGEs are inappropriately shaped for the "hole," which means they simply won't fit and their function is therefore lost.

Many of the negative consequences from AGEs don't present themselves until people are in their 30s and beyond. Our bodies are equipped with mechanisms to correct the faulty proteins, but those mechanisms function less optimally as we age, and the lifetime effects of exposure to radiation, poor eating habits, toxins, oxidative stress, and hormones begin to take their toll until we're simply unable to prevent AGEs from damaging our bodies.

Damage from AGEs occurs in one of three ways: less functional proteins, impairment of the proteins when they link to other impaired proteins, or an increase in free radicals (the AGEs become a production source of free radicals). It's important to note that our modern diet is one that drastically increases the production of free radicals. Glycated proteins (AGEs) increase free radical production by a factor of 50! High-carb diets also increase glycation, but sugar seems to be particularly problematic. High-fructose corn syrup is an even greater source of free radical production, with a production rate 10 times higher than plain table sugar. Eating excessive carbs and sugar therefore damages tissues, fats, and proteins, and can even damage our DNA through the process of oxidation. It can also impact our DNA expression by turning the epigenetic switch on or off. Put another way, changes in the expression of DNA can result in the presentation of a disease that might otherwise not have expressed itself.

To fully understand the process through which glycation causes cell damage we have to first understand the aforementioned free radicals and oxidation. Oxygen is the final electron acceptor in metabolic pathways within the body. When metabolism goes awry, oxygen is left with an incomplete or excessive number of electrons, which changes its energetic capabilities. Free radicals are sometimes referred to as reactive oxygen species, because, well, they're a species of oxygen that is no longer benign; they're reactive. Therefore, it's in our best interest to eat antioxidants so as to combat reactive oxygen that is capable of cell damage via oxidation. Antioxidants essentially neutralize free radicals and prevent them from damaging (oxidizing) our cells.

Then there is the issue of inflammation. Dozens of degenerative disease such as diabetes, cataracts, atherosclerosis, emphysema, and dementia have been linked to inflammation that occurs as a result of deformed proteins. Remember that glycation results in misshapen proteins? Well, high levels of glycation have been linked to many of these same diseases, which is indicative of a link between glycation and inflammation. Future research will explore this link further, but for now it provides a direct explanation as to why sugar can actually be such a toxic substance. So keep in mind that when you eat sugar you're effectively impairing your proteins on some level.

Cystic Fibrosis and Our Journey with June

Cystic fibrosis (CF) is a genetic disease in which a person's DNA codes for faulty CFTR (cystic fibrosis transmembrane conductance regulator) proteins. Improper coding (from the mutated DNA), thus improper manufacturing of the CFTR protein, prevents the protein from performing its job within the body. CFTR proteins are responsible for regulating the movement of sodium chloride (salts) in and out of cells. There are around 1,900 different disease-causing mutations that result in a protein that is either inadequate in numbers, misshapen, nonexistent, or has a faulty opening. Such a seemingly simple function results in a domino effect of health consequences for individuals who carry the CF genes. Scientists are learning that these faulty CFTR proteins have cascading effects on the regulation of other substances in and out of cells, but the primary malfunction lies with the salt issue. Improper salt movement results in abnormally thick and sticky mucuses throughout the body. CF is a multi-organ disease and can impact every individual differently, but the primary organs to suffer include the lungs, pancreas, liver, and intestines.

The role of mucus in the lungs is to remove varying substances—dead cells, bacteria, spent DNA—but these substances instead get "stuck" when the mucus is too thick. Combine these dead substances with the warm, moist, and oxygenated environment in the lungs and you have the perfect breeding ground for unwanted bacteria. People with CF can have a variety of organisms grow in their lungs, organisms that would not be problematic for you or me, but it's very difficult for them to remove these organisms given the viscous nature of their mucus. Routine treatments and therapies are therefore aimed at thinning the mucus and helping to prevent bacteria from taking hold.

In the pancreas, CF results in thick mucus that traps digestive enzymes. Under normal circumstances these enzymes are exuded into the small intestines during digestion. Bile from the liver can also become abnormally thick in people with CF, preventing bile from reaching the intestines as well. People with CF can therefore have extreme difficulty digesting food and require digestive enzymes at every meal. Skipping the enzymes causes intense discomfort and, more important, severe malnourishment. While the inability to gain weight could seem like a blessing to some, the curse of constantly fighting malnourishment is a major struggle for some individuals with CF. Maintaining a healthy body weight is especially important because stored energy is needed to fight any major infection in the lungs.

Since CF is genetic, it's not contagious; it's something you either have for a lifetime or you don't. It

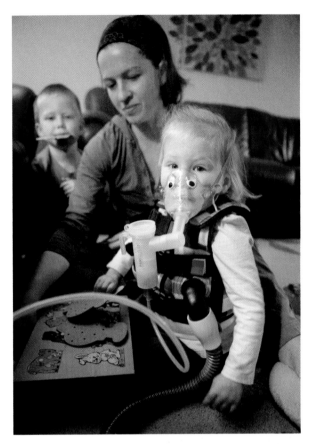

June performs airway clearance twice per day, every day, and more often when she has a cough. These treatments involve inhaled mucolytics and a vest that helps to keep her lungs clear. This is just one form of airway clearance.

impacts approximately 30,000 people in the United States and over 70,000 people worldwide. My daughter is one of such individuals, but she's one of the lucky 10 percent who are considered pancreas sufficient—the enzymes from her pancreas successfully reach the small intestines, making digestive enzymes unnecessary for her. I cannot even begin to express the blessing of this scenario. Her lungs, however, seem to be more affected. My daughter takes frequent antibiotics during cold and flu season to help keep her lungs clear of infections, and she's been admitted for IV antibiotics when oral doses didn't do the trick. She wears a vest to perform airway clearance and dislodge any stuck mucus, two times per day, 20 to 30 minutes each session. Airway clearance techniques vary from country to country, but this is currently the most common method in the US. She inhales mucolytic drugs while wearing her vest in order to help thin the mucus, making airway clearance therapy more effective.

My friends all know that their children aren't allowed at our house when they're sick. I've even pulled my daughter out of preschool multiple times to prevent her catching colds from other classmates. When she has a cough, we increase treatments and therapies to three or four times per day, which is a huge investment of time. Not only this, but every cold has the potential to turn into a severe infection for her. She takes antibiotics under circumstances that most people wouldn't dream of taking such a thing, but it's to prevent the lung damage that occurs from bacterial overgrowth in the lungs.

Life expectancy for someone with CF is a moving target these days. It's hard to say for sure where that number currently lies, but the most recent suggestion puts it around 40 years of age. I expect this number will continue to rise, but had my daughter been born 30 years ago, we wouldn't have expected her to live into her teens. There are, of course, many individuals who have far surpassed that expectation with much gusto and fight, but the overall increase in longevity is a result of improved drugs and aggressive treatment with antibiotics.

My daughter is among the first to have a protein-modulator drug available starting at the age of two. These protein-modulators are expected to be game changers for people living with CF, especially for those who start the drugs early in life and can prevent lung damage and bacterial colonization. Placing my child on a new drug at such a young age was a difficult decision, but I can already guess the long-term consequences of not having it. We'll take our chances and hope that the trajectory of her life is improved as a result.

Microbes, pH, and Mood

Now that we understand the process of glycation let's investigate some of the other negative outcomes associated with sugar consumption. One of the most prevalent issues that I see as a health coach is that a diet high in processed carbs and sugar influences the microbial diversity in the large and small intestines. For example, many people suffer from chronic yeast infections, a symptom that is treatable through fervent diet and lifestyle adjustments. Keep in mind that yeast infections can appear on any surface on the body; this isn't an issue unique to the female population. I've seen yeast overgrowth on people's trunks, faces, and limbs—it can happen anywhere. In fact, most any skin condition appears as a result of a microbiota imbalance or excess inflammation in the gut, which is why many doctors treat skin conditions such as acne with antibiotics. Of course we can much more holistically treat acne and other skin conditions by simply improving diet and learning to manage stress.

Sugar consumption effectively lowers the pH of the body, making the internal environment more acidic. The goal is to maintain a relatively neutral pH in the body, but the American diet, which leans more toward acidity, encourages a high consumption of processed foods, sugar, excess carbs, and poor-quality meats. An acidic environment further contributes to the overgrowth of yeasts and other less desirable occupants in our gut. It also impacts our bones. Dr. Annemarie Colbin does a fantastic job of explaining the role of diet in bone health in her book *The Whole-Food Guide to Strong Bones*. She explains that the strength of our bones isn't limited to our calcium consumption but is a more complex process that involves numerous minerals and proteins. When our blood is acidic, our bones are prompted to release minerals in an attempt to balance the pH, which can ultimately weaken our bones. We should therefore aim to consume alkalizing diets that include very limited amounts of sugar, reasonable consumption of carbs, and high intakes of fresh fruits and vegetables, healthy fats, and healthy proteins in order to better care for our bones.

I'm sure we've all recognized that sugar impacts our mood, especially when we're feeling a bit addicted. (I'll talk more about the addictive properties of sugar in a moment.) Many people and animals demonstrate symptoms such as depression and anxiety when deprived of sugar. Sugar further impacts our moods by contributing to variable blood sugar, which can lead to mood swings, irritability, and anxiety. A study in mice showed that sugar may be particularly problematic for adolescents who are developing the brain pathways responsible for their stress response. Adolescents are prone to feeling depressed or anxious until these pathways are fully developed, thus sugar consumption can heighten these emotions. If you look back at table 1.1 on page 3 that documents sugar intake based on sex and age for children, you'll see that adolescents are eating more than three times the recommended limit for sugar. When you consider that suicide is the second leading cause of death in the United States for people ranging from 10 to 34 years old, I often wonder how these numbers would change with improved diets that involved far less sugar consumption, although I haven't seen any supporting data yet.

The Diabetic Crisis

Weight gain and obesity are some of the most widespread results of excess sugar consumption. Centers for Disease Control and Prevention (CDC) data shows that 36.5 percent of US adults and 17 percent of US children are obese. (Remember that excess glucose is stored as glycogen, but excess beyond storage capacity is converted to fat. As you can see, we've got excess!) Some experts argue that even fruit sugars can be problematic for individuals who are especially sensitive to sugar, and that these sensitive individuals should eat very limited fruit and must drastically reduce their carb intake in order to better manage their blood glucose levels.

We often assume that diabetes is limited to those who are overweight, but that's not always the case. Adults with a normal weight suffer from it as well. The average insulin level for men living in the United States is 8.8 micro international units per milliliter, and the level is 8.4 for women. Some specialists argue that two micro international units per milliliter is a more desirable number, and that anything over five is problematic. The incidence of diabetes in the United States has continued to increase since the early 1960s, with a drastic increase that began in the mid-1990s. From 1980 to 2012 the number of adults with diabetes nearly quadrupled, and in the last 10 years we've seen a 70 percent increase in adolescent diabetes. Adolescent diabetes is particularly problematic in that the progression of complications in youth is much faster than in adults, which can lead to premature metabolic and cardiovascular difficulties.

An important distinction exists between type 1 and type 2 diabetes. Type 1, also called insulin-dependent diabetes, is an autoimmune condition that reveals itself early in life. Type 1 diabetics produce inadequate levels of insulin, the hormone responsible for delivering glucose to our cells. These individuals are therefore dependent on insulin injections to lower blood glucose levels and deliver glucose to the cells within the body. While little can be done to prevent type 1 diabetes, type 2 diabetes is a condition that is largely preventable through diet and lifestyle choices. Type 2 diabetics are insulin resistant, meaning that the pancreas manufactures insulin, but chronically elevated insulin levels cause cells within the body to become resistant and blood sugar levels remain high even in the presence of insulin. Type 2 diabetes was

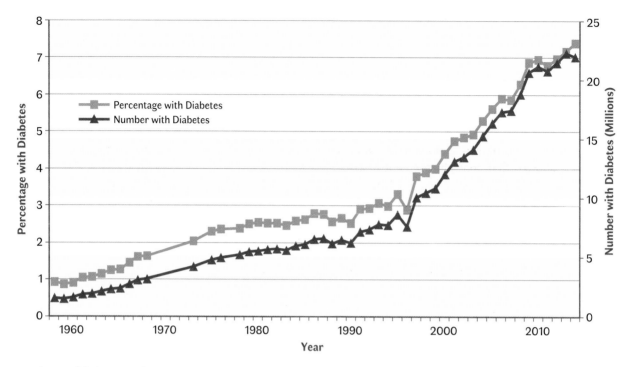

Incidence of diabetes in the United States, 1958–2014. Data from the Centers for Disease Control and Prevention.

formerly known as late-onset diabetes since it was historically only seen in an aging population, but it's now a disease that affects both children and adults. In 2000, less than 3 percent of all new cases of diabetes were type 2. Fast-forward to 2011 and we find that 45 percent of all new cases are type 2. Type 2 diabetes now accounts for 90 to 95 percent of all diabetes in adults living in the United States. Even more troublesome is that approximately 37 percent of all adults are considered prediabetic, but only a fraction of those people are aware of their condition. Diabetes is clearly a disease that is on the rise, and prevention includes the elimination of sugar from the diet and reducing carb intake.

Increased blood sugar, such as the condition created in diabetics, is responsible for the release of pro-inflammatory compounds called cytokines. While this is

certainly problematic for diabetics, the release of cytokines occurs even when blood sugar is elevated for short durations—a condition that easily occurs in any individual upon the consumption of sugar. These increased levels of inflammatory compounds can suppress the immune system and also result in inflammation throughout the body including the brain.

Your Brain on Sugar

One of the more surprising effects of sugar consumption is related to cognitive ability. In his book *Grain Brain*, David Perlmutter cites a study showing that developing diabetes before the age of 65 resulted in increased risk of mild cognitive impairment by 220 percent. A study in rats showed that a diet containing high-fructose corn syrup impaired learning and memory. Surprisingly, these effects could be prevented by omega-3 supplementation, an essential fat that is lacking in the American diet.[1] Studies of this nature demonstrate that insulin is able to pass through the blood-brain barrier, thus impacting the way in which all cells of the body utilize glucose. It is believed that because of this, thoughts and emotions are likely impacted by insulin resistance as well.

A large 2012 study of over 3,000 elderly (mean age 74.2 years) showed that poor glucose control associated with diabetes substantially increased the rate of mental decline.[2] Twenty-three percent of test subjects had diabetes, and two groups (diabetic and nondiabetic) were followed over the course of nine years. Not only did diabetics demonstrate greater decline in cognitive function, but their baseline cognitive scores were significantly lower at the beginning of the study. Researchers point to AGEs, inflammation, and other mechanisms as the drivers behind mental decline.

Can't Stop, Won't Stop: Addiction at Its Finest

The negative health outcomes associated with sugar intake are even further complicated by the fact that sugar has very addictive qualities, meaning our good intentions to consume less sugar can be easily overridden by our intense physical desire for the substance. Blood glucose levels immediately spike when consuming sugar, but levels soon dip since very little actual digestion takes place from the time sugar hits your stomach to the time glucose levels rise. Eating fruits or other whole foods that contain varying forms of sugar doesn't have this immediate spike because fibers and other more complex structures must be broken down before the sugar is released into your blood. However, the large spikes associated with sugar of any kind (natural sweeteners like maple syrup included) result in elevated levels of insulin, which then drives cravings for more sugar.

Even as sugar drives cravings through a physiological need to satisfy insulin levels, it also drives cravings through the release of feel-good hormones. Sally Fallon Morell writes in *The Nourishing Traditions Book of Baby & Child Care* that sugar "produces dopamine and endorphins that mimic cocaine, morphine, opium, and heroine: sugar stimulates the production of adrenaline and norepinephrine, which mimic methamphetamine; and sugar feeds yeasts that control ethanol and acetaldehyde, resulting in symptoms of inebriation and hangover." She continues to say that you simply can't expect positive behavior from a child who is constantly overloaded with such an overabundance of mood-impacting hormones. As I discuss in chapter 2, in the section *Marketing of Kid-Friendly Foods*, many of these foods also contain food dyes—yet another substance known to impact behavior. If your child (or yourself) suffers from emotional or behavioral problems, the most effective approach is to tackle the problem from a dietary standpoint while also seeking psychological and behavioral help as needed.

A number of studies using mice have clearly shown the extent of sugar addiction. One such study showed that when given the choice between cocaine or saccharin, the majority of mice chose saccharin.[3] The researchers saw the same results when using sucrose (table sugar). These sources demonstrate that the desire for sweets goes beyond our physiological need for calories, since it doesn't seem to matter if the source of sweetness has calories or not. The results from the study are interesting in that while cocaine more effectively releases dopamine into the brain, something about the sweet taste of sugar delivered a greater reward than the neurological effects of cocaine.

Sweetness triggers the pleasure center of the brain using a series of chemical reactions that involve taste receptors. This series of reactions produces dopamine and other pleasure hormones that leave us wanting more. Over time, our brains become immune to a certain level of dopamine and we need more of a stimulus to experience the same level of pleasure. Serotonin, a feel-good neurotransmitter, is also released during sugar consumption. Studies show that frequently eating sweet foods can deplete serotonin reserves, thus leading to depression.

Grains, Grains Everywhere, but Are They Good to Eat?

According to the Food and Agriculture Organization of the United Nations (FAO), "cereal grains are the most important food source for human consumption." Yet many people argue that not only are grains unnecessary, but they can actually be harmful, especially when consumed in large quantities. A true grain is produced from a grass such as wheat, rye, oats, or barley, and pseudo-grains from the seeds of broadleaf plants such as quinoa and buckwheat. A grain itself is a seed comprised of a shell (bran), embryo (germ), and endosperm (starch). The bran and germ store the most nutritious components of a grain, but these parts also contain many of the components that are detrimental to health.

Consumption of grains increased in the 1970s as the low-fat craze drove consumers away from fat and toward carbohydrates. Since then the way in which we consume grains has drastically changed. This is due to a number of factors. The increased availability of fast food is one. That more women joined the workforce, thus leaving their home kitchens, is another. In the early 1900s, 90 percent of all flour products were prepared in the home, but by 1990 less than 10 percent were prepared at home. The majority of grains now being consumed are in the form of packaged and processed foods.

As most people are well aware, grains are primarily comprised of carbohydrates, which are broken down into glucose. Insulin is produced as a result of increased blood glucose levels upon digestion, and a diet high in carbohydrates results in a high production of insulin, which can eventually lead to insulin resistance and associated diseases. Some experts even claim that elevated insulin resulting from a diet high in grains and sugar is the number one cause of overall disease. But it's not just the carbohydrate content of grains that can be problematic.

Our First Offender: Phytic Acid

Grains and pseudo-grains contain a large amount of a substance called phytic acid, an antinutrient that binds with minerals such as calcium, magnesium, iron, and zinc. When bound to phytic acid, these important minerals are unavailable for uptake and assimilation throughout the body. Even when eating a nutrient-rich diet, malnutrition from the overconsumption of phytic acid can result in mineral deficiencies, leading to bone loss and tooth decay. Phytic acid also inhibits digestive enzymes such as pepsin, amylase, and trypsin, which leads to incomplete digestion, thus causing digestive upset and further limiting nutrient availability. A diet rich in phytic acid is especially problematic for children who have underdeveloped digestive systems, because they require a highly nutritious diet for proper growth and development.

The highest concentration of phytic acid is found in the bran and germ part of a grain. Surprisingly, white rice and white flour are both low in phytic acid because they've been stripped of both the bran and germ. Eating white rice or white bread may actually cause fewer problems when it comes to impaired digestion and mineral absorption; however, overprocessed bleached white flours and nonorganic white rice that are completely void of nutrients and contain toxic chemicals should be avoided. Phytic acid levels can be affected by the growing conditions of a plant, because phytic acid is a phosphorus-containing molecule. Higher levels of phytic acid are therefore found in greater concentrations when crops are grown using chemical fertilizers that have high phosphorus availability.

Nuts, seeds, and beans also contain relatively high concentrations of phytic acid. However, eating nuts is often only problematic for individuals who frequently consume products made from nut flours or nut butters. They consume a larger volume of nuts than recommended, which is simply eating a handful of nuts once or twice a day. The same problem of overconsumption is true for diets that are comprised of excessive quantities of seeds or beans. Even so, you'd be hard-pressed to find an individual who eats quantities of seeds or beans in the same way that many individuals consume grains—for breakfast, lunch, dinner, and snacks. Moderation is key when it comes to phytic acid–containing foods. If you happen to consume a large amount of beans, nuts, or seeds, you may want to consider soaking, sprouting, fermenting, or all of the above as a way to minimize phytic acid consumption. Soaking and sprouting alone can increase the amount of phytase, the enzyme responsible for phytic acid neutralization, by three- to fivefold. It's also important to note that a vegetarian diet is extremely high in phytic acid. A vegetarian diet, especially for a child, needs careful monitoring in order to prevent malnourishment. Vegetarians will truly benefit from soaking, sprouting, and fermenting nuts, seeds, beans, and grains before consumption.

You may be thinking that phytic acid doesn't initially appear to be a problematic component of grains since it also exists in other foods, but recall that it's our excessive consumption of grains that seems to be the problem. The human body produces a small amount of phytase, the enzyme responsible for phytic acid neutralization, yet our consumption of phytic acid exceeds what our bodies are capable of neutralizing. Grains inherently contain small amounts of phytase, which also aids digestion, but phytase is destroyed when grains are pulverized to produce the fine flours we've grown accustomed to enjoying. After processing, such flours are left with high levels of phytic acid and very little phytase to aid in digestion, which makes breads and cereals (specifically those high in bran or germ) especially toxic.

Moving On to Lectins

Grains contain lectins, carbohydrate-binding proteins with their own negative consequences. Not all lectins are inherently bad, however, as their unique structure allows them to embed within cell membranes and help regulate communication and movement of substances between cells. The protein portion of a lectin embeds itself within the membrane while the carbohydrate portion extends outward to perform its duty. However, some lectins such as prolamins and agglutinins cause harm to the digestive system and wreak havoc on the body's natural immune defenses. These types of lectins are responsible for reducing the body's ability to recognize hunger, blocking proteins responsible for building tissues, interacting with the gut barrier and mucosal lining in a negative way, allowing undesirable particles to cross the gut lining, and stimulating a pro-inflammatory response from the immune system.

In order to truly understand the undesirable effects of lectins, we must first understand what it means to have "leaky gut," a profoundly simple yet damaging condition. The digestive tract relies on tight junctions between cells to regulate the absorption of nutrients across its membranes. Digestion begins in our mouths with mastication (don't forget to chew!), and digestive enzymes in saliva help to further prepare our food for the journey into the stomach where it is "attacked" by large amounts of acid. The acidic mixture is somewhat neutralized before making the long journey through the small intestines, an intricate winding tube covered in fingerlike projections covered in more fingerlike projections that are lined with digestive cells called enterocytes. As if this wasn't enough, enterocytes are coated in glycocalyx, a layer responsible for supplying

Soaking Seeds and Beans

Beans and seeds serve as an important food source for a number of animals, including humans. However, plants have adapted traits in their reproductive structures (seeds) to resist consumption and digestion by hungry vertebrates. Take mistletoe as an example, a semiparasitic plant whose seeds are dispersed after being consumed by a bird, passing through the digestive tract unharmed, and being deposited onto a new host branch via bird droppings. The name *mistletoe* comes from two Anglo-Saxon words quite literally meaning "dung on a twig." (You can think of that next time you get smooched under a hanging branch of mistletoe.)

Mistletoe is not unique in that it is set on survival. Plants need successful reproductive strategies, but this means they are equipped with mechanisms to resist chewing, extreme acidic conditions in the stomach, digestive enzymes in the small intestines, and aggressive bacteria in the colon. They can resist all of the above through the use of hard-to-digest compounds such as phytic acid and other recalcitrant substances.

Traditional preparation methods for beans, seeds, and even grains made use of soaking, sprouting, and fermenting—processes that help to degrade undigestible compounds. The Weston A. Price Foundation has a number of valuable resources on their website, or you can look into purchasing one of the resources noted at the end of this sidebar to help you better implement these strategies. In the meantime, I recommend that you simply start by *soaking* your beans and seeds. When a seed is soaked (a bean is nothing more than a seed from a legume), it is prompted to grow. Proteins become "unlocked" since the growing embryo will soon need to access these nutrients, and sugars break down into more digestible forms. Growth-inhibiting compounds will start to degrade since the seed is no longer in survival mode—it believes it has found suitable habitat.

digestive enzymes. Without all of these brilliant folds, creases, projections, and enzymes our intestines would have to be four and a half miles long to ensure adequate surface area for nutrient absorption. The remaining digestive slurry makes its way into the large intestines where it is feasted upon by billions of bacteria and yeasts that are responsible for extracting the last bits of usable nutrition from our food.

The genius of our digestive tract relies on two very important assumptions. First, our intestines and the flora within are capable of breaking down food into its smallest components. Second, our intestines are able to selectively absorb the nutrients that can be safely and effectively incorporated into tissues, while simultaneously forcing larger particles to continue their journey through the great tube until they, too, have been broken down into their smallest parts. When this "filtration" system is incapable of recognizing appropriately sized particles, one is said to have leaky gut, a condition in which a faulty discrimination process allows particle entry from the interior of the gut into the rest of the body.

When I say that lectins are capable of harming the tight junctions in the intestines, I mean that they destroy the cells and mechanisms that filter particle penetration and absorption. The particles that pass into the bloodstream are recognized as foreign invaders (called antigens), and the immune system signals

Use the instructions in the Roasted and Salted Walnuts recipe (page 173) for soaking seeds and nuts. These are best soaked in a light saline solution for 12 to 24 hours before cooking. You'll notice that I've used raw sunflower seeds in a few recipes including Plantain Muffins and Plantain Blender Pancakes. I've made an exception in these instances since the seeds are pulverized into a flour followed by baking. Both of these strategies improve digestibility.

Beans are similar to seeds in that they, too, require 12 to 24 hours of soaking. They contain varying recalcitrant constituents, the most noticeable of these being oligosaccharides, which are complex sugars that are impossible to digest in the human digestive tract and are instead fermented in the colon by specialized bacteria. The byproducts from this anaerobic digestion are none other than carbon dioxide and methane gases, ultimately earning beans their nickname, the musical fruit. Soaking helps to break oligosaccharides into more digestible forms of sugar, helping to improve and mitigate the flatulent effect of beans. Place your beans into a bowl, large jar, or pot and add enough water for the beans to be completely submerged with an additional four to six inches of water on top. The beans will rehydrate and expand as they soak, so be sure to use an adequate amount of water (too much is better than not enough). Some cooks recommend changing the water halfway through, but this is something I can never remember to do. Strain and rinse the beans when the soaking period is complete, and cook the beans as instructed.

ADDITIONAL RESOURCES

Nourishing Traditions: The Cookbook That Challenges Politically Correct Nutrition and the Diet Dictocrats by Sally Fallon and Mary Enig
The Art of Fermentation by Sandor Katz and Michael Pollan
Wild Fermentation by Sandor Katz and Sally Fallon Morell

for an attack. This attack leads to the release of pro-inflammatory cytokines and systemic inflammation. While this response is a perfectly reasonable way to cope with a foreign invader, the body's own defense strategies inadvertently further attack the lining of the gut. The result is a cycle of damaged cells, immune responses, more damaged cells, and so on.

The issue of leaky gut is complicated by lectins because they not only damage the enterocytes and other cells that line the gut wall, but also bind to sugars and other molecules to aid in their movement across the intestinal barrier. So not only are lectins causing damage that enables gut permeability, but they also act as transporters through the gut lining.

Once in the body, lectins can be a difficult thing to get rid of. They're nearly impossible to digest and are highly resistant to changes of temperatures and pH. It's an incredibly stable molecule. Moreover, because they're able to effectively bind to many different cells and tissues, they can also accumulate in the gut. This makes for a lengthy healing process for those with leaky gut. Lectins are also present in beans and other foods such as tomatoes, but again, we don't typically consume these foods in the same quantities as grains. Soaking, sprouting, fermenting, and prolonged cooking can deactivate some lectins such as agglutinins, but these preparation methods are no longer common practice in our modern society.

Where Are the Omegas?

Grains are also responsible for contributing to fatty acid imbalance, a hallmark of the Western diet. Grains are high in omega-6 fatty acids, a fat that elicits an inflammatory response. By contrast, grains lack the anti-inflammatory counterpart, omega-3. The two omegas work in tandem in the complex process of immunity and healing, but problems arise when omega-6 intake is far greater than its anti-inflammatory companion. Ideally, we would have a relatively balanced intake of the varying omegas, but that's often not the case. Most processed foods or foods prepared at restaurants are not only grain-based, but made using vegetable oils such as safflower, soybean, peanut, canola, corn, and others high in omega-6 fatty acids. But the story doesn't stop with the direct consumption of grains and oils. Conventionally raised animals are fed grains because they're an inexpensive and convenient source of food. This practice affects the fatty acid profile of the meats that we consume. Under natural conditions (such as grass-fed cows living in a pasture for their entire lives) cattle raised for meat have a 1:1 or 1:2 ratio of omega-3 to omega-6 fatty acids. But the ratio for grain-fed cows is closer to 1:10, a ratio that contributes to systemic inflammation in those who consume these meats.

Wheat: The Grain in the Spotlight

Some experts argue that there is little inherently wrong with consuming grains. They believe that the health-degrading characteristics of grains aren't an issue, but that the issue instead lies in our farming practices and our preparation methods. One such grain has received more controversial attention than any other grain in existence—wheat. Per capita consumption of wheat in the United States far exceeds the consumption of any other food, and wheat is the third largest crop in the world after rice and corn. This gluten-filled grain contains a form of sugar that is extremely easy to digest, giving wheat a higher glycemic index than straight-up table sugar. This means that the most commonly consumed food in the United States has a more profound impact on blood glucose levels than plain old sugar, yet our diabesity epidemic remains a mystery. Is it just me, or is there a blatantly obvious connection here?

A look at wheat history shows that wheat hasn't always been available as the processed, fluffy breads that we know today. The first of many changes to wheat occurred in 1869 with the invention of the steel mill. While the modern milling technique produced an improved flour texture compared with the traditional stone mill, the problem was that such intense grinding destroyed the beneficial components of the bran and germ. The result was chronic vitamin B deficiencies that led to diseases such as pellagra and beriberi. But fear not, the experts caught on and started to fortify wheat flour in the 1930s. To this day, much of the nutritional value of wheat flour is accomplished from the addition of synthetic vitamins. While supplementation with synthetic vitamins is necessary in some instances, these vitamins are generally poorly absorbed when compared with their naturally occurring counterparts that exist in whole foods.

The Broadbalk Winter Wheat Experiment was started in 1843 as a way to monitor and document changes in the production and nutritional value of wheat over time. Despite the nutritional loss from the new milling methods of the late 1800s, the nutritional value of wheat in its whole-food state remained relatively constant until the 1960s when a dwarf variety was selected for improved cultivation. The mid-1900s were a period in agriculture known as the Green Revolution, when a multitude of improved farming methods were developed in areas such as irrigation, crop management, hybridization, and chemical fertilizers and pesticides. The hybridized wheat was pest resistant, was easier to harvest, had better drought resistance, and was higher in gluten—a trait that produces the gorgeous bleached, nutritionally void, chewy bread products that are available everywhere. Data from the Broadbalk Experiment shows that the shallow root system of this new dwarf variety was unable to penetrate deep enough into the soil to access adequate minerals, thus producing a grain with overall lower mineral content. Remember how phytic acid binds with minerals to inhibit mineral absorption? Well, the phytic acid content of the dwarf variety remained constant, which ultimately translated into even fewer minerals available for uptake.

Another major issue with the production of wheat is the widespread use of glyphosate, the main ingredient in an herbicide better known as Roundup. Glyphosate is not only sprayed to control weeds but also applied to many crops including wheat, barley, oats, canola, flax, peas, lentils, soybeans, and dried beans before harvest in a process called desiccation. Glyphosate effectively kills the crop, which according the Roundup *Preharvest Staging Guide* allows for earlier harvest, more uniform crop maturity, and increased combine efficiency. Roundup was certainly not intended for this purpose, yet the measurable increase in crop yield made this practice common in the 1990s. Glyphosate is now present in the majority of conventionally grown wheat as well as many other crops that are sprayed before harvest. Even more disturbing is that some reports state that glyphosate has made its way into our water cycle and can even be found on organic crops as a result of precipitation residue. In fact, the most interesting research happening right now in regard to our current epidemic of chronic illness is around glyphosate and its effects on the microbiome.

In 2015 the International Agency for Research on Cancer classified glyphosate as a probable carcinogen, and its use is banned in the Netherlands and El Salvador. Varying interest groups worldwide have called for glyphosate bans, but governing bodies have not supported the requests.

Glyphosate is known to suppress the function of one of the most important detoxification mechanisms in the body, cytochrome P450. Without this mechanism, the body cannot effectively rid itself of metals and other toxic compounds that are capable of damaging our nervous system. A 2013 review published in *Interdisciplinary Toxicology* demonstrates a strong correlation between the application of glyphosate on varying crops (primarily wheat, soy, and corn) and incidence of celiac disease, death from intestinal infections, thyroid cancer, acute kidney injury, and deaths from Parkinson's disease.[4] The bottom line is that we're not entirely clear on the long-term effects of widespread use of glyphosate. But this much is clear to me: I'm not willing to use my body as part of an experiment to find out.

Diets Void of Nutrients

Now that we've explored some of the toxic highlights from eating grains, including overprocessing, phytic acid, lectins, omega-6 fatty acids, glyphosates, and issues specific to wheat, I want to briefly explore the greatest problem of all: consumption. Our substantial consumption of grains leaves little room for other foods. If we eat cereal or pancakes for breakfast, sandwiches for lunch, crackers and muffins for snacks, and pasta with bread for dinner, then when do we eat all of the other nutritious foods that are readily available to us? Sure, grains like rice, corn, and wheat have been staples for thousands of years, but people weren't eating these foods in the quantity (or form) consumed today. Have you ever grown your own grain, collected the seed, ground it into flour, and then made your own bread? There's a reason why very few home gardeners are this ambitious. I've grown a variety of interesting vegetables that require a bit more attention than, say, lettuce, but I have no interest in growing grains in my

What Constitutes a Healthy Fat?

There's much confusion when it comes to dietary fat. For decades, people have believed that less fat is best and that high-fat diets will eventually lead to cardiovascular disease (CVD) and other health complications including obesity. However, the greater availability of low-fat foods that became popularized in the 1970s did nothing but fan the flames on what is now a modern-day public health crisis. When you remove the fat, you remove the flavor. And how do you make those foods flavorful once again? You load them up with sugar and refined carbohydrates, embellishments with clear negative health consequences.

A 2016 article published in the *Journal of Food and Nutrition Research* compiled dietary data from 42 European countries in an attempt to identify the nutritional factors most influential on cardiovascular disease in Europeans.[5] The results of the study showed that diets rich in carbohydrates, specifically those from cereal grains, potatoes, and alcohol, were correlated with a higher risk of developing CVD compared with a diet high in fat. In fact, high fat consumption was negatively correlated to CVD. Does this mean that fats offer a protective effect? Not necessarily. It's not so much that fat is protective as that a high-carb diet is disease causing.

Saturated fats have received an especially large amount of negative attention, yet there's a lack of evidence proving these fats are the culprit in the development of CVD or coronary heart disease (CHD). Take France as an example. The French consume greater quantities of animal fats (a major source of saturated fats) than any other population, yet they have the second lowest worldwide CVD mortality.[6] The saturated fat hypothesis influenced the widespread use of trans fat, a chemically manufactured fat that is commonly used in packaged foods due to its stable shelf life and high smoking point. A 2015 meta-analysis compiled data from 12 different studies, concluding that saturated fat intake was not associated with all-cause mortality (all deaths that occurred, regardless of the cause), CVD mortality, total CHD, ischemic stroke, or type 2 diabetes.[7] However, consumption of industrial trans fats, even in extremely small amounts, was positively associated with all-cause mortality, CHD mortality, and total CHD. In other words, when we stopped eating saturated fats and replaced those fats with trans fats, refined carbohydrates, and sugar, we started getting sicker.

Fats are an essential part of the diet that should come in varying forms. They fill a number of vital roles in the body. Fats are an excellent source of energy in that they are the slowest of all the macronutrients (carbs, proteins, and fats) to be metabolized. Some vitamins and minerals such as vitamins A, D, E, and K are fat soluble, meaning that you simply cannot absorb these nutrients without the presence of fat. The best source of these vitamins happens to be fatty foods.

The human brain is comprised of about 60 percent fat. Indeed, fat, including cholesterol lipids, are essential for cellular metabolism throughout the body. Cholesterol controls the fluidity of cell membranes, which impacts the movement of substances in and out of cells, and influences the proteins that are embedded within. Fatty acids build cell membranes and myelin sheaths, the protective coverings on most nerve cells that form an electrically insulated layer. Without fats, our bodies are incapable of proper blood clotting, hormone production, muscle movement, or initiating an appropriate inflammation response. Fats are clearly an important component of a good diet. But the question is, "What constitutes a healthy fat?"

All fats are comprised of long carbon chains with attached hydrogen atoms. The shape, length, and configuration of these chains translate into different functions throughout the body. Saturated fats are fully *saturated* with hydrogen atoms. The carbon chains are holding as much hydrogen as possible, a structure allowing for molecules to be tightly stacked, thus resulting in a substance that's solid at room temperature. There are varying types of saturated fats, such as lauric acid in coconut oil, that has gained much attention for its antimicrobial and heart-healthy benefits. Indeed, a number of different saturated fats exist in varying foods with their own unique health benefits.

Unsaturated fats are either monounsaturated or polyunsaturated. Each is different based on the number of attached hydrogen atoms and double carbon bonds. These fats can be further divided into types such as omega-3 fatty acids, found in cold-water fish and walnuts; omega-6 fatty acids, found in vegetable oils; omega-9 fatty acids, found in avocado oil; and others. Distinguishing the difference between these types of fats isn't necessary for understanding what constitutes a healthy fat, but in general, each of these fats is beneficial when found in a whole-food source. The problem with unsaturated fats arises when the fats are extracted from the food, such as in corn, vegetable, soybean, peanut, and safflower oil. These fats are unstable, meaning that they can degrade in the presence of light, heat, oxygen, and pressure. Processing mechanisms often employ many of these techniques, yielding an oil full of chemical constituents that are harmful to the body. To make these oils more stable, scientists have turned them into hydrogenated oils, the major source of trans fats. The FDA concluded in June of 2015 that hydrogenated oils can no longer remain classified as GRAS (Generally Recognized as Safe), and therefore set a ban on their use starting June 18, 2018. Companies were granted a three-year compliance stage to make necessary changes to their products to reflect these new regulations. But don't be fooled. The FDA ended up extending the compliance date to January 2020, saying that companies needed more time to ensure a smooth transition. Furthermore, these processed oils most likely will be replaced by other toxic options such as Monsanto's Vistive Gold soybeans, a high oleic, GMO, Roundup-resistant soybean that became available to farmers in early 2018. These toxic alternatives are far from an improvement.

The best fats to use for cooking include fats that are stable when heated. Good choices include saturated fats such as lard, tallow, coconut oil, and other fats reserved from cooking meats. Using a variety of sources is best since each of these fats has a different fatty acid profile. The aforementioned fats are not comprised of 100 percent saturated fats; they're a mix and fulfill varying physiological functions throughout the body.

Olive oil and avocado oil are other good options for cooking. The paleo movement popularized the belief that olive oil (well known as a source of heart-healthy monounsaturated fats) should not be used for cooking since these molecules aren't considered to be stable at high temperatures. However, this belief was debunked by Sarah Ballantyne, aka The Paleo Mom. What I love about Sarah's work is that she has a doctorate in medical biophysics; the woman knows her chemistry! Dr. Ballantyne argues that the presence of varying phenolic antioxidants in extra-virgin olive oil protect the oil from oxidation, thus making it stable at temperatures as high as 410°F (210°C). In fact, extracts from olive oil and avocado oil can be added to canola oil to use for frying, and the antioxidant benefits make the canola oil more stable. Avocado oil is thought to have an even higher smoking point, possibly as high as 570°F (299°C).

Cooking with avocado oil and olive oil is best when using extra-virgin or cold-pressed versions. Extra-virgin indicates that the oil was derived during a single press (the term *extra-virgin* is unique to olive oils). Cold-pressed indicates that the oil extraction process did not involve heat. Heat causes the food to release a higher quantity of oil, but the heating process also destroys the beneficial constituents of the oil.

In summary, it's best to limit your cooking oils and fats to animal fats, unrefined coconut oil, extra-virgin cold-pressed olive oil, or cold-pressed avocado oil. Other oils such as cold-pressed walnut or flaxseed oils can be used in dressings, but avoid using such oils for cooking. Vegetable and soybean oils that are expeller pressed or highly processed, especially if they're not organic certified, should be avoided entirely.

limited space. Grains provide a relatively low yield, especially traditional nonhybridized varieties, and the transformation of plant to edible product is incredibly labor intensive. Our ancestors were consuming grains when they were available, but I guarantee this didn't mean grains for breakfast, lunch, and dinner, 365 days a year.

Even if you're reading this chapter as someone who's not ready to buy into the belief that all grains are bad all the time, then you should at least consider the fact that when you fill your belly with bread (or whatever grain-based food you frequently consume) you're wasting calories on a less nutritious food. Comparing the nutrient density of a grain to that of almost any vegetable, nut, seed, fruit, or whole-food animal product reveals that grains are an inferior choice. The fact that flour is fortified alone should be an indicator that you're eating a nutritionally subpar food. Luckily, better choices exist and are often readily available.

Dr. Sarah Ballantyne (aka The Paleo Mom) compared essential vitamin and mineral content of the 30 most frequently eaten vegetables to eight whole, unprocessed grains. She found that "when compared to vegetables, calorie for calorie, vegetables contain double or more of every single vitamin . . . [and are] higher in most essential minerals."[8] Hands down, grains simply aren't worth eating in such large quantities.

The Dairy Debacle

Oh, dairy. What to do? While it seems to be crystal clear that sugar is slowly killing the Western dieter and that we can all benefit from eating far fewer (if any) grains, it is less clear as to whether dairy is problematic for the average individual. I'll present arguments both against and in favor of dairy and tell you a bit more about my own family's decision to eliminate dairy, but I'll first start by talking about bones and politics—the driving forces behind dairy's long-standing residence on the USDA's Food Guide Pyramid.

David Ludwig and Walter Willett coauthored a 2013 article titled "Three Daily Servings of Reduced-Fat Milk: An Evidence-Based Recommendation?" In this article, these leading nutritional experts state that "humans have no nutritional requirement for animal milk, an evolutionary recent addition to diet."[9] Keep in mind this is coming from two well-known, mainstream nutritionists. How can this be true? We've been told for decades to eat and drink dairy as a staple for bone health maintenance. The problem is that good science has very little actual influence on dietary recommendations. The National Dairy Council promotes high dairy intake, and research dollars are therefore poured into studies that support its consumption. An analysis of data quality from studies involving soft drinks, juice, and milk showed that financial sponsorship heavily influences the study's outcome.[10] In fact, researchers found that unfavorable conclusions from consuming the beverage of study were completely absent from studies sponsored by interested parties. They concluded that industry funding results in a four to eight times greater likelihood of favoring the financial interests of the sponsor when compared with studies without conflicting funding sources. I believe this is a primary example of something we call bias. But in the unfortunate case of dietary recommendations, this bias is costing millions of people their health.

Bone Health

When we think of milk we think of calcium, and calcium is indeed what keeps our bones strong. We had to find a way to maintain our bones without consuming the dreaded fat, especially artery-clogging saturated fats, so the USDA recommended that most age groups consume three cups of reduced-fat milk per day in order to prevent osteoporosis and other bone-related diseases. This unfortunate recommendation stripped dairy of one of its finer qualities—rich, creamy, nutritious fat. No matter, the important thing was to supply our population with enough calcium to create strong bones.

While Americans consume more cow's milk and dairy products per person than most other worldwide populations, American women over the age of 50 have one of the highest rates of hip fractures. Fracture rates for Europe, New Zealand, and Australia are even higher. These populations just so happen to consume even more milk per capita than the United States. Do you know what causes hip fractures in older women?

Osteoporosis. But I thought we were preventing that with our three servings of milk per day. If milk isn't the solution to bone care, then what is?

Bones are a complex matrix with a variety of functions. In the center is marrow interlaced with connective tissue, stored minerals, and fats. Vitamin A and specific bone-building enzymes are responsible for bone growth early in life, which is why a deficiency in vitamin A can cause stunted growth. Bones have an intricate composition that involves a collagen matrix with dynamic mineral deposits throughout. The collagen matrix is a lattice protein structure that comprises approximately 35 percent of our bones. Collagen is built from proteins and helps to provide our bones with flexibility. Our bones are not like wood or rocks, which don't flex; they have an inherent ability to bend as needed in response to muscle movements and impact.

The collagen matrix is responsible for "trapping" mineral salts such as calcium phosphate to make up the other 65 percent of our bone structure. But it's not just calcium that is trapped within the matrix. Bones store magnesium, sodium, potassium, and other minerals in the process of mineralization. Minerals are continually flowing in an out of our bones in response to our body's needs, qualifying bones as highly dynamic organs that are continually being rebuilt. This is great news for those who suffer from weak bones. Adults regrow 5 to 10 percent of their bones every year, meaning that a full replacement can occur in about 10 years. Conditions such as osteoporosis can therefore be improved through dietary approaches, but once you're over the age of 30 or so, your bones can never be as healthy as they were in your youth. Rates of bone deposition can't keep up with reabsorption once you're over 30, which results in a small amount of bone loss over time. However, this information should by no means discourage you from improving your bone health via diet.

Now, here's what interesting—if you dissolve a bone in an acid bath, the minerals dissolve away but the collagen (protein) matrix remains. That is, you're left with a matrix that cannot be broken; it bends. Alternatively, if you remove the collagen matrix from a bone, leaving only the minerals behind, you're essentially left with a structure that mimics chalk, a rigid yet easily broken substance. If you consider that populations who are consuming the greatest quantities of calcium are also suffering from the highest rates of fractures, then you can assume that calcium recommendations are only targeting the breakable, mineral component of our bones. A better approach would be to focus on the varying components of bones and how bones are created, degraded, and made rigid yet flexible.

The question then becomes, how do we improve and maintain bone health if we don't eat loads of dairy? First off, we certainly need calcium, but not in the quantities found in dairy. Leafy greens and cruciferous vegetables such as kale, cabbage, broccoli, cauliflower, and brussels sprouts are all excellent sources of calcium. Additional food sources of calcium include oysters, soft-shell crabs, and foods with edible bones such as sardines and homemade bone stocks. Our bodies also require the help of two essential vitamins in order to properly assimilate calcium—vitamin D and vitamin K_2. Vitamin D is actually a hormone, and it is found in very few foods with the exception of mushrooms, some fatty fish, and egg yolks. Dairy is a source of vitamin D, but only because it has been fortified with a synthetic vitamin. The absolute best source of vitamin D is from the sun, so getting outside every day is an easy way to get what you need. However, taking a vitamin D supplement during the winter months isn't a bad idea, especially if you live in a northern climate. Vitamin K_2's role in bone development has been much ignored until recently, but it is responsible for depositing calcium into places like bones and teeth rather than into arteries. Foods high in vitamin K_2 include natto (a fermented soy product), hard and soft cheeses, egg yolk, butter from grass-fed cows, chicken liver, salami, chicken breasts, and ground beef. Experts also speculate that some organ meats are especially high in K_2, but this has yet to be verified.

Beyond calcium, vitamin D, and K_2, there are a number of other factors that help encourage strong bone development. Some of the other important bone-building vitamins, minerals, and macronutrients include saturated fats, phosphorus, vitamin A, magnesium, vitamin C, boron, manganese, zinc, copper, silicon, vitamin B_6, folate, and many others. Annemarie Colbin, author of *The Whole-Food Guide to Strong Bones*, writes that "if we add up all these nutrients necessary for bone health, pretty soon we'll end up with . . . food!" But she also points out that it's not just food that enhances bone health, but also exercise and time spent outdoors. I already discussed the need for us to get vitamin D from the sun, but exercise stresses the bones in a way that positively encourages growth and development. Even the simple action of walking generates vibrations when the heel strikes the ground, and these vibrations move through the bone structure to stimulate growth. The healthy approach to developing and maintaining strong bones is much like the approach to overall health—eat a healthy, balanced diet, exercise, and spend time outdoors.

Dairy for Children: Is It Really Necessary?

Dairy is promoted as being especially essential for children, who "need" milk for proper growth and development. The American Academy of Pediatrics recommends that children should avoid cow's milk until age one, at which point whole milk should be introduced, but children over the age of two should be switched to 1% milk or skim milk. This recommendation to slowly wean a child from full-fat milk is a result of the low-fat craze that holds little scientific support. In fact, multiple studies have shown that children who consume lower-fat milk actually have higher BMIs (body mass index), which is a measure of body fat based on weight and height. A 2013 study of 10,700 children age two to four showed that the lower the percentage of fat in the milk they consumed, the greater their BMI and greater their risk for being overweight.[11] A 2005 study followed 12,829 children age 9 to 13 and found that children who consumed three or more servings of milk per day had greater increases in BMI over the course of three years than those who drank less milk.[12] This study also confirmed that the intake of 1% milk and skim milk had significantly greater impacts on increased BMI.

There are a number of theories as to why we see increases in BMI and weight with greater consumption of milk, especially lower-fat versions. Perhaps this is the old tale of the chicken and the egg—maybe it's that the kids that drank lower-fat milk were larger to begin with and the low-fat milk was an attempt to prevent these larger children from further increasing BMI. Or perhaps it's because the hormones in the milk actually stimulate growth beyond what is normal. The fact that lower-fat milk had greater impacts on increased weight upholds the well-supported theory that decreased fat intake decreases satiety. These hungry people turn to other foods to find the calories they crave. People who consume low-fat milk are likely getting those additional calories from other low-fat foods that are often full of sugars and processed carbs, which, as we know, increase insulin production and fat storage. Whatever the trend, the recommendations from the American Academy of Pediatrics need to be revised.

Parents should also be reserved about serving dairy to their children because it's a commonly ill-tolerated food, especially by infants and toddlers. Many young children suffer from reflux, colic, and eczema, which often result from food allergies and intolerances. The most common culprits are milk, eggs, soy, wheat, peanuts, tree nuts, fish, and shellfish. Milk and egg allergies don't often persist into adulthood, which indicates that there's something about the immature digestive system that simply can't properly digest milk or egg proteins or both. My son just so happened to be one of those individuals with both a transient milk and egg allergy. We discovered that he had a milk allergy when he was around four months of age. I hadn't yet served him dairy, but the milk proteins that I was consuming were being passed on to him through breast milk. His weight gain came to an abrupt halt and the doctor detected small amounts of blood in his stool, which is actually more common than you would think. This condition is known as occult intestinal blood loss and it occurs in 40 percent of normal infants. You're reading that correctly, milk is actually harmful to the gut of nearly half of all infants. Remember my discussion about leaky gut in the section about grains and how cells of the intestines need to be sealed tightly together in order to prevent the escape of partially digested proteins? Well, the infant gut is leaky by design, and the cells of the intestines don't fully seal until a child is around two years of age. This evolutionary advantage allows for the passing of hormones and other important molecules from breast milk into our baby's bodies, but it also means that we have to implement great care when introducing foods to an already sensitive system. The good news is that occult intestinal blood loss usually subsides as a child grows older. While it is beyond the scope of this book to discuss an indepth healthy approach for introducing solids and early feeding habits, an early introduction of dairy and rice cereal as first foods are outrageously terrible recommendations (see *My Family on GAPS*, page 33). Both foods should be saved for much later in life, when a child has a more developed gut.

Lactose Intolerance and Problematic Proteins

Lactose intolerance is estimated to be present in approximately 75 percent of the worldwide population. There's great variation among ethnicities, with only 5 percent of Northern Europeans demonstrating lactose intolerance, but a prevalence as high as 90 percent for Asians and Africans. In the United States alone, it's estimated that 30 to 50 million people are lactose intolerant. People who are lactose intolerant lack lactase, the enzyme responsible for breaking lactose down into glucose. The lack of lactase (say that five times fast) is often a result of genetics, but can also occur in response to diseases such as Crohn's, celiac, ulcerative colitis, gastroenteritis, and also in response to infections and chemotherapy. Lactose intolerance causes a slew of symptoms that resemble irritable bowel syndrome (IBS)—gas, bloating, nausea, stomach pain, and diarrhea. Some people who are lactose intolerant claim that while they can't tolerate pasteurized milk, they can tolerate raw milk. Milk naturally contains lactase, which is lost during the pasteurization process. The presence of lactase makes raw milk a more digestible source of dairy for those who can't tolerate lactose. Pasteurization is responsible for preventing a number of diseases such as tuberculosis, salmonella, giardiasis, and many other bacterial and parasitic infections. The presence of disease-causing pathogens in milk is more prominent in large factory farms or farms where a lack of proper sanitation and cleaning methods exist. That said, raw milk sourced from a reputable family farm is unlikely to be a source of such diseases. My family sourced raw milk from a friend in Vermont whose family owned a small dairy. They'd been consuming raw milk for decades without issue; their farming practices prevented the spread of undesirable bacteria and parasites. If you decide to go the family farm route to get your raw milk, just be sure to inquire about the dairy's sanitary practices.

Milk contains whey and casein proteins that can be problematic for certain individuals whether it is caused by a sensitivity or an actual allergy. If you suffer from IBS, I highly recommend eliminating all dairy for a minimum of three weeks to see how your body responds. One study showed that 84 percent of people with IBS tested positive for milk protein antibodies, indicating a milk allergy. For others, either casein or whey (or both) can simply be irritating to the gut.

Dairy and Autoimmune Disease

One of the more unfortunate consequences of consuming milk, especially at a young age, is its role in the development of autoimmune diseases. Cow's milk is a source of proteins that mimic our own. At times, these proteins are recognized as harmful invaders, and the immune system responds by releasing antibodies. The problem is that the body loses its ability to distinguish between normal cells and milk proteins, and begins to destroy them all. When your body attacks its own healthy cells, you're considered to have autoimmune disease. Some examples include hyperthyroidism, rheumatoid arthritis, hypothyroidism, anemia, multiple sclerosis, type 1 diabetes, lupus, and others.

People who are type 1 diabetic have an immune system that mistakenly attacks healthy pancreas cells that produce insulin. A strong link between early-childhood milk consumption and development of type 1 diabetes demonstrates that cow's milk is extremely difficult to digest for the immature system of an infant. These improperly digested proteins leak into the bloodstream, where antibodies are formed to attack the invaders. Unfortunately, these invaders look an awful lot like the body's own pancreas cells. Once this response is initiated, an individual's immune cells remain confused and the individual will be diabetic for a lifetime.

A 1992 Finnish study cited within *The China Study*, a famed project that explored the relationship between diet and disease risk, measured milk antibodies in diabetic versus nondiabetic children. Diabetics consistently had higher milk antibodies. Additional studies since that time have shown that early weaning, early introduction of milk-based formulas (or milk), and childhood viral infections that compromise the immune system are all risk factors for developing type 1 diabetes. Genetics also play a small role in the development of diabetes, thus the American Academy of Pediatrics strongly recommends that infants with a family history of diabetes avoid milk until the age of two. An infant has a 13.1 times greater chance of developing type 1 diabetes when there's both a family history of the disease and not being breastfed for a minimum of three months, implying that the child was instead fed a milk-based formula. Not being breastfed for a minimum of three months alone increases risk 11.3 times. The authors of *The China Study* offer perspectives for comparison, stating that smoking increases likelihood of developing lung cancer only 10 times. The risk of developing diabetes from early introduction of milk is therefore extremely profound and should be discussed more often.

Multiple sclerosis (MS) is another autoimmune disease for which a documented trend in development is similar to that of type 1 diabetes. The difference is that rather than attacking the pancreas, antibodies attack the cells of the myelin sheath, the coating that lines the nerves. Some of the initial studies of MS development focused on the consumption of saturated fats, but more recent studies suggest that dairy is the more likely culprit in disease onset and severity.[13] Regardless, a change in diet that reflects the elimination of dairy can substantially improve disease outcome.

Take It or Leave It

All in all, there are certainly risks associated with consuming dairy, but these outcomes appear to manifest on an individualized basis. Personally, I've found that my family members are among the individuals who benefit from dairy exclusion. My son clearly has symptoms of leaky gut and systemic inflammation since he suffers from both asthma and allergies. The same is true for my husband since he, too, has asthmatic tendencies. Individuals who suffer from any type of inflammatory condition should avoid dairy as part of an anti-inflammatory approach aimed at disease management. We also avoid dairy with my daughter because of its mucus-forming capabilities, as CF is characterized by excessive mucus. Quite simply, the consumption of dairy is counterproductive in the treatment of her disease. As for myself, I personally notice very little difference whether I choose to eat or not eat dairy.

There's evidence that supports that dairy can be beneficial in some instances. Studies supporting dairy intake have shown that consuming full-fat and fermented dairy can help protect against metabolic disease, type 2 diabetes, and cardiovascular disease. It can lower an individual's risk for stroke and coronary heart disease. Dairy from healthy, grass-fed cows offers an excellent source of fat-soluble vitamins, calcium, and anti-inflammatory fats such as linoleic acid. Further studies support the consumption of dairy as a beneficial source of calories for malnourished children. Despite evidence showing that dairy consumption may actually be beneficial, it's important to keep in mind that these benefits are only observed for individuals who can tolerate and digest dairy without issue, and there's much evidence showing that these rules simply don't apply to everyone.

The best way to determine whether you can tolerate dairy is to embark on an elimination diet for a minimum of two to three weeks. Most of us never even question the foods we eat, which is why it's important to question our habits by trying something new and unconventional from time to time. I've known numerous individuals (myself included) who felt that certain foods agreed with their body until they tried eliminating these foods for an extended period of time. Sometimes we can't recognize what a food does to our body because we have no basis for comparison. We've only known how our body feels while eating that food, because we've always eaten it.

Whole Foods to the Rescue

We now know that sugar is toxic, overconsumption and processing of grains is harmful, and dairy isn't well tolerated by numerous individuals. Consumption of these foods can lead to serious health consequences. But what do we eat if we avoid all of these staples of the Western diet? Salad? Cardboard? What's left if we take away our grains, sugar, and dairy?

I could use this section to implore you to eat beets because they contain high quantities of detoxifying pigments called betalains. Or I might try to convince you that anthocyanins in dark purple fruits such as blueberries are going to save you from the dangers of oxidation. Our society is obsessed with "superior" foods like spinach, acai berries, and turmeric that declare above-average nutritional benefits. (Okay, I admit that I kind of buy into the whole turmeric thing.) Maybe we could take a scientific approach and construct a diet of only the foods with the highest-ranking nutritional values. We'd surely be preventing heart disease, cancer, diabetes, obesity, arthritis, and numerous other chronic diseases that we could combat with a specific formulation of the perfect foods. The problem with extreme dietary activities is that most of us are busy with other concerns; personally, I don't have time to weigh out every dietary question that pops up. Should we eat cabbage or cauliflower tonight? Which will optimize our calcium intake for the day? Have I eaten enough antioxidants? Should I squeeze in a cup of blueberries before bed? My strategy is to eat real, whole foods and forget about the magic-bullet health claims.

When I consider all of the evidence against sugar, grains, and dairy, what stands out is that these foods, especially the highly processed versions, are disease promoting. Repeated studies show that a change in diet corresponds with a change in health status. When you eat Western foods, you get Western diseases. While some experts point to genetics as the driving force behind disease etiology, the reality is that genetics contribute to less than 10 percent of disease. The author Chris Kresser described it best when he wrote, "Genes may load the gun, but the environment pulls the trigger." Less than 2 percent of all diseases result from a true genetic defect. Unfortunately, CF is one such disease, but this is all the more reason to protect the rest of my daughter's genetic profile, and I do this by providing her with good fuel for her system. What we're learning is that genetics are far more complicated than we previously thought and that a single gene simply cannot cause something like diabetes, heart disease, or cancer. It's instead the interaction of these genes and how the environment affects their expression. Studies of identical twins demonstrate this principle perfectly. Two individuals have identical genes, so you would expect the same disease outcome for both twins if genetics were the sole driving force behind disease development. Yet when we look at an identical twin that develops diabetes, the second twin has only a 13 to 33 percent chance of contracting the same. Yes, the genetics for diabetes are present, but it's the environment and the interaction of genes that trigger the response. Some experts have estimated that 50 percent of worldwide early deaths are caused by three factors alone—diet, indoor and outdoor air pollution, and smoking. Allow me to translate this for you: We're making ourselves sick (or, really, the companies in charge of our food supply)! Our diets (and air) are slowly killing us!

But let's go back to the acai berries and turmeric. Yes, these foods prevent disease for varying reasons, but I'm arguing that it's less important that these foods *prevent* disease and more important that the alternatives (processed, Western foods) are *causing* disease. If you look at it that way, knowing what to eat then becomes really simple—you eat *real* food! When you take away the grains, sugar, and dairy you're left with options like fruits, vegetables, nuts, beans, seeds, meats, eggs, fish, and the like. Hopefully, I've stressed that overconsumption of most any food can be problematic, so we need to eat a variety of these things.

A Broken System with Poor Advice

When deciding what and how to eat, we simply can't count on the government or the medical community to give us sound advice regarding the correct combination of nutrients. Yes, there are some amazing individuals out there who are rising above to lead the way to positive change, but by and large we're at the mercy of a broken system. Agriculture subsidies fund crops like wheat, corn, soybeans, rice, and cotton, which drive the low costs for such commodities. It's a system that encourages overproduction and prevents farmers from implementing more environmentally sound practices or growing more nutritious foods like fruits and vegetables. The USDA spent almost $13 billion on farm program payments in 2016 and none of this money subsidized vegetable production. This money is instead keeping costs low for a loaf of bread.

The sad truth is that money informs policy and unfortunately this doesn't mean that our health is being protected. A 2009 article published in the *New York Times* discussed extreme bias in medical schools throughout the United States and the astronomical amount of funding for medical schools that originates from pharmaceutical companies.[14] The American Medical Student Association rates medical schools based on their conflicts of interest and the amount of money provided by the drug industry. Harvard Medical School, one of the most prestigious schools in the United States, received an F because millions of dollars in direct payments to professors and in research funds came directly from interest groups such as pharmaceutical companies. One Harvard professor was noted to have 47 affiliations with different companies. It would seem that our doctors are being trained to treat disease in a way that brings financial gain for drug companies. As a rule, doctors aren't being taught that avoiding milk until the age of two can help protect against type 1 diabetes. Instead, they're being taught that type 1 diabetes is treated with a lifetime of insulin injections. Prevention doesn't pay, and the system is set up to generate payees.

We can't forget that making people sick is good for business. Dr. Mark Hyman said it this way in a *Huffington Post* article: "The basic fact is that one-third of our economy profits from making people sick and fat. The food industry sells products scientifically proven to kill more people than cigarettes, while our health care industry profits from providing more volume of care focused on medication and procedures, not better health." Corporations are allowed to make unlimited campaign contributions to politicians, and these contributors are informing important policy when it comes to health care and how we prevent disease. I can only imagine what these corporations are getting in exchange for their campaign dollars, but I doubt it's anything to provide the taxpayers with improved health.

Politics is certainly one of the reasons that a low-fat, high-carb diet gained such popularity. We were told for decades that saturated fats and cholesterol would cause heart disease, but the resulting dietary changes created an upsurge in diabetes, obesity, and associated diseases. Drinking more milk led to more osteoporosis. Luckily, the growing body of scientific literature is starting to lay these myths to rest, and we're slowly watching the pointed finger move away from fats and rightfully toward sugar and processed carbohydrates.

The Approach That Works

I've really only described the tip of the iceberg when it comes to conflicts of interest and poor nutritional and medical advice. Nonetheless, hopefully it's clear to you that we need to change our diet and that we need to use a commonsense approach to enacting this change.

We need to eat real food. The question then becomes "How do we do it?" You can start by making it your goal to eventually eat a nearly 100 percent whole-food diet that is free of sugar and processed foods, with very little (if any) grains or dairy. You start by going through the chapters of this book and learning how my own family made this change, and to become inspired by its long-term benefits and sustainability.

Anytime you make a major change, especially one that involves the elimination of an undesirable habit or food, it's helpful to focus more on what you're getting than on what you're taking away. If you decide to start implementing a grain-free, sugar-free, dairy-free diet and all you think about is deprivation and how you're losing all of these fabulous foods, then you're focusing on subtraction, what you're giving up. A better approach is to focus on the positive health possibilities you are getting and the opportunity to experience some amazing foods that you've likely been missing out on. For example, I eat vegetables at nearly every single meal. Have you ever tried eating vegetables at nearly every single meal? Do you know how remarkable you start to feel when you eat like this? If I were eating sandwiches all the time I wouldn't have space in my diet for all of these other nourishing foods. I don't feel deprived of bread, I feel gifted by vegetables and the nourishment they give me.

I encourage you to think about the benefits of dietary change, the possibilities in health, and the incredible additions you're going to be making to your diet as you change the way you eat. All of these whole foods are coming to the rescue.

chapter two

Feeding the Kids—
Get Your Game Face On!

When it comes to human health, children rank as one of my top priorities. Children are growing and developing the bodies, minds, and habits that will propel them into their future bodies, minds, and habits, and they need the right fuel if they're to develop to their fullest potential. Diseases that were once unique to an aging population such as obesity, heart disease, and diabetes are now developing in young children at alarming rates. The youngest child to have developed type 2 diabetes in the United States is three and a half years old. Behavioral and spectrum disorders are at an all-time high, and the number of drug-dependent children continues to grow. Varying theories exist as to why these conditions are steadily increasing, including that of diet. And with that in mind, I'm most interested in the growing body of evidence supporting the benefits of a healthy diet. Among that evidence are the stories of families who have experienced relief from varying symptoms and conditions through dietary interventions.

As parents we have a responsibility to help our children learn and understand how to fuel their bodies in a healthy way. Feeding our kids the proper foods takes effort, but the payoff is substantial. Recall how you feel after eating entirely too much sugar. Personally, I've noticed that I'm far more irritable and my emotions are less stable. As an adult I'm able to stuff my emotions into an internal compartment and go on with my day, but children don't filter their emotions in this same way; a bad sugar binge can lead to explosive emotions that leave everyone in the family feeling drained. Although I'm using sugar as an example, chemical-laden processed foods can generate similar effects, especially in small children. Taking the time to feed your children real food will drastically help improve their mood, behavior, and overall health, which are all powerful motivators in the journey to achieve a better diet.

Marketing of Kid-Friendly Foods

Foods marketed toward children are often brightly colored, void of nutrients, and contain more sugar per serving than what should be consumed by an adult. The Center for Science in the Public Interest (CSPI) has reported that 43 percent of children's foods contain food dyes, stating this is problematic since dyes are associated with hyperactivity and other behavioral problems in children. CSPI has petitioned the Food and Drug Administration (FDA), requesting a ban on the following dyes: Red 3, Red 40, Yellow 5, Blue 1, Blue 2, Green 3, and Orange B (a dye permitted only on sausage casings). They support their request saying that "the European Union requires a warning label on most dyed foods indicating that such products 'may have an adverse effect on activity and attention in children,' encouraging manufacturers to switch to natural (or no) colorings."

Why is it, exactly, that we need food dyes in our children's foods? Somehow we've become caught in a trap of believing that our children won't eat the same foods enjoyed by adults. The efforts to market kid-friendly foods have successfully created an entire line of processed junk for our children, which is supported by our belief that colorful food equates to kid food. Unfortunately, this assumption isn't entirely false. I have yet to buy my kids one single packaged, kid-friendly food, but my son asks me to buy some form of superhero gummies almost every time we're at the grocery store. The brightly colored foods in flashy boxes adorned with Ninja Turtles are enticing to his young mind—a testament to the food industry's successful propaganda. Of course your child *wants* the flashy sugar-loaded cereal rather than eggs and home-made muffins, but does this mean that your child won't eat the healthier alternative? They won't if you allow them to choose. I simply don't buy the sugar-laden kid food, which eliminates the choice altogether and ultimately saves us an argument.

Grocery stores also do their part to enhance purchasing of kid-friendly foods by lining checkout aisles with candies, lollipops, chips, and other unhealthy foods that spark children's interest. We drag our children through the grocery aisles as they relentlessly ask for a variety of products, and we reach the checkout aisle feeling tired, run down, and ready to abort mission. I now understand why my mother often left the three of us girls at home. While I stick to my guns when my kids start asking for the candy bars, I see how many parents get tired of the fight and give in at this point in their shopping adventure.

My advice to you is that if a food is marketed as a kid-friendly food, don't buy it. Run in the other direction. The same goes for many of the "all natural," "organic," or seemingly healthier children's products. Many of these products aren't much better when it comes to nutritional value. Although I will say that buying organic is definitely better than the conventional option.

The bottom line is that your child is a human, and humans need real food. Healthy foods aren't usually sold in flashy boxes covered in Disney princesses. Don't let food marketers fool you into thinking that your child won't eat food unless it's packaged like a toy.

Aborigines and Dinosaur-Shaped Chicken Nuggets

Consider children who grow up in remote societies that consume meat, blood, organs, bitter roots, and seasonal fruits, vegetables, nuts, and seeds. Imagine a mother serving a dish to her child, but the child snubs whatever food has been offered, saying, "I don't like it." The mother rushes back to her primitive kitchen and throws a pile of dinosaur-shaped chicken nuggets into the microwave. The parents eat the nutritious meal prepared from fresh ingredients, while the child stuffs their face with a fake chicken product that's likely loaded with soy protein isolates, wheat, fillers, stabilizers, preservatives, food dyes, and of course just enough chicken to actually market the product as "chicken."

The scenario I just presented may seem absolutely absurd, yet how many families across the developed world have fallen into this pattern with their own version of dinosaur-shaped chicken nuggets? When children refuse to try a new food, parents are quick to offer the kid-friendly foods that their child will willingly eat. Or even worse, most parents won't even try to offer new foods simply because they're tired of battling their children over picky eating. I get it; we choose our battles. As we parents slump over in complacency and exhaustion, our kids consume frozen pizza bites, fish sticks, fruit snacks, processed meats and cheeses, muffins, cookies, crackers, and whatever other convenient, kid-friendly foods they've grown accustomed to.

I'm sure you're wondering how this feeding cycle has developed. The answer is quite simple: Parents provided these processed foods to their children, for whatever the reason, and now their children have developed a taste for processed foods. Trying to get children to eat anything other than these foods then becomes a major challenge. I'll offer suggestions for changing these habits momentarily, but I'd like to first help you understand a loving, logical argument that just might persuade you to stop offering dinosaur-shaped chicken nuggets (or whatever) to your children.

Love Your Kids with Food

One of the mistakes that we often make as parents is when we fail to respect the boundary between nourishment and a child's personal preference. Our kids are picky eaters because we've given them choices that satisfy our immediate desire for them to eat. And our reaction is to replace our initial offering of nutritious food with a more tantalizing food that will likely encourage them to eat, even at the risk of endangering their long-term health. We need to readjust our boundaries so as to focus more on nourishment and less on preference.

When I offer my child something to eat and they refuse, I'm tempted to rush back to the kitchen and offer a different, more appetizing choice. This is especially true for my daughter, whose disease is characterized by malnutrition, improper growth, and an impaired ability to absorb nutrients. I'm so overly invested in the number that appears on the scale that I literally lose sleep over the subject before our quarterly clinic visits. To be perfectly honest, I have even loaded her up with food and water immediately before entering the doctor's office in hopes that those extra few ounces she consumes before stepping on the scale will guarantee a positive response from her CF team. I can't even tell you the number of times I've been tempted to load her up with unhealthy foods just to make that number grow at a rate beyond the normal growth curve. Yet I constantly remind myself that the foods I offer to my children are nourishing choices. If they choose not to eat, it's because they're not hungry. My long-term objective is to help my daughter grow and develop in a way that prevents the devastation of her disease—this is the *loving* choice I make for her each and every day—and I won't let my goal be overshadowed by a short-term investment in my desire to see her eat.

I should note that my daughter is certainly not undernourished. In fact, I'd say she's thriving. I'd hate for you to think that I'm refusing to feed my child because I'm so darn stubborn about health food that I'm watching her waste away. She is currently around the 90th percentile for height and weight, and follows a normal growth curve—all signs that she's growing as expected. We've had issues in the past because she's tall and thin. In the world of CF, children are expected to maintain a BMI above the 50th percentile. Although her numbers seem perfectly average for a "normal" child, our previous CF team felt that her weight wasn't adequate for her height. They'd like for all CF kids to mimic little Michelin Men with rolls covering their bodies. Unfortunately, neither of my children adopted this trait. I blame my husband who's over six feet tall and has never weighed an ounce over 160 pounds in his life.

I also want to add that some families with CF are not as fortunate as us; for them malnourishment is a major, life-threatening struggle. These families have had to make a few more exceptions than they would have liked simply because of their situation. While it's beyond the scope of this book to dive into the multiple reasons a child may develop into a picky eater, certain medications and medical conditions can completely zap a child's appetite. Many of these families are just doing their best to get anything into their child's belly. I'm oversimplifying the issue, because the majority of people fall outside of these special circumstances. The important point is that getting your kid to eat, whatever the circumstances, can often be a complicated issue. So please don't judge your neighbor whose child has severe autism when you see that all he eats are fish sticks and crackers. Our fellow parents could use a bit more grace, and chances are that we don't understand the full story.

Okay, so back to loving our children with food. I encourage you to reflect on what it means to love your children through nourishment. Does it mean filling their bellies with processed, sweetened, kid-friendly foods that will most likely contribute to poor eating habits or disease? I believe that we've somehow missed the mark, and in order to hit that mark we need to take a step back and understand the long-term consequences of our actions. None of us want our children to develop juvenile diabetes or other chronic diseases normally seen much later in life. Can you imagine how heartbreaking that would be? Please know that I'm not condemning any choices you've made. Trust me, I've made (and will continue to make) my own mistakes. I simply encourage you to understand that love is expressed in numerous ways, and that one of those ways is by offering healthy foods to your children that will ensure that they continue to thrive.

The GAPS Diet and Early Foods for Baby

Gut and Psychology Syndrome (GAPS) refers to a combination of symptoms that are speculated to arise from severe gut dysbiosis (abnormal flora conditions within the intestinal tract). Dr. Natasha Campbell-McBride, author of *Gut and Psychology Syndrome*, noticed that several autistic children often developed one or more additional symptoms and conditions including dyspraxia, ADD, ADHD, asthma, allergies, dyslexia, depression, and schizophrenia. These same children often exhibit digestive issues such as gas, diarrhea, bloating, constipation, or frequent upset stomachs. She concluded that the condition within the gut was the cause of these varying conditions. If she could heal the gut, she could heal the condition.

Dr. Campbell-McBride formulated the GAPS diet as an approach to correct gut dysbiosis, thus correcting any associated symptoms. The diet has varying stages, all with a focus on nutrient density and avoiding foods that could potentially irritate the bowels. Stage one involves the simplest foods—homemade bone broths, boiled meats, healthy fats, and boiled nonfibrous vegetables with seeds and peels removed. She recommends ferments and probiotics as an integral part of the healing process, saying that homemade raw fermented dairy and fermented vegetable juice (the actual fermented vegetables are added in later stages) are both excellent choices during this first stage.

Raw organic egg yolks are added during the second stage. Soft boiled eggs that include the whites are added once the raw yolks are well tolerated. The second stage allows for the addition of herbs, more probiotic foods, and ghee. Avocado, pancakes made from nut butters, egg scrambles, and fermented vegetables are added during the third stage. The fourth stage expands preparation methods for meat, such that roasting and grilling may be added to the boiling method. Olive oil is added, as are freshly pressed green juices. The fifth stage begins to incorporate a few cooked fruits (apples, mangoes, and pineapples; citrus is not yet allowed) and some raw vegetables. The sixth stage allows for raw fruits and a few GAPS-approved baked goods that use fruit as a natural sweetener.

A patient can move through the six stages of the GAPS diet in varying amounts of time, using the consistency of their stool as the primary indicator. Dr. Natasha Campbell-McBride has seen it take as little as two weeks or as much as one year's time. The idea is that you're slowly allowing the digestive system to heal and repair itself while simultaneously flushing out undesirable bacteria and replenishing the remaining bacteria with a healthier population. A GAPS patient who has successfully introduced all foods in stage six can then move on to the full GAPS diet, a protocol that is followed for at least two years. The full GAPS diet is grain-free, allows very few legumes, omits all processed foods, and focuses on quality and the addition of ferments. A GAPS patient then continues to eat healthy meats, fats, homemade broths, probiotic foods, vegetables, fruits, nuts, raw dairy, herbs and spices, and green juices. Overall, I'd have to say that the GAPS diet is not very restrictive, other than those initial stages that are necessary for rapid healing and transformation.

My Family on GAPS

I chose to use portions of the GAPS diet when introducing solids to my daughter in order to encourage healthy gut development. I opted not to introduce dairy due to its mucus-forming characteristics. I also avoided raw eggs since my son was allergic to eggs and I was concerned that my daughter, too, might have some of the same issues. Other than that, I followed the stages, slowly introducing one set of foods after another until my daughter was on the full GAPS diet by the age of 18 months. We started with bone broths and healthy fats (primarily animal fats), and slowly added boiled meats and vegetables. I chose to leave the peels and seeds of vegetables intact for the sake of time, but I stuck to non-starchy, nonfibrous vegetables in the beginning and then slowly branched out. I would boil the vegetables and fats in bone broth and create a puréed soup out of the mix that could be eaten for multiple meals. These soups could even be frozen and thawed to switch it up for some diverse combinations. I offered her small pieces of meat that required minimal chewing because it had been pressure-cooked or extensively boiled in broth. Allowing her to pick up the small bits of meat with her fingers also helped her develop the coordination and mouth skills she would need for more advanced feeding.

I didn't know about the GAPS diet when I was introducing solids to my son. Though I'll never know for sure, I believe some of his allergic tendencies may have been at least partially mitigated had I implemented a gentler approach. Introducing solids to a baby in a safe and cautious way is accomplished using the GAPS diet and I wouldn't recommend doing it any other way.

Healthy Eating Habits Start Early

My hope is that mothers of young children will read this book and implement the following strategies in order to prevent the picky eating trap. I have now introduced many foods to two healthy, adventurous eaters and I believe my strategies can work for the majority of parents. There are certainly circumstances for which developing healthy eating habits (medical conditions, sensory issues, or medications) will be a bit more complicated and may even require professional intervention. I encourage families with these circumstances to seek early intervention.

My approach boils down to one thing, and one thing only: I fulfill my obligation to feed my children by offering them a nourishing choice. If they refuse this choice, there's no other option. Dinner is dinner; I don't cook to order.

When my son was around 18 months of age, he was on the path to becoming a picky eater. He would eat only cheesy macaroni, an odd homemade kale bread concoction, and puréed vegetables that were hidden in puréed sweet potatoes. It wasn't the worst diet, but he was eating the same foods at every meal. When I offered him something different, he would refuse, and so I'd replace that food with something that he was sure to eat.

Our pediatrician gently pointed out that my own behavior was at the root of our picky eating situation. I had trained my son to know that I would *always* offer a familiar, tasty food. There was no incentive for him to try something different; the familiar foods were always available. She also pointed out that I would have to break the cycle if I were to make any improvements to his eating habits.

The weeks that followed our conversation were challenging to say the least. I would offer my son the food that my husband and I were eating for a meal, and when he would refuse I wouldn't offer a replacement. He was clearly hungry and incredibly emotional, but he refused to eat what was placed before him. Our standoff was miserable for all of us. I was offering foods that he loved for snacks, such as fresh fruits and other healthy options, and every few days I'd offer a familiar meal that gave some reprieve. But for the most part, I offered the meals that I wanted him to eat and nothing else. Our standoff lasted somewhere between two and three weeks, but then something clicked and he just started eating whatever I gave him. He finally realized that there was one and only one food choice—take it or leave it. He chose to take it. While this may seem like an abrupt approach to conquering the picky eating trap, it's the approach most often recommended by professionals. Children need firm and consistent boundaries if they're expected to alter any behavior. The short-term discomfort that we all experienced during those few weeks has paid off thousands of times over. I am certain that my son's medical condition would not have improved so drastically if his diet had remained so limited. Taking a hard stance on food

was the loving choice that my son needed if we were to avoid further deterioration of his health.

When it came time to introduce solids to my daughter I knew I didn't want to repeat the picky eating cycle, which meant I was going to need a different approach. When she turned six months of age, I chose to implement many features of the GAPS protocol for introducing her to solids. The GAPS diet is designed to help an individual develop healthy digestion and immunity (or to heal digestion and thus the immune system). Knowing that my daughter had CF motivated my search for preventive strategies such as diet that could be part of her complementary care. The GAPS diet could benefit any individual, and I believe it to be an unsurpassed approach for introducing solids to a baby.

Not only did I use an entirely different diet when introducing solids to my daughter, but I had already learned what happens when you offer the same foods repeatedly—you get a picky eater. I offered my daughter whatever nutritious GAPS foods I wanted her to eat, allowed her to eat as much as she needed, and very rarely offered an alternative choice. And can I just say again that I highly recommend this approach to any parent introducing solids to a baby? This approach worked wonderfully!

One of the greatest benefits to our food introduction approach with my daughter was that we established healthy expectations surrounding food from the beginning, which meant there was no backpedaling or need for corrective behavior down the line. Furthermore, using the GAPS diet ensured that we were only introducing the most easy-to-digest and nourishing foods, which ultimately avoided unexplained tummy pains or rashes. My daughter very rarely developed diaper rash, which was much different from my son who was always having his irritated little bum lathered in thick white cream. Even though some pediatricians won't support my claim, I'm confident that the majority of diaper rash incidents can be

Converting a Picky Eater

If you feel that your child is a mildly picky eater, you'll likely be able to tackle the issue on your own as long as you're willing to make a plan and implement a bit of tough love. If your child is young, as my son was when we corrected his picky eating, you can simply refuse to offer an alternative food. Your child will eventually catch your drift. But if you feel that your child is picky above and beyond what you consider to be within a normal range, I recommend recruiting the help of a pediatrician, speech pathologist, occupational therapist, nutritional therapist, or alternative care provider with experience in whole-food nutrition and behavioral change. These providers can help assess your child's situation, implement nutritional interventions, and work with your family to formulate a strategy to meet your specific needs.

One of the most important aspects of correcting picky eating is that a child must be repeatedly offered new foods in a low-pressure environment. Studies show that children won't even try a new food until it's been offered 8 to 15 times, but parents often stop offering after the child has refused that food just 3 or 4 times. Knowing that your child will likely reject a new food repeatedly should at least offer you some perspective and help you adjust your expectations.

Experts agree that kids eat more new foods when those foods are paired with something familiar. Hunger will be a key motivator in your success, so try to avoid filling your kids up with snacks and calorie-rich beverages that will curb hunger at mealtimes. When you do offer new foods know that you're not forcing your child to eat; you're instead providing them with ample exploration opportunities, which lessens unfamiliarity and increases curiosity. Try to pick healthy options that will

guarantee success, especially when you're just starting out. Offer those foods, along with a familiar option, and nothing else. Do not waiver in your expectations. This will only confuse the child and ultimately make this change more challenging.

Some experts recommend the use of Applied Behavior Analysis (ABA), a system based on work and reward, but its use is often limited to eliciting behavioral change in autistic or spectrum children. For example, the child will get *this* (insert highly desirable item) after you try *this* (new food). Most experts agree that using a system of reward is not ideal for all kids, but there are instances in which this approach would be useful.

If nothing else, please realize that change begins with you and that the effects will cascade down to other family members. Don't hold your children to an expectation that even you can't meet. Everyone has to be on board. Correcting the way our children eat also means correcting the way *we* eat. Be part of the solution, implement the strategies in this book for getting your kids more involved in the meal process, and commit to being consistent and upholding clear expectations. The struggle to change your child's eating habits will be well worth the payoff.

ADDITIONAL RESOURCES

Gut and Psychology Syndrome: Natural Treatment for Autism, Dyspraxia, A.D.D., A.D.H.D., Dyslexia, Depression, and Schizophrenia by Natasha Campbell-McBride

Food Chaining: The Proven 6-Step Plan to Stop Picky Eating, Solve Feeding Problems, and Expand Your Child's Diet by Sheri Fraker, Mark Fishbein, Sibyl Cox, and Laura Walbert

avoided through diet. I saw it with my son and again with my daughter, and I've talked with numerous parents who have experienced the same.

One thing to keep in mind when introducing solids to babies is that their appetites are always in flux. Don't interpret their refusal to eat as a dislike for a particular food—they're simply not hungry enough to eat it. Don't force them to eat by providing a "better" choice. Yes, there are days when my daughter, and son for that matter, barely eats, but I allow her the space to respect the ebbs and flows of her metabolic needs. Isn't that a positive attribute to encourage in our young kids anyway? I certainly wish I were better at listening to and honoring my needs, especially when it comes to hunger level. I give you my word that your child will eat when they're hungry; they won't starve themselves. Your only job is to offer food; you don't need to cater the food to their preference. Implementing this strategy in my own family has created a positive culture surrounding healthful foods. Both my daughter and my son will eat almost anything put before them and, as a result, we have minimal conflict surrounding mealtimes. Some coaxing and dislikes certainly happen at times, but it's not our norm by any means.

Getting Your Kids in the Kitchen

Children are capable of far more than we sometimes give them credit for. My son has been responsible for a variety of household tasks since he was three and a half years old. Now at age five, his tasks include things such as washing and putting away his own clothes, folding his sister's cloth diapers and wipes, clearing the table after a meal, cleaning his room, brushing his teeth, carrying groceries, unloading the silverware from the dishwasher, taking out the compost, sweeping, vacuuming, and a variety of other self-care and household chores. Does he do these tasks willingly each time? Certainly not, but these chores are his

responsibilities, he's perfectly capable, and the completion of his duties provides him with a sense of independence, self-reliance, and proud involvement. Children need to feel purposeful, and asking for their help with household tasks allows just that.

In the same way that I expect my children to participate in household chores, I expect them to participate in food preparation. My goal is to raise competent humans who are capable of cooking for themselves and their families someday. I also want to inspire their interest in food, and the best way to get kids interested in anything is to let them be involved.

I once managed a children's learning garden, where a small group of four-through-eight-year-olds was responsible for planting and maintaining an organic vegetable garden. The kids enjoyed their work, but more important they loved eating the fruits of their labor! I remember having a small argument over who got to eat a handful of raw brussels sprouts, which certainly isn't your everyday battle. The kids were interested in the food because they were involved.

While my kids are far from capable of cooking a meal from start to finish, they're qualified to participate in smaller tasks during the food preparation process. I should note that it was not convenient to teach my children how to perform certain tasks. In fact, it made meal preparation much slower at first, but now that my son is more knowledgeable, capable, and efficient he's actually quite helpful with certain tasks. Again, not all tasks; he's just five. For example, I let him cook scrambled eggs on occasion, but I have to hover over him like a hawk to make sure the eggs don't burn. While it would be far easier for me to cook the eggs on my own, my thought is that this small investment of time will help him develop skills that enable him to contribute to the household in the future. How awesome will it be when I can ask my seven-year-old son to make us scrambled eggs and he can do it from start to finish? That's the goal, and we're on the path to accomplishing it.

Jobs for Kids in the Kitchen

Cracking eggs

Whisking eggs

Cooking scrambled eggs in a pan
(supervision may be required)

Stirring

Opening cans with a can opener

Scooping nut butters or dips onto
a plate

Adding preportioned spices and salt

Measuring ingredients

Pouring measured ingredients into
dishes or batters

Pouring batters into pans

Sautéing vegetables (supervision
may be required)

Washing fruits or vegetables

Chopping vegetables

Gathering vegetables from
the garden

Mashing tuna for tuna salad

Serving their own food

Reheating foods on the stovetop,
like soups (supervision may be
required)

I bought my son a nylon kitchen knife set when he was three and it was a great introduction for unsupervised chopping. The knives obviously can't cut foods like carrots or winter squash, but he could use them to chop cucumbers, celery, bananas, plantains, and other soft fruits and vegetables. Now that he's older, I allow him to use real knives, but the nylon set was a good primer. We both especially liked the fact that he could be left unattended while chopping with the nylon set. Mr. Independent felt that my peering over his shoulder was less than desirable, and I felt that my time could be better spent on a different prep task. My two-year-old daughter now uses the nylon knives to chop bananas, avocados, red peppers, or cucumbers while I work in the kitchen. The knives are safe enough that she can do this unattended, and she always eats whatever she's chopping. Allowing young kids to experiment with a set of nylon knives and a few healthy foods is a great way to get them interested in eating a more diverse diet.

One of the simplest yet most exciting things for my son to do in the kitchen is to operate appliances such as the food processor or blender. What can I say? Kids like buttons. I don't allow him free rein with the appliances since he would likely turn my $400 blender off and on as quickly as his little fingers could muster, so I have to do a bit of monitoring.

My list of *Jobs for Kids in the Kitchen* (see sidebar) is a basic introductory list and is by no means exhaustive. The best way to figure out how your child can help you in the kitchen is by observing yourself in the kitchen and making time to teach your child how to do your most basic tasks. As your children grow older you'll be able to slowly entrust them with bigger tasks. I can't wait for the day when I can assign dinners to my children and remove myself from the kitchen entirely. Will they fail at times? Of course. But I wouldn't want it any other way. I want them to be experimenting with foods and flavors so they can develop their own style of cooking. I certainly wouldn't want to raise a child that's afraid to try something new out of fear of missing the mark.

If you happen to have a small vegetable or herb garden, get your child involved. My two-year-old daughter is interested in helping with nearly every gardening task I perform, but the problem is that she's not actually all that helpful. The trick is to give her a job that makes her feel as if she's working alongside me, while not disrupting the actual work that has to be done. I give her a handful of the cheapest and biggest seeds I have (usually peas) and tell her to plant the peas. No additional instructions are provided. Random pea plants pop up all over the garden, but there are worse things in life. My children are also given their own pots to plant when I'm planting my seed starts. I used to have my son help with the flats that we use in the garden each year, but this was extremely frustrating for both of us. Providing him with his own pots, soil, and inexpensive seeds was a much better solution for everyone. He has the freedom to work at his own pace and I have the freedom to get the job done the way that I like.

The last thing to remember is that kids aren't actually all that helpful in the kitchen when they're small or if they're inexperienced. There are days, weeks, and even months that go by when I haven't asked for my kids to help, not even once. I try to ask for their help on a semi-regular basis, but sometimes it's a hard thing to do; I don't always have the patience or time to deal with it. However, taking the time to teach your kids how to do even the simplest tasks in the kitchen will be hugely beneficial for the whole household. My son can now prepare the majority of the Plantain Muffin batter with minimal assistance. I still do the pouring, but it's a task that I should probably let him do now that he's older. Dealing with a mess is part of having kids. Don't let the mess deter you from teaching your child how to be a fully competent and functioning member of society. Your kids need experience in the kitchen in order to eat healthy for a lifetime. Don't deprive them of this skill.

Kid Foods Outside the Home

For many of us who try to avoid grains, sugar, and dairy in the home, challenges arise from school functions, social gatherings, and grandparents or other family members who don't necessarily support (or know how to support) our decisions. We need to start by having a conversation regarding the nature of reward and how we can better celebrate our children without overloading their little systems with unhealthy foods and sugar. This conversation may need to include parents from your child's school, teachers and administrators, grandparents, or even your co-parent. I'm not opposed to indulging every now and again, which is exactly why I included a selection of recipes called *Sweet Treats*. But, as a society, the frequency of our celebrations and the general quality of the foods that we serve have far surpassed a moderate approach. We wouldn't have three-and-a-half-year-old toddlers developing type 2 diabetes if we were approaching food from the angle of optimal health.

Start by encouraging your children and their caretakers outside of the home to think about celebratory events and activities that aren't food-related. Instead of sugary treats, children may instead want a small toy, a couple of stickers, some temporary tattoos, a superhero mask, some cool sunglasses, a small amount of money toward buying a larger toy, a visit to the park, a trip to the library, an evening of being a sous chef, helping Dad or Mom during a carpentry project, or any other special-occasion reward. Candy and sweets aren't the only items that kids appreciate. My son received a pen for Valentine's Day that allows you to select varying writing colors. It was taped to a card saying "I have just the 'write' friend!" The pen was a showstopper. We need to start brainstorming better ways to reward and celebrate our children, and start sharing this conversation with others.

A great challenge presents itself when thinking about how to shift group thinking when it comes to healthy celebrations. I believe the first step is helping the appropriate parties (teachers, administrators, and parents) understand the scope of the issue—diabetes prevalence, obesity statistics, recommended sugar consumption versus actual sugar consumption—and understanding where sugars are hidden in the foods being provided to our children. Proper education surrounding the issue is largely absent unless you're actively seeking out this information. It's up to the enlightened parents to bring this information to everyone else's attention. The next step is to offer suggestions on how to change the typical mode of celebration. Sure, you can restrict people from bringing treats into the classroom for birthday celebrations and tell them to celebrate in other ways, but what would these other ways be? We're not trained to know how to celebrate without cupcakes covered in brightly colored icing. Parents are going to need solutions.

Before I continue, I'd like to point out that there's a very clear distinction between celebrations in the classroom and celebrations at home. It's unfair to ask a child to celebrate without special treats and there's no reason to do this for a party at the house, especially when you have access to all of the wonderful sugar-free *Sweet Treats* recipes in this book! Food has been an integral part of celebrations for centuries and I'm not about to suggest that we change this custom. I've even offered two separate meal plan suggestions for parties in *Holiday Meals and Healthy Celebrations* (page 283). But the culture around food in schools is one that's not easily conformed to healthy celebrations, which is why I'm suggesting that we readjust our customs. Shared foods brought into schools by parents are most often required to be prepackaged so that children with food allergies and other food restrictions can be protected. Teachers and administrators can easily verify that a food is safe for a child with a food allergy if that food is still in its original package and therefore comes with an ingredients list. Sure, preparing a batch of my Chocolate Banana Cupcakes topped with Chocolate Icing would be a great alternative to store-bought treats, but these homemade foods just aren't allowed in schools anymore.

Healthy celebrations in schools could incorporate a fun food project such as building the Strawberry Santas, Banana Snowmen, or Apple Slice Monsters, but preparing more complicated recipes might not be possible. My argument is to replace the candy, packaged junk food, and store-bought cupcakes laden with food coloring and hydrogenated oils, which likely means saving the sweet treats for the home when parents can have more control over the ingredients.

My best advice is to generate a list of celebration ideas that are appropriate for classrooms and share those ideas with your child's teacher, assuming that they're on board. Don't just show up with the list. Instead, have a conversation with your child's teacher beforehand and make sure alternative celebrations are something your child's teacher is interested in implementing in the classroom. You can find numerous ideas online, but I'll briefly share a handful of suggestions. One of my favorite ideas comes from a local Montessori school that has the tradition of letting the birthday child walk around a large sun placed on the ground for each year of the child's life (a five-year-old has made five trips around the sun in their lifetime, thus walks five circles). They sing "Happy Birthday" to the child, and the parents send in one photo from each year of the child's life. The child then has the opportunity to share these photos with their friends.

Other ideas include volunteering on the day of your child's birthday and reading a special book to the class in honor of your child. Do you know how special it would make them feel to have a parent participating in the classroom for a small part of the day, especially if it was a surprise? If you can't take time away from work to volunteer in the classroom, you can instead put together a relatively easy craft for the teacher to use that day for a celebration. You'll obviously want to ask the teacher first, but they'll likely be much more inclined to incorporate a craft into a celebration rather than hold a cupcake party. My last idea is primarily for

Lunch Boxes for Whole-Food Meals

When it comes to packing lunch for your kids, you'll want to invest in a good lunch box that allows flexibility and freedom to pack whatever foods you'd like without having those foods leak into your child's backpack. I tested a number of lunch box styles and I'm happy to report that there are some really great and relatively affordable options out there. Numerous foods produce small amounts of moisture (such as tuna salad or sliced tomatoes) and you simply won't be able to pack these foods without an accommodating lunch box.

I compared the Yumbox Tapas, Bentgo Fresh, Goodbyn Hero, and PlanetBox Rover. I'm happy to report that the Yumbox Tapas was my top pick, with the Bentgo Fresh sliding in as a close second. Really, you can't go wrong with either of these models, and they're both leakproof. I like the bento-style boxes, because they allow you to easily pack a variety of foods without those foods mixing together—dry foods can remain separated from wet, and small foods like nuts can be contained without getting lost among other foods. The bento-style boxes also allow a child to view their lunch in its entirety, meaning that they'll be more likely to sample each food. The silicon seal prevents leakage, even for foods that have watery dressings. I packed a thick soup in the largest compartment and there were no leakage issues. I wouldn't pack something like Chicken Noodle Soup with an extremely thin broth, but it worked well for Not Quite Your Mama's Chili. Just a side note: The manufacturer does not recommend packing liquids.

The entire box is dishwasher safe, which makes for easy cleaning. However, it takes up quite a bit of space in the dishwasher, especially if you have more than one kid, so you may want to wash the outer shell by hand. Yumbox says that this handwashing will also help to preserve the seal.

teachers—the children can sit in a large circle and each take a turn saying something kind about the birthday child.

I'm only listing a handful of ideas here, but none of these ideas involve junk food and junky little toys that will likely make their way into the trash by day two or three. Let's start adding some actual depth and value into our children's celebrations!

When it comes to day-to-day foods at school, I pack all of the foods that my children will eat for the day. I didn't come to this decision lightly, because while I want to establish healthy eating habits, I don't want to create a culture of severe restriction. The children in our preschool eat a shared snack every day (and treats during celebrations) that's provided on rotation by different parents. Some of these foods are healthy options, but some are not, and I don't want my kids eating an unhealthy food every day of the week when they're at school. I instead pack something that my kids enjoy, and they do because they've never known any differently. My hope is that by having early discussions about our food choices and continuing to have open conversations, my children will develop a greater understanding of the many issues surrounding food and food culture. Just the other day I was telling my son that we only buy sweet corn when it's available at the farmers market and I know I'm purchasing non-GMO. While he certainly can't grasp the science behind

The Yumbox Tapas is a fairly large lunch box, holding 4.2 cups (995 ml) plus a dipper. While this may be slightly too large for a younger child, I would still buy this model so that it can grow with your child. At $30 per lunch box, you don't want to have to buy another one in a few years. The Tapas comes in a four- or five-compartment design. I slightly prefer the five-compartment model. For an additional $14 you can buy a second insert that will fit into the same outer shell, therefore having the option of either a four- or five-compartment tray.

The clasp is easy enough for my five-year-old, although it's a bit challenging for my two-year-old. I would imagine a three- or four-year-old could operate the clasp with no issue.

You can purchase an insulated sleeve ($12) for the Yumbox Tapas, but it's not necessary unless you plan to keep foods cold using an ice pack. Simply slide the lunch box into the insulated sleeve along with a thin, flat ice pack and your child's lunch is guaranteed to stay cool for at least five or six hours. Larger insulated bags that can accommodate the Tapas plus a snack and/or water bottle are available at a slightly higher cost, and may be more desirable for sending multiple meals and water with a child.

The dipper container is what sets the Yumbox apart from the Bentgo—I often pack dips or other foods in small quantities that don't necessarily warrant a large compartment. The design of the Yumbox Tapas accommodates foods in large quantities in the largest compartment, yet also accommodates dips like peanut butter, hummus, guacamole, or even small amounts of nuts, seeds, or trail mix without needing an additional container. The Yumbox Tapas is a truly all-in-one lunch box.

My last thought on lunch boxes is that you may want to purchase a stainless steel insulated thermos for packing hot soups, and you'll likely need a few containers for snacks. If you're looking for some ideas for foods to put in your child's lunch box, head over to my suggestions for *Packed Lunches for Kids* (page 280).

GMO, he'll at least be familiar with the term and we can have deeper discussions about it down the road.

I also tend to pack foods when my kids will be staying with their grandparents or any other caretaker for extended periods. I'm extremely fortunate in that everyone in my family is supportive and certainly agrees that this diet seems to be working for my family, though it can be somewhat of a challenge for others to feed my kids since most people are unaccustomed to our way of eating. Rather than continue to have discussions about food options, I pack the foods to take away the guesswork. However, you may be in a situation in which this isn't possible. In that case I recommend that you compile two lists. One list will include the foods that you *don't* want your child to eat. You need to be up-front about what you're avoiding. You don't even need to offer an explanation; just offer the list. The second list should be more extensive and offer numerous foods that you *do* want your child to eat. People have a tendency to think that restrictive diets equate to a complete lack of choices, but that's not the case. Drawing the caretaker's attention away from the restrictions will empower them to know that even with limits, choices abound.

If you feel the need to offer an explanation for your restrictive diet, try to develop a short and sweet justification that focuses on positive outcomes. For example, don't ramble on about leaky gut and lectins.

You're going to immediately lose your listener because you're speaking in terms that aren't relatable. Instead say something like "Olivia's temperament is much better when we avoid these foods. I appreciate your help in this endeavor." Now, that's something that people can understand. Will they agree? Who cares? The decision to eliminate certain foods from your family's diet is a personal choice and outsiders are only going to dwell on your choice if you feel the need to influence their opinion. Keep it simple, own your choice, and don't try to make everyone a convert.

I'm most relaxed about food when it comes to parties outside of school, where I believe the majority of parties need to be held. I want my kids to understand that perfection isn't the goal; the goal is health. In order to stay well, they have to eat healthy foods most of the time, but eating a crummy hot dog and a bunch of chips with highly processed oils at a party a few times each year isn't going to be the end of the world. Party indulgences are where I make the most exceptions, although I have been known to pack our own healthy treats when others are enjoying a store-bought,

Crisco-filled cake. You'll just have to make a decision that feels right for your family.

My approach to feeding my kids outside the home might not be for everyone. We all set our own limits and decide how far we're willing to go with this type of diet. Personally, we're in a position that requires us to follow this diet for specific health needs. I put a lot of work and effort into feeding my family, and I don't want those efforts to be wasted on the frequent consumption of unhealthy foods when we are away from the home. This diet has been hugely beneficial for my family, and I feel that adherence to it is necessary in order to maintain positive results. Keeping my son on track has been fairly easy since he has an anaphylactic allergy to wheat. This alone has made every one of my choices much easier because there's often no choice at all; he simply can't eat what others are eating. My daughter is in a slightly different situation in that this diet is important for her preventive care, thus her devotion doesn't feel as imperative. Regardless, I still mostly follow the same set of principles for both children and try to uphold a food standard that works for our family.

chapter three

Get Prepared, You Can Do This!

I've witnessed numerous successful health transformations. Success usually boils down to three essential steps:

1. **Make a plan.** Simply saying that you want to achieve something isn't enough; you have to know *how* you're going to achieve it. Good intentions will only get you so far; you need guidelines and a solid strategy.
2. **Be patient.** We create habits over the course of our lifetime as our experiences mold our practices. You can't expect to change a lifetime development overnight. Permanent change takes time and you need to adjust your expectations.
3. **Commit.** You won't get it all right every time, but your commitment to a healthier lifestyle is what keeps you coming back for more. When you fall off the health wagon, forgive yourself, honor your commitment to make a change, and get back to it. I like to say that life is about progress, not perfection.

This chapter will help you get prepared so that you can achieve success. The most practical approach may be to tackle one section each week until you feel that you're ready to start getting in the kitchen in a more organized way. Be patient with yourself and only take on what you can handle. Create a checklist with a goal of accomplishing one task each week. Breaking larger tasks into smaller, more manageable tasks can often elicit massive progress over time.

When Change Feels Overwhelming

There may be a number of necessary changes you need to make in order to slowly yet successfully transition your family to a grain-free, sugar-free, dairy-free diet made from whole-food ingredients. Start by recognizing that these are big changes that require an investment of time, energy, and often money. Do yourself a favor and start by admitting that you can't do it all at once. But you can do it with persistence, patience, practice, and a plan (did I just develop the four P's?).

In order to better understand modern-day human nature, I'd like to point out that we live in the age of free two-day shipping; we're an instant gratification kind of society. Popular diet and exercise plans boast titles such as the 21 Day Fix, the 10-Day Detox Diet, the 7-Minute Ab Workout, and 21 Pounds in 21 Days. The list of quick-fix titles is quite extensive, but hopefully you see my point in that we're obsessed with the quick (and easy) way out. We want results and we want them now!

Our anticipation of immediate satisfaction is partly influenced by marketing efforts that lead us to believe we can achieve greatness without actually putting in the time or effort. My encouraging words to you are that by reading this book and making a series of small and continual yet impactful steps toward a healthier diet, you can make changes that will last. Know that there's nothing immediate about big change. Choosing to feed your family differently is no small accomplishment and requires more patience and persistence than you may have ever known. But many families have gone before you and they, too, have successfully made these changes by persevering, sticking with a plan, and continuing to make small steps forward. Change doesn't happen overnight; don't hold yourself to an unrealistic expectation. Slow and steady wins the race.

When I feel myself getting overwhelmed by a daunting long-term project, I try to think back on when I started the task. For example, I was overwhelmed with the inundation of CF information when we first got our daughter's diagnosis, and I have a long way to go before I know as much as I'd like. My ability to fully support her in this illness is partially dependent upon my deeper understanding of the disease. I frequently read CF literature and feel confused by the unfamiliar medical terms and gaping holes in my knowledge. So, what do I do? Do I just give up because it's too hard? No, I think back to the day of her diagnosis and how I wouldn't have even known to look for certain articles or bits of information, but now I have a better sense of direction when it comes to doing research and seeking understanding. Life is a long journey and I've got nothing but time. I do what I can today, forgive any perceived shortcomings, and keep moving forward. As a result, I'm substantially more knowledgeable about CF now than I was two years ago. Just imagine where I'll be in 20 years.

The same is true for you and your family regarding a major change in diet. More than likely you're reading this book because you've recognized that there is a benefit from following a diet free of grains, sugar, and dairy. Think of how far you've already come! You can

only keep moving forward from here. Be patient, be persistent, and commit to making it work, because it takes time.

Making Time for Real Food

I often hear people say that they can't cook from scratch because they don't have the time. While time limitations are often a major constraint, solutions exist. You just have to figure out what works for you. I challenge you to stop saying that you don't have time for cooking, because the truth is that we make time for what matters most. Instead, see how it feels to say, "I don't prioritize cooking."

Prioritizing what's most important is the first step in finding time to get in the kitchen. I often encourage people to do a time study. This is a diary of sorts in which you record what you do throughout the day and for how long. What people usually notice is that they spend more time than they'd like to admit on social media, electronics, and TV. Setting boundaries around these activities can often help us find an extra 30-plus minutes in the day. In this age of technology, installing a tracking app on your phone can shed some light on the amount of time you actually spend piddling away on electronics. I have one such app and I'm often shocked at how much time I waste on technology alone.

Another benefit of a time study is to learn if you spend too much time performing unimportant tasks. For example, being a parent to two young kids has taught me that there is always cleaning to be done. Always. I could clean from the time I wake up to the time I go to sleep and I would still have a mess. I've learned to be a little more comfortable with the clutter, so that I'm not spending every waking minute tidying up. I should also be clear that I'm not the overly tidy type to begin with, so this wasn't a major hurdle for me. But I know that cleanliness in the home can be a major time sink for some individuals. You just have to decide what's worth your attention and what you can let go.

Finding more time also means simplifying your life. I've been exploring a minimalist approach to living and I love the message. The hard truth is that we invest time, lots of time, in our material possessions—time spent buying things, comparing reviews, working to pay for things, removing things from their packaging, disposing of the packaging, putting our things away, and keeping them clean. Acquiring and possessing material goods requires time, and each of us has to decide whether we want to spend our time with our things or if that's time that could be better spent, say, cooking a wholesome meal for the family.

I'm continually reevaluating our material possessions. The grandparents bring the kids thoughtful little goodies more often than I'd like. While these precious little tokens bring the children joy for about five days, the kids are quick to throw them to the wayside and forget them. I don't mean to sound harsh, but these small gifts are unnecessary, teach bad habits and expectations, and quite frankly are a waste of precious time, energy, and resources. Of course I have material possessions that I truly value, but the majority of my possessions I could probably do without and not even notice.

Finding time to cook means that you have to spend time removing, not just overcoming, hurdles that prevent you from living your most fulfilled and healthiest life. Cooking from scratch has such great rewards and is worth the time investment, but you have to decide where your other priorities lie along that spectrum and how you can make better use of this limiting resource. And don't sell yourself short; apply this lesson of time management to all things in your life. We may have a finite number of resources, but we're in charge of how to use those resources. People claim that they don't have enough money for a gym membership. This is true under some circumstances, but how many coffees,

alcoholic beverages, or other unnecessary drinks did that person buy in a month? Do you see my point? We're in control. We have the power of choice, but we may have to give up one thing if we really want another.

Finding time to cook doesn't mean that you have to make time *at* mealtime. I actually do far less cooking at mealtimes since that's usually the most chaotic time of day. Washing and chopping vegetables, roasting, sautéing, and cleaning are pretty much the last things I want to be doing at a time when everyone is tired and hungry. Instead, I cook or prep when it's convenient. I'll get more into specific strategies in the next chapter, but know that finding time to cook means finding *any* time to cook! For now, start evaluating your priorities in order to identify some shifts that can be made over the coming weeks and months. Don't sacrifice necessary activities like sleep and exercise; instead consider reducing activities that are not health promoting such as TV and screen time.

Kitchen Equipment Essentials

When it comes to preparing ingredients in new and exciting ways, having access to a variety of handy tools will be an asset. For example, spiralized zucchini noodles are a unique alternative to grain pastas, but you can only eat spiralized zucchini if you have a spiralizer. There's just no way to re-create these delicate little noodles with a knife.

Kitchen basics, such as knives and cutting boards, will certainly get you started, but I highly encourage you to consider setting some funds aside to purchase a few specialty pieces of equipment. If I were to splurge on only two items, I'd go for a high-powered blender and an electric pressure cooker. These tools are versatile and make healthy eating more creative and achievable. I use both of these appliances a few times each week, and I am slightly embarrassed to admit that I even bring the blender along when we travel.

I happen to own two high-powered blenders—a Vitamix and a Blendtec. I honestly don't think you can go wrong with either one. The Vitamix operates with more finesse, but the Blendtec just really pounds the heck out of whatever you're puréeing regardless of the quantity. I like that there's no plunger involved with the Blendtec, but that means foods often get lodged while blending. In my search for a minimalist life, I've often considered that owning just one of these high-powered blenders would be more than enough, yet I can't bring myself to part with either one. Each has its strengths and weaknesses: The Blendtec does batters slightly better, but the Vitamix does smoothies and frozen desserts slightly better. I will say, however, that there are a number of individuals in the CF community who prefer the Vitamix. Many individuals with CF require a feeding tube at some point in their lives due to malnourishment, and tube-fed meals must be blended into an extremely smooth liquid in order to pass through the tube without obstruction. My understanding is that the Vitamix does this far better than the Blendtec.

Both blenders are extremely pricey, ranging from $230 for a refurbished Blendtec to $800 for the professional series. Refurbished Vitamixes start at $330 and their top-of-the-line products max out around $620. Both come with excellent warranties, although their policies change from year to year, so be sure to understand the warranty that comes with your exact model.

One of the most exciting applications for a high-powered blender is its ability to turn almost any whole-food ingredient into a batter. For my Plantain Muffins and Plantain Blender Pancakes, I start by grinding sunflower seeds into a fine flour, a feat that would not be possible without the horsepower and blade of a superior blender. I then add chopped plantains and all of the other necessary ingredients to blend a smooth, delicious, and naturally sweetened batter from unsuspecting ingredients. Preparing frozen fruit desserts such as the Mango Lime Ice Cream or Chocolate Ice Cream is only possible if you have the right equipment. Blending dates into batters to create an Apple Spice Bundt Cake or Chocolate Icing is made possible by this dynamic and powerful piece of kitchen equipment. Conveying the necessity and versatility of a blender to the blender layperson is challenging, because they've never witnessed the efficiency and creativity that such a machine allows. But converts unanimously agree—we can't create food without our high-powered blenders! Smoothies, soups, sauces, desserts, and more are all possible because of this one (extremely expensive) machine. Is this a good item to place on your wedding or baby registry? Yes, I think so.

I also recommend that an eight-quart electric pressure cooker make its way onto your registry or wish list. Many people will skimp and buy the six-quart version, but remember that it holds eight quarts in total and you have to leave headspace for cooking. This reduces the overall cooking volume to about six quarts. The six-quart model can only prepare four quarts at a time, which is entirely too small for batch cooking. I definitely overfill mine at times, but my eight-quart model will not hold any more than six and a half quarts, even when completely maxed out. The most popular brand of pressure cooker is the Instant Pot, but many other quality brands exist. I initially bought a GoWise USA brand pressure cooker ($90) and was extremely pleased with the gadget until it broke twice in two years. I suggested this brand to friends, and they have been using the GoWise USA for over a year without issue. Nevertheless, I ended up splurging on the eight-quart Instant Pot for $150 (I believe they have a less expensive model, but I was unaware of it at the time). The quality is outstanding thus far, but only time will tell. Larger models are available, such as the 14-quart model from GoWise USA, but the size of the unit and the inconvenience of storing and washing such a large piece of equipment wouldn't be worth the benefit to me.

The greatest advantage to owning an electric pressure cooker is that it can cook recipes or components of recipes in a fraction of the time it would take using other cooking methods. I can steam sweet potatoes under pressure for Coconut and Cinnamon Sweet Potato Mash in just 15 to 20 minutes. Compare this with the hour or so it would take in the oven. Spaghetti squash and other winter squashes suddenly become convenience foods because the cooking time can be as little as 6 minutes for a squash that would take at least 45 minutes to bake in the oven. Most impressively, preparing hard-boiled eggs in the pressure cooker takes all of five minutes and renders an egg that is *always* easy to peel! The peels just flop right off. Another advantage of an electric pressure cooker is that it doesn't generate any heat, so it's an excellent tool to use during the summer months when you're doing your best to keep the house at a reasonable temperature. In the winter months, the electric pressure cooker will be a lifesaver when you want to create rich, flavorful, and nutrient-dense broths in just 2 hours compared with the 24 hours it would take on the stovetop. The bottom line is this: An electric pressure cooker offers you a quick and convenient way to prepare some of your most essential meal components.

While I'd like to say that my high-priced blenders have replaced my need for a food processor, it's simply not true. I use it for certain recipes for blending (such as Lemon Coconut Date Balls), for grating (Cauliflower Hash Browns or Coconut Lime Cauliflower Rice), or for shredding (Dill Pickle Kraut). I own an 11-year-old Cuisinart and it is still going strong. I wouldn't recommend one of the cheap off-brands, simply because cheap products rarely perform well, but there are plenty of good brands out there.

If you don't have the space for all of these gadgets and don't want to spend the money, I'm sure you could get by with just a high-powered blender, but you'd have to learn how to use it in a way that hasn't been necessary for me. While I approach most areas of my home from a minimalist perspective, I tend to go overboard when it comes to kitchen gadgets.

The other gadgets listed in the sidebar *Kitchen Equipment Essentials* (page 48) aren't nearly as pricey as the gadgets I've already mentioned, so I don't go into detail regarding specific brands. Know that I certainly didn't acquire all of these items at once. I slowly accumulated theses gadgets, and I requested most of them as gifts. Many of the items will make perfect holiday gifts from relatives who are never quite sure what to buy for you. Make a list of the items that you'd like to get over time and be sure to share that list with your loved ones.

I'm sure you already own a set of pots and pans, but I want to add a quick note about those essential kitchen items. I do not support the use of nonstick pans regardless of the quality, because the coating will eventually wear off and you'll be ingesting small amounts of toxins when it does. There are nonstick pans with longer life spans and even some that can be resurfaced by the manufacturers, but none that are guaranteed for a lifetime. Stainless steel and cast-iron pans are your best bet, not only because of the longevity of the pans but also because leaching of toxins won't even be a possibility. Moreover, the pans can be used on both the stovetop and in the oven. A variety of quality pan brands are available, but beware that many well-known brands manufacture lesser-quality versions offered at prices that aren't worth paying. I settled on a German brand, Fissler, for all of my pot and pan needs. These are extremely expensive products, but they're accompanied by a 50-year warranty. The worth of a product can often be measured by the extent of the warranty, and 50 years is about as good as it gets.

The size of your pans will be a major limiting factor in your ability to double or even triple some recipes. I

Kitchen Equipment Essentials

2-gallon stockpot
3-gallon stockpot
Large frying pan
Large oven-safe pan such as cast iron or stainless steel
High-powered blender
8-quart electric pressure cooker
Food processor
Immersion blender
Wooden cutting board
Plastic cutting board for meat
Chef's knife
Wooden spoons

Metal spatula
Silicon spatula
Whisk
Grater
Spiralizer
Silicon muffin molds (24) or two muffin pans
Bread pans (4)
Sheet pans (2 large)
Large Pyrex (or other material) baking dish (11 × 15 inches; 28 × 38 cm)

Medium Pyrex (or other material) baking dish (8 × 12 inches; 20 × 30 cm)
Vegetable peeler
Can opener
Large glass jars for fermenting and food storage
Airlock lid for fermenting (optional)
Glass, Pyrex, stainless steel, or BPA-free plastic food storage containers

use a 10-liter (nearly three gallons) pot for bulk cooking, even when preparing sautés like the Probiotic Pork and Vegetables or the stuffing for Cottage Pie. I double or triple these recipes to reserve some for future meals, which would be impossible using my largest frying pan. Bulk cooking for freezing requires the use of a pan or pot that can accommodate an enormous quantity of food. I also own a five-gallon pot that I picked up for a mere $45. I press it into service when I'm serving a large crowd, but it's rare that I ever need something so large; the 10-liter pot usually does the trick.

The *Kitchen Equipment Essentials* sidebar list reflects multiples of some items, such as muffin and bread pans, because baking four loaves at a time can maximize time spent preparing bread. The same principle applies to sheet pans, food storage containers, Pyrex baking dishes, and fermenting jars. You can only be as efficient as the size a vessel allows.

Stocking Your Pantry and Freezer

A well-stocked pantry and freezer makes cooking easier and more convenient. I don't have a huge diversity of foods in my pantry or freezer, but there's a rather large quantity of the things I do use. I buy as much as possible in advance for the items I store in the pantry and freezer, which means that my weekly purchases are primarily limited to foods that I buy fresh.

Stocking your pantry and freezer serves three purposes:

1. **Some of the items that I use on a regular basis could be hard to find,** such as coconut aminos or grain-free tortilla chips. If necessary, you might have to buy a few items online. Knowing that I already have hard-to-find ingredients in the pantry allows me to prepare whatever recipe my heart

Pantry Essentials

Canned skipjack tuna
Canned wild Alaskan salmon
Sardines
Peanut butter
Almond butter
Nuts: pecans, almonds, walnuts
Seeds: raw sunflower seeds, hemp
  seeds, and pumpkin seeds
Dried fruit: mulberries, goji
  berries, raisins, and dates
Dried unsweetened coconut flakes
Dried unsweetened shredded
  coconut

Green and black olives
Organic full-fat, unsweetened
  coconut milk
Organic unsweetened
  coconut cream
Coconut aminos
Applesauce
Organic olive oil
Avocado oil
Lard
Organic cold-pressed coconut oil
  (unrefined)
Raw apple cider vinegar

White vinegar
Balsamic vinegar
Red wine vinegar
Salsa
Mustard
Dried beans
Canned diced tomatoes
Canned crushed tomatoes
Tomato paste
Tomato sauce (sugar-free)
Coffee
Tea

desires. There's no ordering that special item and then waiting five days for it to arrive.

2. **Many items that store well in a pantry or freezer can be bought in bulk,** which saves money. For example, I buy cases of coconut milk, coconut cream, and SunButter, and huge bags of nuts and seeds, which saves us hundreds of dollars over the course of a year. I purchase bulk meat from local farms and stock up on freezable items when I find them on sale.

3. **When you buy items in bulk, you're saving time.** There's a small investment of time that goes into each item on your grocery list. Buying multiples of those items allows you to save time in the long run.

In the *Pantry Essentials* and *Freezer Essentials* sidebars, I list items that I like to keep stocked in my pantry and freezer. You'll have to figure out which items are most cost effective and convenient for you to keep on hand. I suggest that you, too, stock up. I can't tell you how many times I've heard people say that they just don't have the ingredients for some of the recipes that cater to eaters with special diets. Don't let this be you! You'll need to have at least a few key items on hand to make a grain-free, sugar-free, dairy-free diet a reality for you and your family.

Freezer Essentials

Meat and poultry
Fish and seafood
Bones and feet for making stock
Frozen fruit
Frozen vegetables

Quality Matters: Where to Source Foods

Figuring out where to buy certain foods at the best price and quality will take some time and effort on your part. Quality makes a difference, so it's worth taking the time to shop around and find a respectable product that's within your budget.

When it comes to animal products, don't skimp. I know this is challenging because the sticker price for grass-fed beef or free-range eggs seems unreasonable. The problem is that cheap food products are cheap calories. They even have a different nutrient profile than their mindfully raised equivalent. For example, grass-fed beef has less overall fat, has a completely different fatty acid profile, and is higher in omega-3s than grain-fed beef. Conventionally raised cattle (grain-fed cattle) have a fatty acid profile that is known to elevate bad cholesterol (LDL) and influence the development of cardiovascular disease. Grass-fed beef doesn't have this negative impact on the body. It's worth the extra cost.

I also urge you to consider the environmental implications of consuming conventionally raised animals. According to the EPA, agriculture accounted for 9 percent of our greenhouse gas emissions in 2014, and has been responsible for several negative effects on water and soil pollution. The health of our future planet will deteriorate if we don't make positive consumer choices. Choosing the right meats is about taking care of your immediate health, and also taking care of our environment and the health of future generations.

I should note that I'm not saying that you have to buy certified organic beef. While organic would be great, you can find sustainably raised, grass-fed beef at many grocery stores or farmers markets. You just need to read the packaging or talk with the farmer to ensure that the beef was actually grass fed (raised on pastures) and doesn't contain hormones and antibiotics. Also be aware that some grass-fed beef is finished with grains, which increases the fat content and thus enhances the flavor of the beef. However, feeding cattle grain during those final weeks before slaughter negates the benefits of raising those cows on grass, and the fatty acid profile for this beef is then similar to that of a grain-fed cow. Cows should be fed grass from start to finish.

The consumption of fish is another major dilemma when it comes to environmental sustainability and personal health. Fish can accumulate heavy metals in concentrations that exceed the concentrations found in their surrounding environment, a process known as bioaccumulation. Furthermore, destructive fishing practices are quickly depleting our ocean resources, which means that we have to choose sustainably harvested (or farm-raised) fish if we want these resources to be available for years to come. The Environmental Working Group (ewg.org) has a fantastic online Seafood Calculator that can help you determine the best fish to consume on a regular basis. You can quickly find the calculator through a Google search. Just plug in the requested information and use the guide to inform your seafood purchases. For canned seafood, Wild Planet brand is a good pick for sustainably harvested fish.

My absolute favorite source for finding fresh, healthy, sustainable foods is our local farmers market. I like to eat a variety of seasonal foods, and shopping at the farmers market guarantees that I'll be selecting from the freshest ingredients around. Shopping at your local market allows you the opportunity to talk with the farmers about their farming practices, which can help you decide on the best-quality produce for the best price. Meeting your farmers and learning about their growing practices is the best way to ensure you're buying an affordable, superior product. I offer a few more farmers market shopping tips in the next section, *Budget-Friendly Solutions*, but don't underestimate the value of local food.

Having a small vegetable garden is another great way to supplement your family's food budget. I have quite a large garden at this point and it supplies my family with a significant portion of our vegetable needs during those peak production months. I still rely heavily on the local farmers, grocery stores, and some online shopping, but my garden is a significant supplementary source of organically grown produce throughout the year. You don't have to have a large amount of space to grow your own food. If you're new to gardening, start extremely small, even as small as a container garden, and just see how it goes. The smaller the garden, the higher your chance of success, and a successful garden is one that is more likely to be recurring and grow over time (no pun intended).

There are numerous products I use in my kitchen that I simply can't find at our farmers market, such as nuts and seeds, some fats, canned fish, olives, and many of the other items I like to keep stocked in my pantry. For those items I look to different stores, and I do the best I can. For example, small health food stores are often a great source for locally sourced products, but unfortunately, this type of store just isn't readily available where I live. I'll also add that I used to do more online shopping than I do now. While I genuinely appreciate the convenience of having food delivered straight to my front door, I don't appreciate the inconvenience and waste of the packaging. Our pantry area transforms into the staging area for recyclables, and online shopping instantly turns this area into a cluttered mess of cardboard. Is the hassle of dealing with the packaging worth the convenience of the instant deliverables? I'm not so sure it is, which is why I often prefer a monthly trip to Costco or a co-op that's 40 minutes away to purchase things like almond butter, coconut oil, avocado oil, seaweed snacks, sardines, frozen fruits and vegetables, and a variety of other affordable and often organic products. When I do need to buy products online I try to order as little as possible to cut back on the amount of packaging. It's important for us to remember that specialty diets can quickly increase our environmental impact if we aren't mindful as we implement them. Shopping in bulk and trying to find ingredients locally can reduce this impact.

Is Organic Really Better?

The short answer is yes, organic foods are a better option, a *much* better option. The complicated answer is that some natural pesticides approved for use on organic crops, such as pyrethrins and rotenone, are equally as toxic for human and environmental health as chemical pesticides. In general, the use of the more harmful organic pesticides is limited to extremely large-scale organic farms where monocropping (growing just a handful of crops again and again, which ultimately encourages pest infestations and depletes the soil of nutrients) is the norm. I'll discuss ways to ensure that you're accessing better-quality food, but I'd like to start by presenting a handful of issues surrounding human health and conventionally grown produce. Keep in mind that I've chosen to focus solely on human health; the environmental implications are a whole other issue.

One of the most pronounced benefits I see to consuming organic products is that the use of genetically modified organisms (GMOs) is not permitted in foods that hold the USDA organic certification. GMOs are genetically designed to possess desirable traits. Genes are inserted into a plant's DNA, and this insertion codes for the creation of varying proteins that can enhance the plant's capabilities. Proponents of genetic modification (GM) claim that it may be the way to end world hunger because it allows for the creation of specialized food crops that can be grown in the desert and other less-than-desirable conditions. There's potential for developing plants with higher yield, greater nutrient content, and the necessary qualities to satisfy a growing world population. However, the Institute for Responsible Technology states that "the only two traits that are found in nearly all commercialized GM plants are herbicide tolerance and/or pesticide production." In short, we're using GM technology to assist in farming methods that more heavily rely on pesticide use. Soy, corn, cotton, and canola make up the majority of GM crops, with most of these plants being resistant to herbicides such as glyphosate (Roundup) and a lesser amount having the ability to produce their own pesticides. The benefit to an herbicide-resistant plant is that you can repeatedly spray that crop with herbicides in order to suppress the weed population, allowing the GM crop to flourish. Other lesser-known GM crops include Hawaiian papaya, zucchinis, sugar beets, and yellow squash. Notice that many GM crops, such as corn, canola, soy, and sugar beets (for making sugar), are ingredients found in processed foods. In fact, up to 80 percent of packaged foods available in the grocery store contain GMOs.

Research shows a wide range of detrimental effects resulting from the consumption of GM foods in animals, such as toxicity in the digestive tract, liver and other organ damage, increased death rates, loss of ability to reproduce, infant mortality, heightened immune responses that can lead to food allergies, and tumors. The FDA has classified GMOs as generally recognized as safe (GRAS), yet there is a complete lack of evidence supporting this classification. In fact, numerous scientists and international authorities have criticized the United States' approval of GMOs, saying that these crops should not be released into the food chain until a safety profile is clearly established, a feat that seems near impossible given the growing body of research proving otherwise.

Another shortcoming of conventionally grown produce is that it's grown using varying pesticides. One such pesticide, glyphosate (Roundup), has received growing attention over the past decade as it is now the most heavily applied herbicide in the world. Farmers have increased glyphosate use by 100-fold since the late 1970s, and its use is only continuing to increase due to wider availability and use of so-called Roundup Ready GM crops. Refer back to the section in chapter 1, *Wheat: Grain in the Spotlight*, page 16, for more information regarding the negative health consequences and usage of glyphosate.

Some experts argue that the negative effects of consuming GMOs and those crops sprayed with glyphosate (among other issues with industrial food) are at the root of most Western diseases, especially those impacting our children. One simply cannot ignore the profound rise in disease incidence over the past few decades. It's clearer than ever that our food is making us sick. The book *What's Making Our Children Sick* by Michelle Perro, MD, and Vincanne Adams, PhD, paints a grim picture of industrial food and its direct implications for the health of our children. This book is one of the most important resources for any family facing medical and psychological challenges, as it's one of the first to clearly link glyphosate and GM foods to deteriorating gut health, thus the development of varying diseases and conditions. The authors are huge proponents of organic foods as part of a comprehensive and integrative approach to managing and reversing disease. Information such as what's provided in *What's Making Our Children Sick* inspires me to take more control over the food that my family eats. I can do this by growing what I can and purchasing as much as possible from small local farmers who are invested in better growing practices. Try starting conversations with your local farmers, and chances are you'll find that some of these smaller farms aren't utilizing toxic, organic pesticides, even if they're not certified organic. The organic certification is costly to maintain, thus is one of the driving factors behind higher costs for organic foods. It's therefore more economical for some small farmers to uphold organic practices without having the actual certification. But without this certification, they can't market their foods as organic despite their implementation of organic practices.

Their choice helps to keep the cost of their produce lower, ultimately meaning that your conversations with these farmers can lead to better food quality for your family at a better price.

I've only focused on two of the major issues surrounding conventionally grown food crops, but believe me when I say that issues abound. Avoiding these toxins and potentially harmful substances needs to be a priority for every individual, although I realize that affordability of organic foods can be a major constraint, especially when your best option is to buy from a grocery store if you have limited access to local foods. The Environmental Working Group (ewg.org) compiles an annual list of foods that are best to eat organic and a list of foods that are relatively safe to eat conventionally. These lists are the Dirty Dozen and the Clean Fifteen, respectively. Use these lists to help inform your decision regarding which foods are best to buy organic and which conventional foods are safer to eat.

Last, remember that your dollars are votes that promote a way of life; make those votes count.

THE DIRTY DOZEN	THE CLEAN FIFTEEN
Strawberries	Sweet corn
Spinach	(non-GMO only)
Nectarines	Avocados
Apples	Pineapples
Peaches	Cabbage
Pears	Onions
Cherries	Sweet peas (frozen)
Grapes	Papayas (non-GMO only)
Celery	Asparagus
Tomatoes	Mangoes
Sweet bell peppers	Eggplant
Potatoes	Honeydew melon
	Kiwi
	Cantaloupe
	Cauliflower
	Broccoli

Budget-Friendly Solutions

Now that you're equipped with numerous ideas on how to turn your kitchen into a grain-free, sugar-free, dairy-free producing machine, I'd like to also help your wallet make the transition. We've been a one-income family for the better part of the past four years, so budgeting was a big factor in this transition. The following tips come from hard-earned experience as my family managed to implement this diet without going completely broke.

Buy a small chest freezer. I never, ever, ever pay full price for meat, poultry, or fish. But in order to do this I need a place to store items when they go on sale.

Never pay full price for meats and fish. Didn't I just say this? I'm saying it again! This is only possible if you implement my first recommendation to buy the freezer. I look for sale prices on meats and fish every time I go to the store or farmers market regardless of whether it's on my shopping list. If it's on sale, I buy a huge quantity and throw it in the freezer for later.

Have an actual pantry area. We have a storage room in our basement and I've designated four or five small shelves there as a "pantry." Having this storage space allows me to stock up on dried goods and canned goods when I find them on sale.

Get to know your farmers and ask about bulk purchasing. I buy beef and whole chickens in bulk from the local farmers, which saves hundreds of dollars every year. I also buy seasonal vegetables in large quantities when farmers are interested in getting rid of their excess supply. For example, this past fall I bought 11 giant Blue Hubbard squash for $20. The farmer was tired of hauling the enormous produce back and forth, so they welcomed the opportunity to unload. Each squash was normally $5 to $8, so even though a few of the squash went bad before I had the chance to use them, it was still a killer deal.

Use less expensive cuts of beef. We don't eat steaks, because it's just not affordable. We instead eat ground beef, stew beef, and varying roasts. Some of the least expensive and most nutritious cuts of meat are organs. If you're feeling adventurous, beef heart can easily replace half of the ground beef in Not Quite Your Mama's Chili. Liver is less easy to substitute since it has a rather strong flavor.

Buy whole chickens. I certainly enjoy cooking with breasts and thighs, but I buy whole chickens frequently because of the greater affordability. You can use whole chickens in the place of most shredded chicken recipes and you have the added bonus of being left with a chicken carcass. I store chicken bones in the freezer to use for bone stock at a later date.

Buy your own bones, save your bones, and sometimes cook them twice. A nutritious store-bought bone stock is nearly impossible to find, and it's even more impossible to afford if you do actually find it. Save and store all animal bones in the freezer to use for making your own stock. I've found that I can actually make two batches of bone broth out of large beef bones that have adequate connective tissues attached. I get twice as much bone stock for the same price this way.

Buy in bulk. I already discussed the advantages of bulk buying in the section *Stocking Your Pantry and Freezer* (page 48), but it's important for me to say it again. Many items are significantly cheaper when bought by the case or in bulk.

Make a weekly meal plan. I make a quick meal plan every week and only buy the items that I need. This way I don't buy excess that eventually ends up in the compost pile. Much more on this in chapter 4, *The Importance of Meal Planning.*

Shop only once each week. Yes, this saves you time, but it'll also save you money. How many times have you gone to the store to pick up just one item and left with $35 worth of groceries? It happens to us all. You didn't even realize that you needed these extra items until you saw them, which makes you wonder how badly you actually needed them.

Check out weekly sales before creating a meal plan. I'm not great at this, but it's always really helpful when I look ahead and plan to incorporate items that are on sale.

Have a flexible meal plan. Let's say you've planned to eat salmon with roasted broccoli, but you see that brussels sprouts are on sale this week. Forget the broccoli and eat the brussels sprouts instead. Be flexible.

Buy beets with greens intact. I know this seems simple, but we eat a lot of beets and they're relatively expensive. Beet greens can be used much like spinach, so buy the beets with the greens and forget the spinach (or other greens) that week.

Buy bags of produce. Items that are available in bags include apples, onions, potatoes, and a variety of other fruits and vegetables. We can easily use a bag of onions in a week and it costs far less than buying individual onions.

Check out bulk food sections, especially spices. I had access to great bulk food buying when my family lived in Vermont. The selection isn't nearly as good or cost effective here in North Carolina, but I do what I can. Bulk spices are almost always more affordable than jarred spices.

Grow your own food. If you decide to try growing a few choice items, choose items that are more expensive. For example, buying organic lettuces can add up pretty quickly, but they're relatively easy to grow and can save you $5 to $10 each week depending on your family's consumption.

chapter four

The Importance of Meal Planning

I cook approximately 90 to 95 percent of our meals from scratch while juggling work, kids, home life, friendships, and exercise. I make time for cooking through efficient meal prep strategies. I've prioritized whole-food meals and have streamlined the process so that I'm not a slave to my kitchen.

Even as I outline the strategies that have turned me into a total kitchen boss, please know that I sometimes fall short and miss the mark. I don't do everything perfectly—nobody does. This is especially so when we're dealing with a family crisis that requires the majority of my energy. My daughter was admitted to the hospital twice while writing this book, and meal planning and prep took a backseat to more pressing priorities. Times of crisis are when your body needs the most support, yet it's often the time when you don't have enough energy to meet those nutritional demands. For this reason I've included a section in this chapter called *Vacation Foods and Major Life Events*, page 65. Staying a few steps ahead is the best strategy, and this section is designed to help you do just that.

When figuring out your own life balance in the kitchen, I'd like you to remember that you and your family eat 365 days per year, and want *at least* three meals per day. You can *always* count on the fact that someone will be hungry. Whoever is taking the lead in the kitchen should be anticipating that next meal. Anticipating the next meal is especially important if you're feeding small children who are not keen on patiently waiting for sustenance. How many times have you found yourself arriving home at dinnertime, panic stricken because you've forgotten to plan dinner—you know, the meal that you eat nearly every single day of your life? I don't understand it, either, but it happens to me more frequently than I'd like to admit.

My peculiar situation of having a severely food allergic child, specifically to wheat, has forced me to anticipate meals in a way that most normal people don't. Quick options are few and far between, which means I always have to be ready. As a result I plan, prep, multitask, cook in batches, and freeze foods. While it takes a bit of extra brainpower when learning to think ahead and get organized in this way, it slowly becomes second nature and ultimately makes meal preparation a less stressful endeavor.

In case I haven't stressed it enough already, learning to implement all of these strategies in an organized way will take time and practice. Do what you can, slowly become comfortable with a few new strategies, and then add another. Gradual forward movement will be the key to success!

Meal Planning 101

I firmly believe that developing at least some semblance of a meal plan for the week will enable a family

Understanding and Preparing for Anaphylactic Reactions

The term *food allergy* has become quite popular these days. It's a catch-all term that includes symptoms ranging from digestive upset and bloating to full-blown anaphylactic reactions. It's my understanding that many people aren't actually "allergic," they're just "intolerant" or "sensitive," yet the loose use of the term *allergy* has made it difficult for parents like myself to convey the severity of an allergy to necessary parties. Clinically speaking, a true allergy manifests as anaphylaxis, allergic asthma, uticaria (hives), angioedema (swelling), allergic rhinitis, or atopic dermatitis (eczema). The response is mediated by a specific immunoglobulin (antibody) called immunoglobulin E (IgE). Non-allergic responses are mediated by different immonoglobulins including IgA, IgG, or IgM, or from T cells. The immune system produces immonoglobulins to fight bacteria, viruses, toxins, and even foods in the case of allergies and sensitivities. There are varying names for these responses and their associated reaction, but the term *allergy* is limited to an IgE-mediated response.

An allergic reaction is a hypersensitive response from the immune system that can occur upon exposure to a food or environmental allergen. The level of response varies from person to person, but some responses can serve as a source of severe discomfort (seasonal allergies) while others are a life-threatening situation (anaphylaxis). The immune system serves to recognize foreign invaders and manufactures antibodies to attack those offenders. However, people with atopy (allergic tendencies) have overreactive immune systems that are programmed to attack when an invader isn't actually all that offensive (such as with wheat, eggs, or peanuts).

Anaphylaxis most often occurs from the ingestion of food or in response to an insect sting. Some people are so allergic to certain foods that even inhalation or contact can elicit an anaphylactic response. The reaction will likely ensue within minutes of exposure, but delayed responses that occur 30 minutes to hours later are possible.

Signs and symptoms of an allergic reaction include skin reactions such as hives or swelling, difficulties breathing, changes in skin color, drop in blood pressure, tightness in the throat, swelling of the mouth, tongue, or lips, repetitive vomiting, severe diarrhea, or feelings of confusion or anxiety. Mild symptoms include mild nausea, runny nose, itchy mouth, or a few hives. A person is said to be in anaphylaxis when two or more of these

to successfully follow a whole-food diet, especially one that requires some creativity. I'm not saying that you have to be 100 percent organized when it comes to meal planning for this diet, but you need some sort of forethought in order to maximize your time usage throughout the week. Your goal is to optimize your time spent shopping, prepping, and cooking. Meal planning equates to efficiency. The sooner you embrace this fact, the sooner you'll be on the path to whole-food success! I'm sure there are people who can shop and cook for the week without implementing a meal plan of any sort; I'm betting they are also either eating more processed foods than they might like to admit or they are eating the exact same thing for every single meal.

Meal planning allows me more freedom throughout the week because I can cater the plan to meet the demands of that particular week. If Tuesday through

symptoms are occurring simultaneously, even if the symptoms are mild. If the response is limited to only one mild symptom (for example, a runny nose), then the reaction does not require epinephrine. But it is recommended to respond with epinephrine if more than one symptom is occurring or if the person is having difficulties breathing. As you can see, anaphylaxis is a multi-organ response and is not just limited to difficulties in breathing.

My son is severely allergic to wheat and barley, although we believe his anaphylactic response is limited to ingestion and does not include contact or inhalation. His last reaction occurred in December 2017 from the ingestion of a gluten-free sandwich wrap that had been manufactured on shared equipment. His typical response upon ingesting wheat had been primarily a GI response (repetitive vomiting) with some swelling and hives, but his reaction had shifted, as allergies often do, and he almost immediately had difficulties breathing. I administered his EpiPen at the house then transported him immediately to the emergency room, where he was given two more doses of epinephrine, IV steroids, IV Benadryl, and four different nebulized breathing treatments, and was placed on oxygen for nearly two hours. I then knew: What used to be a mild anaphylactic reaction was now a severe life-threatening situation.

My experience with Owen taught me that you always have to be prepared for the worst when it comes to anaphylactic allergies. If you have a child with minor to moderate allergies, their response to the allergen can advance without notice. We always knew this was a possibility, but I'm not sure what would have happened to my son if I hadn't been there to respond during the reaction. I had been trained by multiple physicians, but I didn't do a great job at conveying that information to the other people who cared for Owen simply because I didn't understand the potential for his reaction to intensify without any notice. *Some advice: If your physician has instructed you to carry an EpiPen for your child, be sure that every person involved in their care fully understands how to prevent a reaction from occurring and how to use the EpiPen in the case of an emergency.*

Every child with food allergies needs an Emergency Care Plan. A template for a plan can be found on the Food Allergy Research & Education website (foodallergy.org). Your emergency plan, along with epinephrine, should travel with that child no matter where they go, a lifelong habit that starts early. The likelihood of your child having a severe anaphylactic reaction may be low, but there are no guarantees. Being unprepared for such a thing could be the greatest regret of your life.

Friday are particularly busy, for example, I plan for meals that can either be prepped in advance or that will take very little effort on those days. Allow me to outline some strategies that can help you create a flexible and efficient meal plan:

Don't plan to eat something new every single meal of every single day. Decide on the meals that you're willing to reheat or eat as leftovers, and then decide how many times you're willing to eat that food in one week. For example, grilled chicken is great when it's fresh off the grill, but it's also great as a leftover when chopped to top a cold salad, made into chicken salad, or reheated and served as a side. I therefore plan to make loads of grilled chicken at a time (enough to take over our entire four-burner grill) whenever it's on the meal plan. Excess can be easily frozen for a later date.

Pick five meals to prepare for the week. These meals will serve as dinners, lunches, and even parts of breakfast. Build the meals to suit your family's needs and preferences. I usually plan for each meal to contain a protein, a vegetable or salad, and another vegetable or starch (in the form of a starchy vegetable like potatoes or winter squash). I don't serve a starch at every meal, but I most always serve one or two vegetable sides depending on the other meal components. Note that this is a general rule of thumb and that some meals don't quite fit this scenario. You'll also have to determine how your particular family likes to eat. It may be that a starch is 100 percent necessary at every single meal.

Pick two to five different breakfasts that can be served throughout the week. My family tends to eat the same meals again and again for breakfast, but I like to have a bit of variety to keep everyone satisfied.

Plan for snacks, even if you eat the same snacks every week. I can get by without snacking, but my children are a very different story. Snacks are essential for their growing bodies. The menus that appear in appendix A do not include between-meal snacks. I've left this up to the individual to decide, because snacking preferences vary greatly depending on the circumstances. Refer to the *Quick and Easy Snacks* on page 170 for a list of my go-to snacks; I always add ingredients for snacks to my shopping list before heading to the grocery store. If you do the same, you'll visit the grocery store with a comprehensive list of your weekly needs (don't forget soap!). It's easy to forget snack-y ingredients, especially when balancing other daily tasks.

Know which meals freeze well and make more servings of those meals. For example, I always make around two and a half gallons of Not Quite Your Mama's Chili or Black Bean and Vegetable Soup since I know both of these soups freeze well. My weekly meal plans regularly incorporate meals or components of meals that are already frozen, because utilizing frozen meals saves time in the long run. For more information about freezing, see *Your Freezer, Your Friend* on page 64.

Mix and match with leftovers. I only prepare five different meals for a week, which means these components are going to comprise an entire week's worth of lunches and dinners. Meals don't have to be fixed combinations of food; you just have to prepare enough of each meal component to last through the week.

Jot down your meal plan and use this plan to make your shopping list. I like to plan my shopping days around the farmers market so that I'm able to get as many fresh, local ingredients as possible. I find the remaining ingredients at the grocery store.

Make a combination of side dishes into a meal. Throwing together some quick sides can often create a meal when you're in a pinch. Obviously, meal planning doesn't go perfectly in the beginning (or even once you've practiced for a while), but a good grouping of sides and snacks can make for a wholesome meal when nothing else is available. For us, these "snack meals" can mean a plate of sliced cucumbers and red peppers with store-bought hummus, whole olives from a jar, sardines in olive oil, a small handful of nuts, and any other leftovers I can scrounge together in a pinch. Organic, nitrate-free hot dogs from the freezer or canned tuna are other good options. (Of course, this is only possible because I've stocked these foods in the pantry and freezer!)

Adjust your plan to reflect your own family's appetites. The menu examples in this book are meant to help you get started, but know that these plans reflect the typical needs of my own family. I'd say that we eat an above-average amount of food due to our high level of activity. Your family's needs may be different, and may change according to the season.

Essential Food Prep Strategies

Time is by far the most limiting resource when it comes to food prep. I discuss ideas for time management in the section *Making Time for Real Food* in chapter 3, page 44, and I highly recommend reading that section if you haven't already. Making time for good food is all about prioritizing. Although this book offers numerous solutions to help you become more efficient in the kitchen, none of these solutions will work unless food prep becomes a priority for you and your family.

The biggest piece of advice that I can offer you is to prep before you actually need to eat. Cooking meals with whole foods requires washing and drying vegetables, chopping ingredients, cooking ingredients, and then cleaning up whatever mess you've created in your kitchen. The whole process can easily take two (or three) hours from start to finish depending on your efficiency and the degree of disarray. If I were to cook from start to finish for every meal, I'd need to plan to be in my kitchen at least an hour or two before it was time to eat, and this is just not realistic, especially for breakfasts.

Weekend mornings and afternoons are often a great time for me to get some food prep done for the week. The same is true for the occasional evening after I put the kids to bed and still have some energy left for tasks like chopping vegetables, cooking beans, or baking plantain bread. This hour or so is often the window that feels most meditative and calm since the low (and sometimes intensely bizarre!) hum of children has ceased for the day. I use this peaceful hour to enjoy some silence and sort through my busy thoughts, but you might find this to be the perfect opportunity to catch up on a podcast or audiobook. (I suggest Barbara Kingsolver's *Animal, Vegetable, Miracle* for a food-inspiring and soothing evening listen while preparing loving meals for your family.)

I look at my meal plan to see which tasks can be performed in advance. One approach is to wash, dry, and chop all of your vegetables for the entire week, and store them in the refrigerator in large Ziploc bags

Suggested Tasks to Perform in Advance

Washing, drying, and chopping vegetables

Washing, drying, and chopping fresh herbs

Preparing an everyday salad to eat throughout the week

Preparing a salad dressing or sauce for the week

Making bone broth

Whipping up a batch of Homemade Mayonnaise

Marinating meats

Making hamburger patties

Baking or pressure-cooking winter squash

Roasting, baking, or pressure-cooking sweet potatoes, potatoes, or beets to be used in varying salads and other side dishes

Preparing a tuna or chicken salad, or at the very least, chopping the vegetables and herbs to be used in those salads

Making a large pot of soup

Baking and freezing multiple loaves of bread

Roasting two or more whole chickens

Soaking and cooking or pressure-cooking beans

(I wash, dry, and reuse these bags until they're falling apart). When I prepare salads I make enough for the entire week, and sometimes I even divide salads into individual portions using small food storage containers. This way I have a quick meal that doesn't even need a plate! I can use these salads as a base for whatever leftover ingredients I choose to put on top—tuna fish or sardines, grilled chicken, guacamole, olives, nuts or seeds, or other toppings of choice.

As you review your menu, consider the suggestions in the sidebar *Suggested Tasks to Perform in Advance*, and then use your prep time, whenever you have it during the course of the week, to complete those tasks. I also recommend lumping similar tasks together because this means you'll only have to clean up once. For example, chopping large amounts of various vegetables includes one or two cutting boards, countertops, and a mess on the floor around the chopping area. It might sound like a lot of work initially, but once you've washed, chopped, and bagged all of your vegetables for the week, you're done. I can't tell you how amazingly satisfying this can be.

I use this same approach when turning on my oven or pressure cooker. Steaming foods in the pressure cooker doesn't actually dirty the insert. Many items can be steamed, including sweet potatoes, winter squash, and eggs (to hard-boil them). Preparing these items one after another without washing the insert in between will ultimately save you time. The same is true for the oven. Once it's on, I tend to pack it full or cook foods in successive order, especially during warmer weather when I don't want to have my oven blasting all the time. Once or twice a week is enough.

The best part about prep work is that it sets you up for success for the week. If you've had a busy day and don't necessarily feel like cooking when you come home, you'll be far more inclined to go ahead and cook if you know that most of the prep work is already out of the way.

Another approach to prep work involves the use of homemade raw and bagged freezer meals. This approach requires a decent-sized freezer and often the use of a Crock-Pot or pressure cooker to cook frozen meals that have not yet been cooked. This isn't a technique that has ever appealed to me, since I tend to freeze items after they've been cooked. I favor the approach where you prepare more than you'll need, eat some now, and freeze some for later, because it feels like a better time-saver and I appreciate the efficiency of storing already cooked meals in the freezer. However, I know a handful of people for whom freezing meals raw has worked well. If this approach appeals to you, start by reading the sidebar *Freezing Meals Before They're Actually Cooked*, and then choose recipes that can be chopped, bagged, and frozen raw. Most people who implement this approach pour the contents of these bags into a Crock-Pot in the morning, allow it to cook throughout the day, and return home in the evening to a piping-hot meal. (Note: You could likely make these meals in a fraction of the time using a pressure cooker.) People who are clearly better planners than myself use this technique to prepare meals for an entire month in one sitting! If this appeals to you, spend some time on Google and you're sure to find a plethora of expert freezer meals. Personally, I don't like to eat Crock-Pot meals every day. I like a variety of grilled, roasted, baked, sautéed, and raw ingredients, and using this technique simply doesn't allow for as much variation as my family prefers. However, I'm sure I could combine this method with what I'm already doing and it would complement it nicely.

I highly recommend doing anything and everything in advance (within reason) when it comes to breakfast meal prep. I'm sure there will be a day when mornings aren't filled with hungry children and school start deadlines, but I don't see this day approaching in the next few decades. I am of the belief that breakfast is the most important meal of the day for my kids

Freezing Meals Before They're Actually Cooked

I know a handful of individuals who simply despise eating leftovers. This would present a major challenge when trying to implement my method of meal planning, since it so heavily relies on bulk cooking, freezing cooked meals, and eating leftovers till the sun goes down. Freezing meals before they're cooked might be your solution if you've already decided that my method won't work for your family of eaters who have an aversion to leftovers. Some of the recipes in this book such as Pulled Mojo Chicken, Turmeric-Ginger Baked Chicken, Mexican Shredded Beef, and many of the soups yield extremely large quantities. The expectation is that leftovers will be frozen. The raw ingredients could instead be divided into one-meal portions and frozen until ready to be cooked.

Meals that serve themselves well for freezing raw are those that require a pressure cooker, slow cooker, or oven. You simply chop and bag the ingredients, label the bag accordingly, and note any additions that need to happen before cooking. For example, the solid ingredients for the 40-Minute Beef Stew could be chopped and bagged, and the label on the bag could read "Beef Stew—add 8 cups beef stock." (Do not include liquid ingredients in the frozen bags; add these just prior to

cooking.) The frozen ingredients could then be thrown into the pressure cooker, Crock-Pot, or large stovetop pot along with the beef stock (thawed, if frozen), and you'd proceed to prepare the recipe as instructed. Other soups that would lend well to this technique include Creamy Cauliflower Soup, Creamy Carrot Ginger Soup, Apple Butternut Soup, Black Bean and Vegetable Soup (only if using cooked beans), White Bean, Fennel, and Sausage Stew (only if using cooked beans), and Chicken and Vegetable Coconut Curry Soup. You'll obviously be skipping the sauté step for all of these soups since you're throwing a frozen block of solid ingredients into a large pot or pressure cooker along with the cooking liquid. Any frozen items that are placed into the oven such as Herb-Encrusted Drumsticks or OMGrain-Free Chicken Tenders will clearly need additional cooking time, but this is something you'll just have to experiment with because it's not a method that I use. Also keep in mind that items such as the drumsticks and chicken tenders will need to be spread out on a parchment paper–lined baking sheet for freezing; otherwise, you'll never be able to separate the frozen items if they're piled together before freezing. Once frozen, they can be lumped together in a bag and stored in the freezer.

because it sets the tone for the rest of their day. Feeding them something sweet and sugary for breakfast sets them on the path to sugar cravings and unstable blood sugar levels. To avoid that I like to start them off with a healthy fat and protein. The problem is that creating healthy breakfasts can take more time than I'm willing to commit in the mornings. Thus the importance of breakfast prep! I prep frittatas, egg

casseroles, and hard-boiled eggs; wash and chop vegetables for egg scrambles; cook breakfast sautés; and prepare breads or muffins in advance. The end result is a more nutrient-rich breakfast that sets a positive tone for the rest of the day. So be sure to account for breakfast foods when planning for prep work. You don't want to be cooking a 50-minute frittata first thing in the morning!

The Multitasker Wins the Race

Think of multitasking as the advanced version of meal prep. Food prep methods including baking and pressure-cooking don't actually require your attention once the foods are cooking, which means that time spent waiting for these foods to cook can be filled with prep tasks for the next day's meal. Furthermore, interjecting unattended tasks (namely pressure-cooking and baking) throughout your day when you plan to be at home can save you time. For example, I often throw something in the oven in the early-morning weekend hours and go about preparing for the day that lies ahead while the food cooks. If you work at home as I do, this is particularly applicable. You can cook numerous foods in advance by simply taking a 15- or 20-minute break from work to complete a task in the kitchen.

If I haven't had enough time to prep foods in advance for the week and I'm cooking a meal from start to finish, I often find that there's some downtime while I wait for an item to cook. Time for multitasking! This downtime can be filled with any number of tasks to make the following night's (or morning's) meal easier to prepare. Something as simple as filling five minutes with a task like chopping cilantro or garlic and storing it in the fridge for the next day's salad saves time in the long run. I've even used five spare minutes to crack and beat eggs for breakfast the next morning.

If you've set aside some time to work in the kitchen, downtime should be nonexistent during that period. Fill that time with as much prep work as you can. If you're stirring a sauté or soup base every now and then, use the time in between to start another meal. You can easily make breads and muffins, chop vegetables, or assemble salads while stirring or completing other simple tasks in the kitchen with a little forethought and planning. Don't underestimate the impact that these small windows of prep time can have on your total weekly kitchen commitment!

Batch-Cooking Basics

Batch cooking happens automatically when you prep in advance and multitask in the kitchen. I'd say the major difference is that batch cookers like to prep the majority of their meals in one or two sittings, rather than spread the workload out over the course of the week. This may be the most realistic approach for someone who maintains an extremely busy or unpredictable weekday schedule. You'd be amazed at how much you can actually accomplish when you set aside time specifically for cooking large amounts of food. The meal plans described in this book utilize Saturdays and Sundays to complete some introductory-level batch cooking. Personally, I love having all meals prepped in advance by Monday, but I often don't make it happen. I tend to batch cook as much as I can handle on the weekends, which then leaves me with minimal prep throughout the week. Minimal prep before each meal offers me a moment of meditation and enjoyment, *especially* when most of the hard work is already done, since my time in the kitchen is often a welcomed change of pace from the hectic day that preceded it. For those who like cooking less or who don't find it deeply fulfilling, I recommend batch cooking to get all of the work out of the way.

Batch cooking is especially popular among fitness gurus who are exceptionally focused on sticking with a calculated diet. They calculate the appropriate number of calories, carbs, fats, and proteins needed for each meal, build meals to reflect those numbers, cook everything for the week in one or two batch-cooking sessions, and then portion that food into individual meal containers. I'll be honest in that I'm in awe of these people and someday hope to become that organized. Not because I want to calculate the calories of every meal, but because it would be amazing to have a fridge full of preportioned, ready-to-eat meals for an entire week! But can you imagine the stacks of containers you'd need to accommodate this type of planning for a family of four? That's four containers per meal, three meals per day, seven days in a week for a total of 84 individually portioned meals. My head spins just thinking about the level of organization and containers this would take! However, if you're cooking for just one or two people, preportioning meals may be both viable and possible.

When I organize my batch-cooking time I start by looking at my weekly meal plan and decide which tasks should be started first. These are the tasks that need my initial attention, but can then be left unattended while I prepare something else. I usually start with prep work that involves baking, pressure-cooking, and boiling. If my meal plan includes Plantain Sandwich Bread, Apple Butternut Soup (which requires a baked or pressure-cooked butternut squash), or Roasted Non-Starchy Vegetables, then I'll start my prep work by preparing these dishes first. First is plantain bread assembly, since this has the longest baking time. I next prep the squash, throw that in the oven, and lastly add in the non-starchy vegetable, let's say broccoli. I start with the item that will bake the longest, and I finish with the item that takes the least amount of time. You have to be choosy about pan size when doing this, and, of course, all the dishes in the oven, regardless of how long they take to bake, need to have the same oven temperature.

You often have to increase your cooking time when you pack an oven full. How much depends on your individual oven. Textures of certain foods, such as the crunchiness of roasted vegetables, may be slightly sacrificed when the oven temperature is adjusted to meet the needs of the other occupants, but I find this sacrifice to be minimal. Baking bread while roasting vegetables may create a more humid oven environment, further altering the crunchy end-point, but I barely even notice a difference. The benefit of having so many foods prepared at once

makes up for the minimal change in texture. You may also have to adjust cooking times since you're cooking a group of foods at one temperature and that temperature may be higher or lower than what's specified in the recipe. (I wouldn't adjust the temperature for things like breads, cakes, or other baked goods, but you can get away with adjusting the cooking temperature for vegetables and sometimes meats.) If adjusting a recipe bothers you, you can cook multiple items at their required temperature and then adjust the temperature to suit your needs for a second round of baking. I've used both techniques and both work perfectly fine.

Once you've started your unattended cooking, such as baking or pressure-cooking, you have a couple of options for the next phase. You can start washing, drying, and chopping vegetables, or you can start preparing a second round of foods to go into the oven. Let's return to the preceding example where I cooked breads, squash, and broccoli during my first bake. For a second bake, let's say I go on to prep an Eat Your Greens Frittata, Kobocha Casserole with Pecans, and Simple Whole Roasted Chicken. Of course, what you choose really depends on how much time you have for prep and how long you're willing to leave your oven on. I'm less inclined to bake large quantities of food in the summer when keeping the house cool is a priority. But if I'm turning on my oven, a second round of baking saves energy since the oven is already warm.

The key to success when batch cooking is to maintain a steady workflow and keep the multitasking going. Some people will even set a timer and work until their allotted time runs out. Of course, this won't necessarily feel natural at first, since you're developing an entirely new skill. You might find yourself fumbling and feeling disorganized and overwhelmed, but practice makes perfect. I have slowly developed a sense of intuition when it comes to cooking, and with practice you, too, will develop the same.

Your Freezer, Your Friend

I highly recommend investing in a small chest freezer if you don't already own one. These small freezers don't take up a lot of room, and they can help you save quite a bit of time and money in the long run. I have two small freezers, which, for a family of four, gets the job done. I store frozen beef in one since I buy bulk meat from a local farm (beef is my largest bulk meat purchase, so it often needs an entire freezer to itself). In the other I store pork, poultry, organic hot dogs and deli meats, and foods that I've prepared and then frozen, including soups, stews, cooked meats, and breads. Miscellaneous items are scattered throughout such as bulk nuts or seeds, dates, frozen fruit, and other items I find on sale. (If you're planning to freeze whole raw and bagged meals and batch cook them for a week in advance, you'll definitely need a sizable freezer.)

One advantage I have to owning a chest freezer is that I can prepare larger amounts of recipes in advance and store the excess for subsequent meals, which greatly reduces time spent in the kitchen. There are so many foods that can be cooked and frozen in advance, but you may not have room for all of these items if you're simply relying on the freezer in your refrigerator.

My daughter is occasionally admitted to the hospital for IV antibiotic treatments, and on the occasions she's unwell we make the unexpected five-hour trip to the specialist. These trips are often last-minute affairs, and they leave me little time to prepare foods for my husband and son before I depart. Sure, my husband is capable of preparing a few meals, but that's not his norm and these periods of crisis are the wrong time for him to take on a whole new workload. We often don't take my son out to eat because of his allergies, so having a number of prepared frozen foods has been a lifesaver for my family on multiple occasions. I realize that if your family doesn't face similarly dire circumstances, this may sound like overkill to you. But there's no reason that your family can't adopt a similar approach and have meals on hand for when unpredictable circumstances prevent you from preparing home-cooked meals.

Organizing Your Freezer and Labeling Food

A freezer can quickly become a home cook's abyss of freezer-burned foods if you don't implement some organization. Like items must be grouped together and have their own designated space. For example, I put poultry on the left, unopened frozen fruits and vegetables are in the center, bacon and pork products go on the shelf area to the right, organic hot dogs and deli meats go in the basket, and prepared foods get stored on top of everything else. My second freezer is reserved for beef (roasts in the back, ground beef in the front, stew beef in the basket), with organ meats, bones, and fish on top. The freezer attached to my refrigerator holds prepared sauces, frozen opened bags of fruits and vegetables, ice, chicken carcasses, nuts, and a plethora of random items such as leftover glow sticks from the last Fourth of July party that we attended. Always storing food in airtight containers—whether it's a Ziploc bag, glass jar, or casserole dish—is your best bet for retaining freshness, in either the refrigerator or freezer.

Proper labeling of freezer items is equally important as organizing the items themselves. You need to record what's in the container or bag and the date that it was prepared and frozen. For example, a label might read "Mojo Chicken 9/3/18." I use a black permanent marker and write directly on Ziplocs or onto a piece of painter's tape or masking tape that's been secured to the plastic or glass container. You could even use different colored tape or markers for different food categories—meats are red, vegetables are green, sauces are purple, and so on. Another idea is to download an app that tracks food storage. While I haven't actually used such an app, I've seen options for pantry, freezer, and refrigerator storage tracking. I actually love this idea, since you could take a look at this app while at the grocery store to know whether you should buy more of a particular item when it's on sale. Whatever system you use for labeling and freezer organization, know that it's an important step in making sure the foods you buy and prepare don't go to waste.

Vacation Foods and Major Life Events

My family doesn't dine out in restaurants due to my son's wheat allergy. The chance of cross-contamination is low, but his reaction is so severe that it's simply not worth the risk. This means that I still have to cook every meal for my family when we go away on vacation, but cooking is often the last thing I want to do when vacationing. We spend some extra money on getting a few more prepared foods than we would normally, like coconut sandwich wraps, natural deli meats and hot dogs, organic chips, and a few other acceptable convenience foods. But the truth is there are very few packaged foods I feel good about eating. Packaged foods only get us so far. The cooking still remains.

Many people like to use vacations and holidays as a time to overindulge and enjoy a variety of junky foods and alcohol. I'd like for you to instead consider that vacation is a time for renewal. The foods you put into your body can help to support that renewal or they can prevent it. How many times have you returned from vacation feeling like you're ready to take a break from junk food? There's a better way, people!

I make a meal plan for vacation week about two months in advance. I build the plan knowing what types of resources will be available for me to use. If we're camping, we'll need foods that can be stored in a cooler and easily reheated on a camp stove. If we're staying in a hotel with a kitchenette or in a house with a full kitchen, I have more flexibility regarding packed

foods. My family doesn't often fly, but when we do I bring food on the plane, or at least enough for travel days when I'd prefer to avoid the overpriced convenience foods in the airport. I've brought salads, muffins, chicken salad, fruits, vegetables, and a variety of other foods. Just be prepared for some smiles and comments about your unusual luggage contents. While I've never done it, I believe families with children with allergies and other conditions requiring a special diet can get a physician's note to make the journey through airport security a bit easier, if necessary. While they still may not allow liquid foods, the note will help expedite the process of luggage scrutiny. I recommend that you call the TSA in advance, describe the nature of the situation, and ask that an agent offer guidance on carry-on limitations. Foods that are even questionably liquid (hummus, for example) should probably be avoided because TSA screeners will likely request that you throw these foods away if you're carrying more than the allotted three or four ounces. Knowing your limitations in advance will help you to develop a meal plan based on the resources that will be available to you while traveling and at your destination.

Once you've created your weekly vacation meal plan you can start to prep and freeze the meals or components of meals well in advance. I simply complete one or two extra recipes each week leading up to vacation, meaning that I have a good part of our meals prepared and frozen by the time we leave. Half-gallon-sized glass jars are great for freezing some foods (but do *not* freeze liquids like soups in glass, because they'll expand and break the jar) since you can easily pack six to eight jars into a medium-sized cooler upright. This prevents the inevitable dilemma of constantly reorganizing the cooler and draining off melted ice water to prevent the water from seeping in through the lids of the now-submerged storage containers. The jars are completely waterproof and tall enough so that melted ice water can't reach the lids. Use these same jars for your nonfrozen items and stagger their storage next to the frozen jars to create a built-in cooling system: The frozen jars will keep the nonfrozen jars cool, while the frozen jars will thaw in a few days, making their contents available for consumption. Just be sure to keep an eye on the temperature of your cooler, because you'll likely have to start adding ice after day three or four depending on the number of frozen items that you started with and the temperature at which you're storing your cooler.

The large jars can also be used to pack cooked components of meals that will need to be assembled later. For example, I usually plan for my family to eat Summer Potato Salad while vacationing. I chop the vegetables and place those in the bottom of the jar. I then place whole, cooked potatoes on top of the vegetables, seal, and refrigerate the jar. When we're ready to eat potato salad, I pour the contents into a bowl, dice the potatoes, add condiments (mayo and mustard), mix, and serve. I then store any leftovers in the original jar. This is a side dish that took all of five minutes to prepare. You can also pack jars with diced vegetables to be used for breakfasts, lunches, or dinners.

If you're going to implement this strategy for packing vacation foods, then you need to be sure that you're starting the process of cooking and freezing well in advance. This allows you to spend those last few days leading up to a vacation preparing the fresh foods. If you're trying to cook an entire week's worth of food in a few days before you depart, you're going to feel completely overloaded.

Major life events, such as the birth of a child, are another opportunity to plan well in advance. I froze a number of meals in the months before the birth of my daughter because we were planning to move from Vermont to North Carolina when she turned five weeks old. I knew that this period would be incredibly stressful and having meals already prepared helped alleviate some of the stress, especially given my son's

dietary restrictions. Major events are times when our body needs its greatest support, which isn't often possible given high stress or high demand. People tend to rely heavily on restaurant or prepackaged foods that don't support the stress response in a helpful way. If you know that you have a major event coming up, do yourself a favor and plan to freeze an appropriate number of meals ahead of time.

A Word on the Recipes and Menus

A complete approach to meal planning and prep, including unusual circumstances such as vacations, is key to making this diet work for you and your family. Meal planning, batch cooking, multitasking, freezing foods, and planning ahead are all important tools in the development of better intuition in the kitchen, an intuition that will help you reach your goals to feed your family a healthy diet made from whole-food ingredients. The following sections combine all of these skills.

The recipes include advice for batch prepping or cooking, storage, and for making it into a meal. The advice for prepping is designed to help you learn how to prepare the recipes in a way that reduces your overall cooking time, whether that time you save is today or in a few weeks when you're pulling leftovers out of the freezer. Storing leftovers is a major consideration in batch prepping, so I've made this information easily accessible using notes and icons. The advice for making it into a meal are suggestions that have to do with using each recipe in the book. You may find that some of the combinations feel out of the ordinary, but this book is about thinking outside the box when it comes to family meals.

The recipes often call for "cooking fat" or "cooking oil." I only designate a specific type of fat when it actually matters. Cooking fats are typically lard, tallow, or reserved fats from cooked meats such as bacon grease, but olive oil and avocado oil can be used instead. The solid cooking fats are generally inexpensive, so use these whenever possible and reserve your more expensive cooking oils (olive and avocado oil) for use when a liquid oil is necessary. Coconut oil is another option for a cooking fat, but I don't use it often unless called for since it adds a specific (sometimes desirable, sometimes not) flavor to a dish.

The four weekly menus in appendix A are to get you started on an efficient and organized path toward creating your own meal plans. (For those readers who want even more meticulous instructions that walk you through the menus step-by-step with prep sequences, please visit deeprootedwellness.com/grainfree where you can download a PDF for free.)

A Note on Natural Sweeteners

Maple syrup, agave syrup, and honey are often presented as healthy alternatives to table sugar since they contain trace minerals and antioxidants, but the benefits of eating these foods, especially when compared with other whole foods, is negligible. Raw honey boasts additional advantages such as its antiviral and antibacterial properties, and it certainly has its place as a natural remedy in the treatment of acute illnesses. However, I don't believe that any of these sweeteners have a regular place in the grain-free, sugar-free, dairy-free diet and have thus removed them from all the recipes. The point of this book is to teach a family how to avoid sugar on a daily basis and instead consume it in extreme moderation as a special treat for special occasions (namely birthday parties and holiday celebrations). When my family left Vermont, we brought with us a gallon of maple syrup. Three years later, we've only used about half. *This* is what I mean by moderation—treating sugar like a limited resource that warrants use only under special circumstances.

Access to sugar, honey, maple syrup, and other natural sweeteners was once a privileged occurrence.

Think back to people who lived centuries before us. Varying constraints (access and affordability) prevented sweeteners from being enjoyed by common folk on a regular basis. The trick now is in moderating consumption of a commodity that is readily accessible (and frequently consumed) by all.

However, I'm well aware that the near-zero approach to sugar isn't practical for many families and that my view on the subject is extreme (see *Slow Death by Sugar*, page 3, for an explanation as to why I take this approach). I have therefore included recipes in the *Sweet Treats* section that are prepared using stevia or dried dates. Stevia is a plant with a flavor that's recognized by our sweet receptors, yet it actually contains zero sugar or calories. Stevia is available in a powdered form (the dried leaves are ground into a powder that has the consistency of confectioners' sugar), as a liquid extract, or mixed with varying artificial sweeteners. Some health food experts disagree when it comes to using stevia as a sugar replacement, saying that it can further disrupt hormone regulation or thyroid function in individuals who are already experiencing health issues, but it seems as though the major reason to avoid stevia has to do with its processing and added ingredients. Powdered forms should contain just the leaves and nothing more. A popular brand of stevia powder is mixed with erythritol, a natural alcohol sugar that can also be used as a sugar substitute, but is not always well tolerated. Liquid stevia should contain stevia extract, water, and perhaps one or two other recognizable ingredients. If you choose to use stevia, be sure to read the ingredient list before purchasing.

The downside to using stevia is that besides being sweet, it has a very distinct flavor that not everyone appreciates. I have found that it can be used along with fruits in dishes like Mango Lime Ice Cream that require very little additional sweetness, but it doesn't make a great substitute for all sweet dishes. Stevia is about 200 times sweeter than table sugar, so start with a very small quantity and go from there. This also helps explain why a small bottle of stevia is so expensive; a little bit goes a long way. Monk fruit extract is another acceptable sugar replacement that, like stevia, is extremely sweet. Monk fruit has not been utilized in the recipes because of my lack of familiarity at the time of writing this book.

Dates are the most common sugar replacement in the *Sweet Treats* recipes. Dates are a whole-food ingredient, have less sugar per serving than maple syrup and honey, and contain substantial fiber to slow sugar digestion. What's more, dates have a legitimate nutrient profile and are a decent source of potassium, calcium, magnesium, vitamin B$_6$, vitamin A, iron, and even a small amount of protein. Our modern society has heavily integrated sweet treats into all sorts of occasions, and I want your family to have the option to celebrate these occasions in a healthier way.

Recipe Icons

Each recipe includes a set of icons to help you organize your prep time and inform you of proper food storage.

The apron describes the amount of hands on time required to complete each recipe.

The timer describes the total amount of time to complete the recipe, including the active time plus any unattended time. Total times are based on multitasking (sautéing onions while other vegetables for the dish are washed and chopped). Cooling times are only accounted for when it's a limiting factor in completing the recipe.

The plate tells you the number of servings or quantity yielded by the recipe. Pay special attention to this number since some recipes yield large quantities that are intended for freezing leftovers.

The refrigerator depicts the duration for which a recipe can be stored in the refrigerator. Recipes that do not store well in the fridge have a slash through the icon. Recipes that have no need to be stored in the refrigerator are missing the icon altogether.

The snowflake depicts the duration for which a recipe can be stored in the freezer. Recipes that do not store well in the freezer have a slash through the icon. Recipes that have no need to be stored in the freezer are missing the icon altogether.

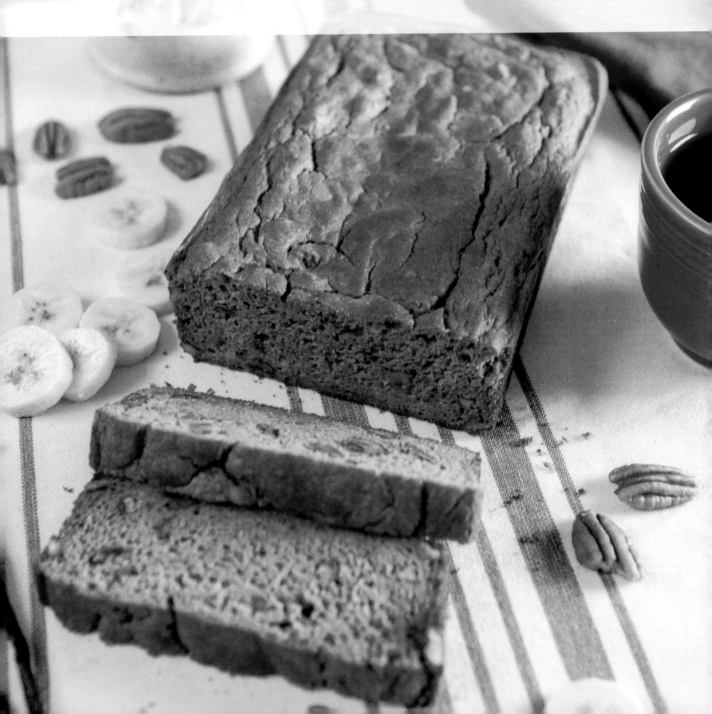

breakfasts and "breads"

perfectly baked bacon

active minutes

total time

servings

days

months

This foolproof method of bacon preparation is almost completely hands-off and makes perfectly crispy bacon every time. Don't forget to reserve the fat after the bacon is finished cooking. I prepare as much bacon as will fit in my oven at a time, use whatever is needed for the week, and then transfer the rest to the freezer. You can adjust the baking temperature on some recipes, but not this one. The bacon will burn if you cook it any hotter.

12 ounces (340 g) bacon
(or desired amount)

Preheat the oven to 300°F (149°C).

Spread the bacon into a single layer on a large baking sheet. Bake it for 25 minutes, drain off any excess fat into a small jar for storage, flip the bacon, and bake it for another 20 minutes. Exact cooking time will vary depending on the bacon thickness. Most bacon will work for the given recipe, but thick-cut bacon will need to cook slightly longer.

Drain the excess fat into the jar and place the bacon on a kitchen towel–lined plate, pat off the excess fat, and serve immediately.

Make It a Meal: Crumble on top of Creamy Cauliflower Soup, add to your Everyday Salad, or serve with Eat Your Greens Frittata.

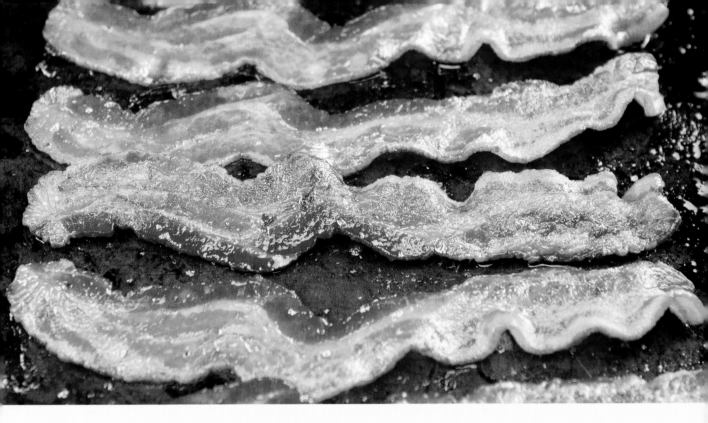

Saving Excess Fat from Cooked Meats

Most people discard fats from cooked meats such as bacon, ground pork, or ground beef. But these fats are an affordable and very valuable option for a healthy cooking fat, especially when you're buying quality meats. Be sure to reserve any solid fats that form at the top of cooled stocks and use them as cooking fats as well. Start saving these fats as an inexpensive way to improve your diet!

Reserved fat from cooked meats or stocks

Strain off the fat from cooked meats including ground beef, ground pork, or bacon by pouring the cooked meat into a fine-mesh metal colander over a bowl.

Pour the collected fat into a glass jar and allow the fat to cool to room temperature.

Once cooled, cooking liquid often accumulates underneath the layer of solid fat. You can remove the fat from the liquid and store the fat at room temperature for up to two months or for six months in the refrigerator. Alternatively, you can leave the fat sitting on top of the liquid, but it's best to store this in the refrigerator and use within two months. The fat keeps for quite some time, but the liquid portion will eventually go bad. You can transfer excess fat to the freezer for storage up to a year.

Use melted, reserved bacon grease from Perfectly Baked Bacon as the cooking fat to prepare Roasted Non-Starchy Vegetables, Red and Yellow Rosemary Potatoes, or a Simple Whole Roasted Chicken.

sage and rosemary sausage patties

10	30m	6–8	5	2
active minutes	total time	servings	days	months

Prep these rich and flavorful sausage patties the night before, and simply throw them in the oven while you get ready in the morning. You'll love this hot and satisfying side that can easily be taken on the go or packed into a lunch box. The Eat Your Greens Frittata would make a nice accompaniment for a grab-and-go, no-mess breakfast that can be reheated at the office. It's perfect for those who don't have time to enjoy a sit-down breakfast at home.

2 pounds (910 g) ground pork
1½ teaspoons dried sage
1½ teaspoons onion powder
1½ teaspoons garlic powder
1 teaspoon dried rosemary
1 teaspoon salt
Pepper, to taste

Preheat the oven to 400°F (204°C).

Combine all ingredients in a medium-sized bowl and use hands to work the spices into the ground pork. Divide the pork into 16 evenly sized balls. Next, form each ball into a small patty.

Place the sausage patties on a baking sheet and cook for 9 minutes, flip the patties, and bake for another 8 minutes.

Remove the patties from the oven and place them directly onto a kitchen towel–lined plate. Lightly press the tops of the patties with the towel to remove any excess fat.

Serve immediately.

Batch Cooking and Leftovers: Reheat on the stovetop or in a microwave.

Spread cooked (or raw) patties on a parchment paper–lined baking sheet to freeze without sticking, then transfer to Ziploc bags for long-term freezer storage.

Make It a Meal: Serve with Hard-Boiled Eggs, olives, sliced raw vegetables, and a piece of fruit.

cauliflower-sausage breakfast casserole

20 active minutes   1h 15m total time   16 servings   6 days   2 months

This hearty casserole is the perfect breakfast for the late fall or winter when you need something substantial to start your day. You'll need a large baking dish (or two smaller dishes, approximately 9 × 7 inches [23 × 18 cm]) to complete the recipe since it has such a large yield (because the dish holds up so well in the refrigerator or freezer). Most breakfast sausage is already spiced, but I often use unflavored ground pork to avoid the added sugars. Experiment with your own flavor profiles if you're using unflavored ground pork.

2 pounds (910 g) ground breakfast sausage

1 onion, diced

1 head cauliflower, chopped

1½ teaspoons salt

20 large eggs (or 16 extra-large eggs), beaten

Preheat the oven to 350°F (177°C).

Brown the sausage and onion in a large frying pan for 8–10 minutes, stirring frequently. Strain off any excess fat and reserve the fat for later use.

Use 2 tablespoons of the reserved sausage fat to grease a 10 × 15-inch (25 × 38 cm) baking dish. Spread the chopped cauliflower into the bottom of the dish to form the base of the casserole and evenly cover the cauliflower with the sausage-and-onion mix.

Whisk the salt into the eggs and pour the eggs evenly over the sausage and cauliflower. This dish appears to need more eggs, but the egg mixture will rise during baking and the casserole will set properly.

Bake the casserole for 50–55 minutes or until completely set and the top is golden.

Cut the casserole into 16 evenly sized pieces and serve immediately.

Batch Cooking and Leftovers: Double the amount of sausage and onions and freeze half for use in a future casserole.

Make It a Meal: Serve with small glass of Beet Kvass with Lemon and top it with Dill Pickle Kraut for a probiotic boost in the morning.

vegetable egg scramble with avocado and salsa

active minutes   total time   servings

There's something about a high-fat, high-protein breakfast contrasted with brightly colored mixed vegetables that sets a positive tone for the day. I used two of my favorite vegetables, but you can prepare this dish using whatever vegetables you have in excess at the time. Try kale, zucchini, or leeks for just a few other options. Just be sure to adjust the cooking time since some vegetables take longer to cook. Adding fresh basil or chives is an option for enhancing flavor.

2 tablespoons cooking fat
  (lard or reserved fat from
  cooked meats)
½ small red onion, diced
½ red pepper, diced
2 large handfuls spinach,
  roughly chopped
8 eggs, beaten
Salt, to taste
Pepper, to taste
8–12 tablespoons Fermented
  Salsa Fresca
1 avocado, diced

Heat the cooking fat in a large frying pan over medium heat and sauté the onion in the fat for about 2 minutes. Add in the red pepper and sauté for another 2 minutes. Add the spinach to the pan and sauté just until it begins to wilt, about 30 seconds.

Pour in the eggs, add your desired amount of salt and pepper, and stir gently and frequently until the eggs are cooked through.

Divide the egg-and-vegetable mixture among four bowls and top each serving with 2–4 tablespoons of salsa and a quarter of the avocado.

Serve immediately.

Batch Prepping and Leftovers: Prep the onions, peppers, and spinach ahead of time and store in refrigerator for up to 6 days.

Make It a Meal: Serve with Carrot Cake Applesauce Muffins.

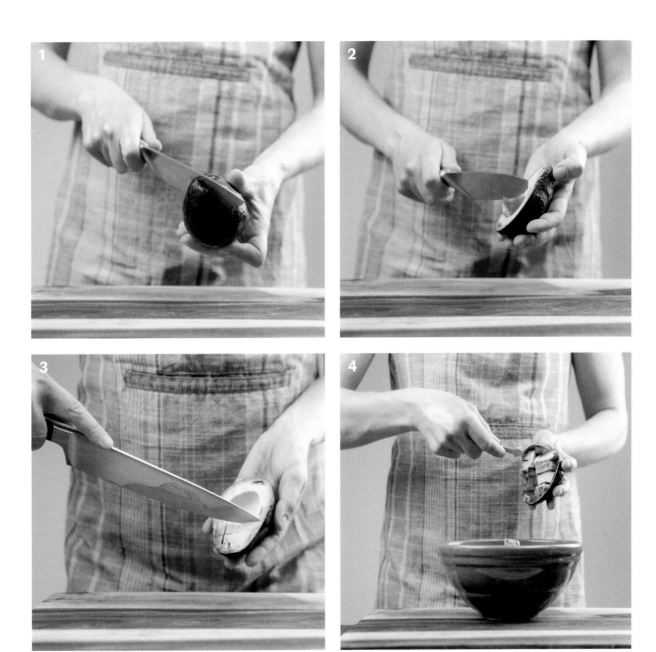

Step 1. Using a sharp knife, cut the avocado in half by moving the knife around the pit, and then twist the avocado apart. The pit will remain in one half. **Step 2.** Hold the pit half of the avocado in one hand and use the other hand to swiftly lodge the knife into the center of the pit. Twist the knife to remove the pit and lightly thump the pit off the blade using a hard surface. **Step 3.** Holding the avocado half in your hand, use a knife to score the avocado flesh into cubes of your desired size. Repeat with the second half. **Step 4.** Use a large spoon to scoop out the diced avocado.

probiotic pork and vegetables

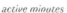

active minutes · total time · servings · days · months

This recipe is a nontraditional take on breakfast, yet it's satisfying, quick to reheat in the morning (I allow my five-year-old son to reheat his portion in a pan for cooking practice), and full of nutrient-dense ingredients that will keep you full most of the morning. You can use whatever fresh herbs you have on hand to replace the dried herbs. I often use fresh tarragon, sage, and parsley since I often have an overabundance from my garden during the summer. You could also use 2 pounds (0.9 kg) of any seasonal green in the place of cabbage in this recipe—kale, collards, chard, or napa cabbage. Zucchini or any other seasonal vegetables of your choice can also be subbed for red pepper. There's a lot of flexibility in this recipe!

2 pounds (0.9 kg) ground pork
1 large yellow onion, diced
1 small cabbage (approximately 2 pounds [0.9 kg]), shredded
2 medium zucchinis, halved and sliced
4 cloves garlic, minced
1 tablespoon dried tarragon
1 teaspoon dried basil
2 teaspoons salt
Pepper, to taste
2 cups (340 g) Dill Pickle Kraut or raw sauerkraut
2 avocados, diced (optional)

Brown the pork in a large frying pan or large pot for approximately 10 minutes. Once browned, strain the pork through a fine-mesh colander over a bowl to collect the excess fat. Set the pork aside.

Using the same pan, add 2 tablespoons of the reserved pork fat to the pan and sauté the onion over medium heat for about 2 minutes. Add in the cabbage and cook for an additional 7 minutes, stirring frequently. Add the zucchinis, garlic, tarragon, basil, salt, and pepper and cook 5 minutes more or until the vegetables reach the desired texture.

Remove the pan from the heat and stir in the cooked ground pork.

Serve each portion immediately topped with ¼ cup (43 g) raw sauerkraut and a quarter of an avocado, if using.

Batch Prepping and Leftovers: Double the recipe and store one-fourth in the refrigerator; freeze the other fourths for quick breakfast meals.

Make It a Meal: Serve with Plantain Muffins and top with Dill Pickle Kraut.

cauliflower hash browns

20	30m	6	5	
active minutes	total time	servings	days	

Don't get me wrong, I have nothing against potatoes, but I do love that you can reinvent a classic breakfast dish using a nutrient-dense cruciferous vegetable. These hash browns could double as a breadlike conduit to lay flat on a plate and top with The Tuna Salad Upgrade or as a bun for Herbed Beef Burgers. Just be sure to shape the "bread" accordingly.

1 head cauliflower, approximately 2½ pounds (1.1 kg)

4 eggs

1 tablespoon dried parsley

1 teaspoon garlic powder

1 teaspoon onion powder

3–4 tablespoons cooking fat (reserved bacon grease preferred), divided

Salt, to taste

Use the grater on a food processor to grate the cauliflower. It can be done by hand, but it's not easy and it takes more time.

Combine the grated cauliflower, eggs, parsley, and garlic and onion powders in a large mixing bowl. Mix until everything is evenly distributed. Do *not* add salt until after the cauliflower hash browns are cooking in the pan, as the salt will pull water out of the raw cauliflower and you'll be left with a soppy mess.

Heat a large frying pan on medium heat and evenly coat the pan with 1 tablespoon of the cooking fat. Using a ⅓-cup (80 ml) measuring cup, scoop the cauliflower mix into the pan and press each scoop into a ¾-inch-thick patty using the back of the measuring cup.

Lightly sprinkle salt over the patties, cook for 3–4 minutes, flip, salt, and cook for another 3–4 minutes until both sides are golden brown.

Repeat until you've used the entire mix. Be sure to add more cooking fat to the pan before adding consecutive rounds of cauliflower hash browns.

Serve hash browns immediately.

Batch Cooking and Leftovers: To save time (but sacrificing the crunchiness), bake the cauliflower mixture in a 400°F (204°C) oven for 25–30 minutes.

If prepping ahead, store grated cauliflower in the fridge for up to 5 days.

Make It a Meal: Serve with Probiotic Pork and Vegetables, or use as a base for fried eggs, Perfectly Baked Bacon, and fresh diced tomatoes.

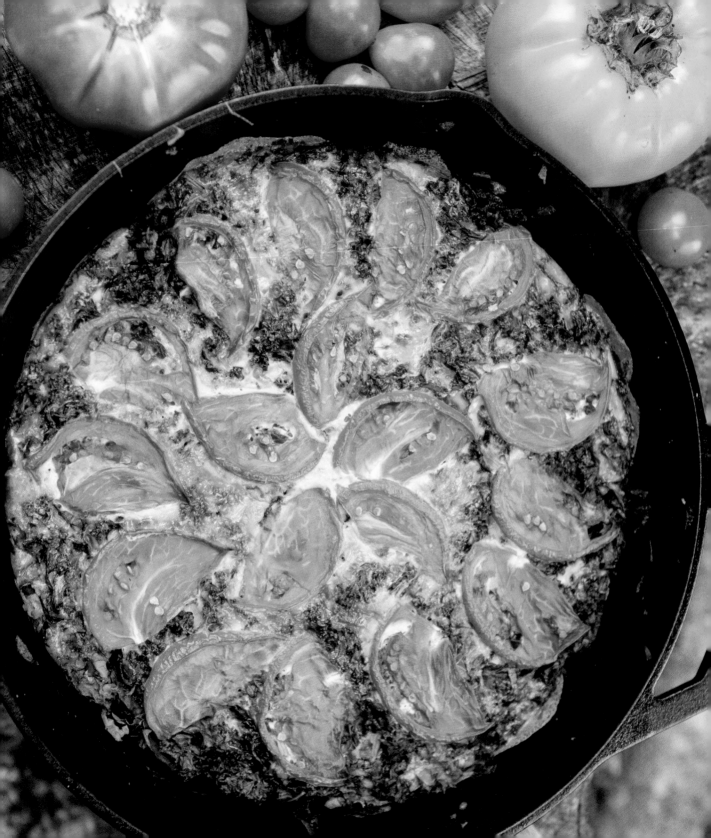

eat your greens frittata

active minutes   total time   servings   days   month

Frittatas and other egg preparations like the Cauliflower-Sausage Breakfast Casserole are my most frequently prepared breakfast dishes since they can be made in such large quantities and store nicely in the refrigerator for the week. This light frittata is loaded with the flavors of summer with its heavy reliance on tomatoes, basil, and garlic. You can sub in any fresh herbs of your liking including dill, oregano, and fresh chives. Vegetable substitutions can also be made: Try using leftover portions of Simple Spaghetti Squash to line the bottom of the pan before adding the other ingredients. The dish has better flavor and texture when the vegetables are sautéed first, but it's not entirely necessary.

12 eggs

2 tablespoons cooking fat
(lard or reserved fat from
cooked meats)

1 yellow onion, diced

2 bunches kale, washed and
chopped, ribs intact

4 cloves garlic, minced

1 cup (50 g) thinly sliced, loosely
packed fresh basil

2 teaspoons sea salt

1 large tomato, halved and
thinly sliced

Preheat the oven to 350°F (177°C).

Whisk the eggs together and set aside.

Heat the cooking fat in an oven-safe pan (such as cast iron or stainless steel) on the stovetop over medium heat and sauté the onion in the cooking fat for approximately 3 minutes.

Add in the kale and garlic, and sauté for an additional 2 minutes until the kale is slightly wilted.

Remove the pan from the heat and mix in the basil and salt.

Pour the eggs evenly over the top of the greens, arrange sliced tomatoes on top of the eggs, and bake the frittata for 45–50 minutes or until the top is golden. Allow the frittata to cool for 5–10 minutes before dividing it into eight even pieces.

Serve immediately.

Batch Prepping and Leftovers: If doubling the recipe, use a greased baking dish, and freeze half for later.

Make It a Meal: Serve with sliced avocados or Banana Nut Bread.

asparagus and mushroom quiche with almond flour crust

25
active minutes

1h 10m
total time

8
servings

6
days

1
month

I love having the option to prepare a creamy and colorful dish for special-occasion breakfasts or even potlucks. You can also prepare mini quiches in muffin tins, which can be good (albeit more time consuming) for special-occasion brunches.

CRUST

2½ cups (240 g) almond flour

¼ teaspoon salt

1 egg, beaten

¼ cup (55 g) melted lard or tallow, more for greasing

FILLING

1 tablespoon cooking fat (lard or reserved fat from cooked meats)

1 small onion, diced

½ pound (225 g) baby bella or shiitake mushrooms, sliced

12 ounces (240 g) asparagus, trimmed and cut into 1-inch (2.5 cm) pieces

4 cloves garlic, minced

1 teaspoon salt, divided

6 eggs, beaten

1 can (5.4 ounces [160 ml]) coconut cream

2 teaspoons Dijon mustard

3–4 cherry tomatoes, thinly sliced (optional)

CRUST INSTRUCTIONS

Preheat the oven to 350°F (177°C).

Mix the almond flour and salt together in a medium-sized bowl. Pour the egg and melted lard into the almond flour mixture and stir until the liquid is absorbed and a dough has formed.

Place the dough into a well-greased 9-inch (23 cm) pie pan and use your fingers to press the dough evenly into the pan. Using a fork, pierce the bottom of the crust about 10 times, evenly spreading the pierces throughout, and bake the crust for 10 minutes.

Prepare the filling while the crust bakes.

FILLING INSTRUCTIONS

Preheat the cooking fat in a medium-sized pan and sauté the onion in the fat for about 2 minutes. Add the mushrooms and asparagus, and continue to cook for an additional 6 minutes. Add the garlic and ½ teaspoon of the salt, and sauté all ingredients for another 2 minutes. Remove from the heat.

Prepare the egg mixture by blending the eggs with the coconut cream, mustard, and remaining ½ teaspoon salt. I use an immersion blender, blending just long enough to combine the eggs with the coconut cream. The coconut cream will *not* mix into the eggs without blending (a whisk will be useless).

Fill the piecrust with the vegetable sauté, spreading the vegetables evenly in the bottom of the crust. Pour the egg mixture over the top. Tomatoes can be arranged on top of the egg mixture, if using. This is primarily for aesthetics.

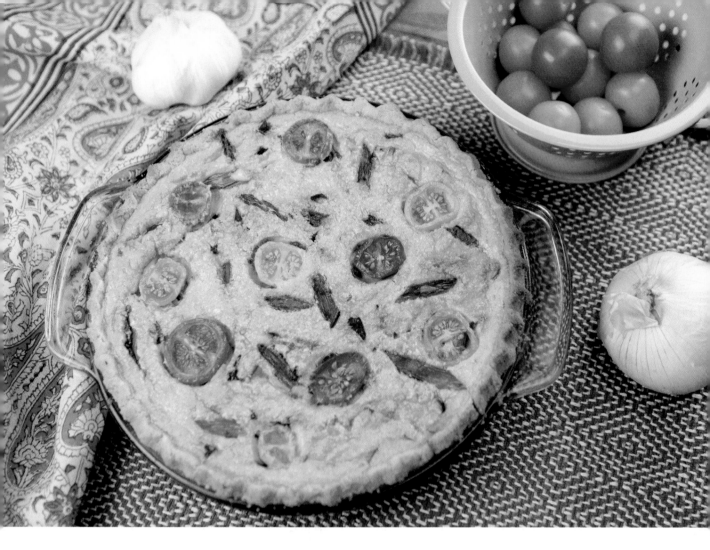

Place the quiche in the oven and bake for 40–45 minutes or until golden and firm in the center.

Allow the quiche to cool for about 10 minutes before dividing it into eight servings.

Serve immediately.

Batch Cooking and Leftovers: Prep the dough and vegetables in advance to save time.

Make It a Meal: Serve for a special brunch with Perfectly Baked Bacon, Cauliflower Hash Browns, Pecan Bread, and Infused Water.

spaghetti squash porridge

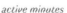

active minutes   total time   servings   week   month

This deliciously sweet and creamy breakfast porridge will hit the spot when you want something that resembles a huge bowl of oatmeal. With far fewer carbohydrates and a greater concentration of healthy fats and proteins than a grain porridge, this is a much better choice to start the day off right. You can sub in any sugar-free dried fruit in the place of raisins. Figs, mango, goji berries, or mulberries are great choices, too. You can also add extra goodies like hemp hearts or pumpkin seeds for an even heartier bowl.

1 prepared Simple Spaghetti Squash, flesh removed and roughly chopped

1 can (13.5 ounces [398 ml]) unsweetened full-fat coconut milk

¾ cup (85 g) chopped walnuts

½ cup (85 g) raisins, packed

1 teaspoon cinnamon

1 teaspoon vanilla extract

Salt, to taste

Combine all ingredients in a medium pot, cover, and bring to a simmer. Turn the heat to low and continue to simmer, uncovered, for 15 minutes, stirring frequently. Try to chop and break up the spaghetti squash as it cooks to form a creamier consistency.

Remove the porridge from the heat and serve hot.

Batch Cooking and Leftovers: Easy to reheat, and tastes better over time! Prep a day or two before serving, and double it and freeze half for later use.

Serve in the same week as Simple Spaghetti Squash and batch prep squashes for both meals.

Make It a Meal: Pair with a contrasting savory beverage, Truly Green Smoothie, or add protein with Sage and Rosemary Sausage Patties.

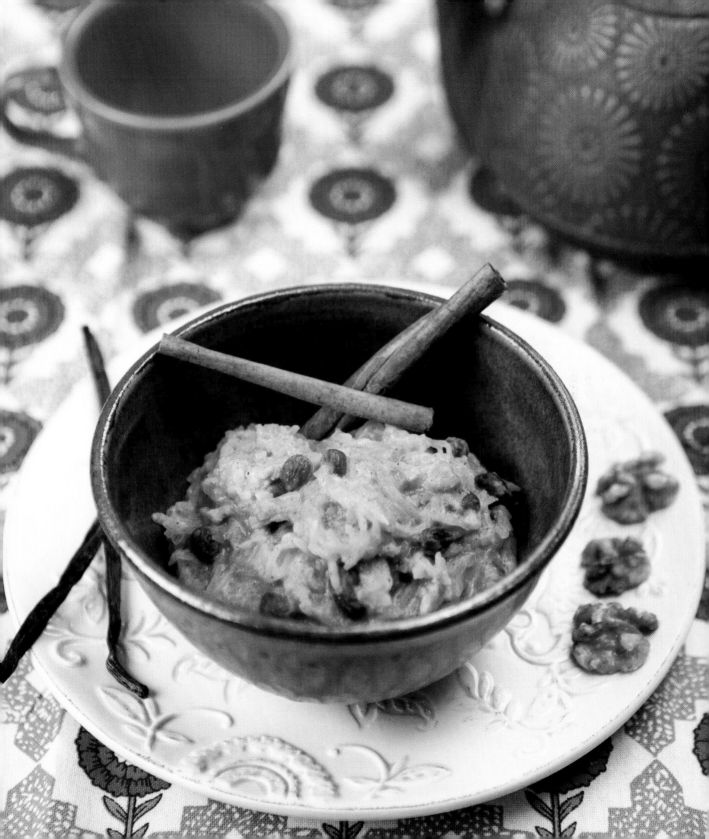

simple spaghetti squash

Spaghetti squash is a surprisingly easy and diverse addition to any culinary repertoire . . . once you learn how to prepare it, that is. Spaghetti squash can be used as an excellent substitute for pasta in a variety of dishes, including "Pasta" Bowls. It can also become a unique breakfast dish, like the Spaghetti Squash Porridge. It's affordable, easy, delicious, and versatile—a real gem among the winter squashes! My family's frequent consumption of spaghetti squash has been made far easier by owning an electric pressure cooker. What takes about 10 minutes in the pressure cooker takes as much as an hour in the oven.

I often prepare two squashes at once and use them for different purposes throughout the week. Leftovers can be stored in the refrigerator in a sealed container for up to 7 days or in the freezer in a freezer-safe bag for up to 4 months. You could even choose to prepare as many squashes as will fit in your oven in one bake, remove the flesh from the squashes after cooking, and store each squash in a freezer bag for quick meals in the following months. Freezing Simple Vegan Pesto, Sun-Dried Tomato Tapenade, and Grilled Chicken Breasts with Basil and Thyme will allow you to pull each of these items from the freezer to create Greek-style "Pasta" Bowls, a delicious and complete freezer meal.

OVEN INSTRUCTIONS

Preheat the oven to 350°F (177°C).

Place the entire whole squash on a baking sheet and place it in the oven for 45–60 minutes or until the squash can be easily pierced with a fork. Cooking time depends on the size of the squash.

Once the squash has cooled enough to handle, remove the stem from the squash using a large, sharp kitchen knife.

Cut the spaghetti squash into two equal halves lengthwise and remove the seeds from the squash using a spoon.

Using a fork, scrape out spaghetti-like strands.

Note: You can first halve the spaghetti squash, remove the seeds, and place it facedown on a parchment-lined baking sheet to reduce the cooking time by 15 minutes.

PRESSURE COOKER INSTRUCTIONS

Remove the stem from the squash using a large, sharp kitchen knife.

Cut the spaghetti squash into two equal halves lengthwise and remove the seeds from the squash using a spoon.

Place the spaghetti squash halves facedown in the pressure cooker on top of the included rack. Add 1 cup (235 ml) of water and cook on high pressure for 6–7 minutes, depending on the size of the squash.

Release the steam as soon as it's done and scrape out spaghetti squash as indicated in the oven instructions.

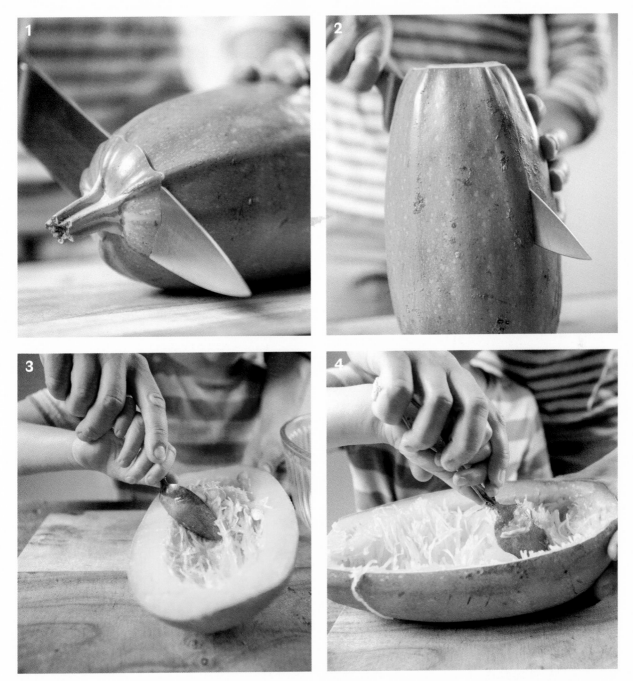

Step 1. Allow whole cooked squash to cool enough to handle, then remove end with a sharp knife. **Step 2.** Cut squash in half lengthwise. **Step 3.** Use a large spoon to remove seeds. **Step 4.** Remove flesh with a fork or spoon to create "spaghetti."

apple walnut crisp cereal

active minutes · total time* · servings · week · month

30 · 1h · 16 · 1 · 1

The sophisticated crunch of walnuts combined with the delicate sweetness from apples and cinnamon makes this breakfast cereal a win for the whole family. It's easily prepared in advance, helping you breeze through the morning before hustling out the door. I suggest serving this breakfast with Homemade Coconut Milk, but you can use Homemade Almond Milk if you prefer. A combination of whatever nuts you have on hand can be used to replace the walnuts. Try raw pumpkin seeds for a nut-free version.

2½ teaspoons salt, divided

5 cups (1.2 l) water, for soaking

1½ pounds (680 g) whole raw walnuts (about 5½ cups), soaked overnight

4 pounds (1.8 kg) apples (about 10 small apples)

1 tablespoon cinnamon

1 teaspoon lemon zest

½ cup (100 g) coconut oil, melted

Homemade Coconut Milk, prepared four times (see *Batch Cooking*)

* plus 12–24 hours for soaking

Dissolve 2 teaspoons of the salt in the water. Combine the salt water and walnuts in a large bowl or glass jar and allow the nuts to soak overnight. Strain and thoroughly rinse the walnuts after soaking. (See *Soaking Seeds and Beans*, page 14, for more information.)

Preheat the oven to 350°F (177°C).

Core and dice the apples into ½-inch (1.3 cm) cubes (do not remove peels), and roughly chop the walnuts.

Combine the apples, walnuts, cinnamon, lemon zest, and remaining ½ teaspoon of salt in a large mixing bowl. Mix everything until well combined. Pour coconut oil over the apple-walnut mixture and mix until evenly coated.

Evenly distribute the apple-walnut mixture onto two parchment paper–lined 12 × 16-inch (30 × 40 cm) baking pans. Bake for 30 minutes, stirring halfway through.

Allow the apples and walnuts to completely cool before placing the cereal in airtight containers for storage. Serve the cereal topped with your desired amount of Homemade Coconut Milk.

Batch Cooking and Leftovers: Make three or four batches of Coconut Milk to guarantee you'll have enough milk for several meals.

Make It a Meal: Serve with a refreshing glass of Infused Water or Hibiscus Zinger Iced Tea.

carrot cake applesauce muffins

active minutes   total time   muffins   days   month

These light yet insanely filling little muffins are densely packed with flavorful ingredients that the whole family will love. I serve these muffins as a breakfast side or a quick snack throughout the week. Make sure to pay attention to rationing since kids will devour these muffins if given the chance.

10 eggs

2 cups (490 g) unsweetened applesauce

1 cup (130 g) coconut flour

½ cup (100 g) melted coconut oil

4 tablespoons cinnamon

2 teaspoons vanilla extract

2 teaspoons baking powder

½ teaspoon salt

¾ cup (75 g) shredded carrots

¾ cup (130 g) raisins

¾ cup (85 g) chopped walnuts

Preheat the oven to 400°F (204°C).

Whisk the eggs, then add in the applesauce, coconut flour, coconut oil, cinnamon, vanilla, baking powder, and salt. Whisk together all ingredients to form a smooth batter.

Using a large spoon, mix in the remaining ingredients.

Use a ¼-cup (60 ml) measuring cup to scoop batter into 24 silicon muffin molds or paper-lined muffin pans. Bake the muffins for 18 minutes or until the tops are just barely set. The muffins do not appear to be cooked through, but they'll continue to set as they cool.

Muffins are best 24 hours later, which allows time for the flavors to meld, but can be served once completely cool.

Batch Cooking and Leftovers: Work in batches if you double this recipe.

Make It a Meal: Pull from the freezer to use in packed lunches along with sliced raw vegetables, Turkey Cucumber Rolls, and Fiesta Sunflower Seed Hummus.

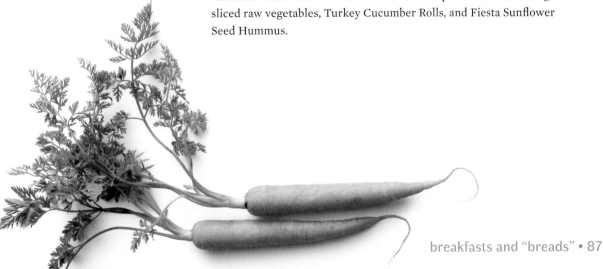

hearty almond flour bread

| active minutes | total time | small loaf | week | months |

Hearty Almond Flour Bread is the ultimate food to power up for a day of intense activity. It is densely packed with healthy fats and proteins, the macronutrients that will sustain energy the longest. I use a store-bought blanched almond flour, but you can make your own using a high-powered blender or food processor. Use caution not to overprocess the almonds or you'll end up with almond butter. The high concentration of nuts and nut flours in this bread will go a long way. I eat very small servings at a time to prevent nut overload.

2 cups (190 g) almond flour

¼ cup (25 g) flaxseed meal (or ground flaxseed)

2 tablespoons coconut flour

½ teaspoon sea salt

½ teaspoon baking soda

5 eggs

2 tablespoons coconut oil, melted, divided

¼ cup (28 g) chopped walnuts

¼ cup (35 g) sunflower seeds

¼ cup (35 g) pumpkin seeds

Preheat the oven to 350°F (177°C).

Combine the almond flour, flaxseed meal, coconut flour, salt, and baking soda and mix together in a medium-sized bowl.

Add in the eggs and 1 tablespoon of the coconut oil, and whisk until a batter forms. Work relatively quickly because this batter will thicken as it sits.

Stir in the walnuts, sunflower seeds, and pumpkin seeds using a large spoon.

Use the remaining coconut oil to grease a 4½ × 8½-inch (10 × 20 cm) bread pan. Place the bread mixture into the pan and smooth it flat using the back of a spoon or spatula. The batter won't pour, so it will need to pressed into the pan to take on the correct shape.

Bake the bread for 30–35 minutes or until the top begins to turn golden.

Allow the bread to cool for about 5 minutes before removing the loaf from the pan and placing it on a cooling rack. Allow the bread to completely cool before cutting.

Batch Cooking and Leftovers: The recipe freezes very well: Double it and freeze half!

Make It a Meal: Top a small slice of bread with Garlicky Greens and a fried egg for a delicious, keto-friendly breakfast.

plantain sandwich bread

active minutes   total time   small loaves   days

You don't have to completely give up sandwiches simply because you've given up on grains! This sandwich bread isn't quite as squishy as Wonder Bread, but it's a big step up from the grain-free store-bought options that taste more like chalk or cardboard than bread, and it holds together well once completely cooled. It's perfect for the occasional sandwich craving or for packed lunches for the kiddos! Try adding in your favorite dried herbs and spices for a more flavorful bread.

6 yellow plantains
(no black spots but not green;
see *A Note about Plantains*,
page 93, for more info)
8 eggs
½ cup (120 ml) avocado or
olive oil, more for greasing
½ cup (65 g) coconut flour
2 teaspoons baking powder
2 teaspoons baking soda
1 teaspoon salt

Preheat the oven to 350°F (177°F).

Peel and dice the plantains into 2-inch (5 cm) pieces.

Place the plantains, eggs, and oil into a blender or food processor and blend until a smooth batter forms. Add the remaining ingredients and blend for another 15–30 seconds, just until evenly mixed.

Evenly pour the batter into two well-greased bread pans and bake for 45 minutes or until an inserted fork comes out clean. Allow the bread to cool for about 10 minutes before removing the bread from the pan and placing it on a cooling rack.

Allow the bread to completely cool before slicing.

Batch Cooking and Leftovers: If you don't eat the bread quickly (within 4 days), halve the recipe and make just one loaf, as it becomes stale and brittle quickly.

Make It a Meal: Top with a scoop of The Tuna Salad Upgrade and fresh heirloom tomato slices.

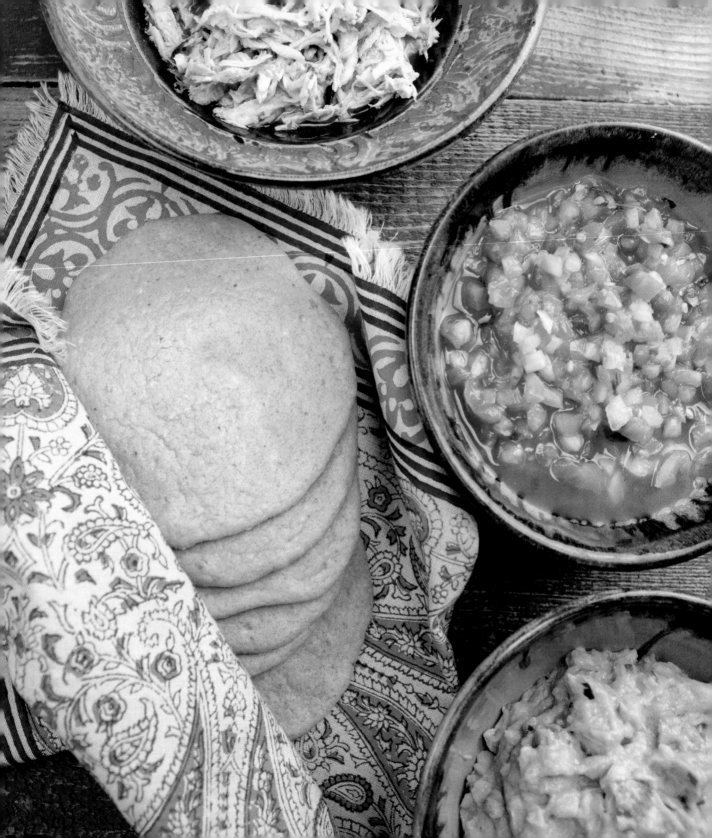

plantain tortillas

15
active minutes

25m
total time

8–10
tortillas

I cannot emphasize enough the excellent quality, texture, and taste of these simple tortillas. Your family will absolutely adore grain-free tacos made from 100 percent whole-food ingredients! Try serving these tortillas to guests along with delicious fillings and sides for a stunning example of how adventurous a restrictive diet can be.

2 plantains (yellowish green, not fully ripe, see *A Note about Plantains*, page 93), peeled and cut into 2-inch (5 cm) pieces
¼ cup (60 ml) avocado oil
1 egg
1 teaspoon vinegar
½ teaspoon baking soda
½ teaspoon salt

Preheat the oven to 425°F (218°C).

Blend all ingredients together in a blender or food processor for about 30 seconds to form a batter. You can add 1–2 tablespoons of water if the mixture will not blend, but be reserved with the addition of water.

Using a ⅓-cup (80 ml) measuring cup, scoop the batter onto a parchment paper–lined baking sheet, allowing for 6 inches (15 cm) of space between scoops, and about 3 inches (7.5 cm) of space from the edge of the pan. You need to leave enough space for each tortilla to be smoothed into a 5- or 6-inch (12.5–15 cm) round.

Using the back of a spoon, smooth each scoop into a flat circle about ¼ inch (6 mm) thick to form the tortillas. Bake the tortillas for 10 minutes.

Allow the tortillas to slightly cool before carefully moving them to a serving plate.

Batch Cooking and Leftovers: Not great for leftovers, so plan to make these on a day you have the time.

Make It a Meal: Taco night! Top the tortillas with Pulled Mojo Chicken or Mexican Shredded Beef with Chimichurri Sauce, Pico de Gallo, and Garlicky Guacamole.

Plantain tortillas shown with Pulled Mojo Chicken, Fermented Salsa Fresca, and Garlicky Guacamole.

plantain muffins
(with pecan bread variation)

active minutes   total time   muffins*   week   month

How often do I prepare these muffins? Every week. Why? Because they're that good. Plus I love having a guiltless bread product to pair with breakfasts or serve as a snack for the kids. These muffins are so moist, fluffy, filling, and flavorful. And I *love* the fact that they're plenty sweet, even without the addition of any sugar. The plantains need to be ripe, which means yellow with some black spots. If the end product isn't sweet enough and is slightly on the dry side, you've used the plantains too early. If it's mushy and doesn't seem to set properly, the plantains were too ripe. You may have to make this recipe a few times to get the hang of it, but it will be well worth the effort!

1 cup (145 g) raw sunflower seeds

1½ tablespoons cinnamon

2 teaspoons baking powder

1 teaspoon baking soda

½ teaspoon salt

4 ripe plantains, peeled and
   sliced into 2-inch (5 cm) pieces

4 eggs

½ cup (100 g) coconut oil

½ cup (120 ml) water

* or 2 loaves of bread

Preheat the oven to 350°F (177°C).

Grind the sunflower seeds into a flour using a high-powered blender or food processor. Do not overblend or the seeds will start to turn into a seed butter. If using a high-powered blender, 5–8 seconds of blending should be adequate, but it will take closer to 30 seconds in a food processor or less powerful blender. The flour will have the texture of almond flour. Scrape down the sides and corners after blending to free any lodged flour.

Add the remaining ingredients to the blender or food processor in the order listed in the ingredients list and blend just long enough to form a smooth batter.

Pour the batter evenly among 24 silicon muffin molds or paper-lined muffin pans, filling the cups about three-quarters full. The exact volume of batter depends on the size of the plantains. If you have excess batter, pour the remainder into additional muffin molds (if available) or into a greased bread pan for a long, flat bread that can be cut into quarters or thirds depending on its size.

Bake the muffins for 25 minutes or until firm to the touch. If you have excess batter in a bread pan, this may take an additional 5–10 minutes to cook depending on its size.

Allow the muffins to cool for about 5 minutes before transferring them to a cooling rack.

For a delicious Pecan Bread variation, add 1½ cups (170 g) chopped pecans and pour the batter into two greased bread pans. Bake the bread for 55 minutes or until completely set.

Batch Cooking and Leftovers: For batch cooking: Grind flour for both batches first. Then proceed in two batches (blenders are too small for a double batch).

Freeze muffins for quick snacks or packed lunches.

Make It a Meal: Serve with Garlicky Greens and diced tomatoes, or fried eggs and Dill Pickle Kraut for a sweet and savory nutritious breakfast.

A Note about Plantains

Plantains are an inconspicuous grain substitute that can be blended and baked into breads, batters, and cakes. Plantains have a slightly higher starch content than bananas, resulting in a bread product with excellent texture and natural sweetness. I don't suggest eating plantains raw. They should instead be blended and baked; or sliced, slathered in coconut oil, and then baked, fried, or grilled.

Bananas can be used in the place of plantains in these muffin, bread, and pancake recipes if you're unable to find this fruit or if you're uncomfortable with using conventionally grown plantains. I see organic plantains on rare occasions (ask your local health food store if this is something they can special order), but organic bananas are often easy to find. To substitute bananas for plantains, replace four plantains with six large bananas, because bananas have a much smaller mass. You can also experiment with adding small amounts of cassava flour to the recipes to help replace any lost starch. This is an unnecessary step that is only recommended for those who like to deviate from recipes and experiment with their own creations. I will say that using plantains yields a superior flavor profile since plantains have less of an actual flavor when compared with bananas, but the bananas work perfectly well. You won't even know the difference if you've never had plantains.

Knowing when a plantain is ready to eat can be challenging and requires a bit of practice and patience. Plantains are much like bananas in that they start out green and slowly transition to yellow. As plantains ripen they develop a number of black spots on the peel. A yellow plantain without black spots is not yet fully ripe, as you would expect. Ripe plantains will have some black spots, and they yield a finished bread product with the perfect balance of starch, natural sweetness, and moisture. The starches convert to sugars as the plantains ripen, ultimately reducing the starch content. As this starch is lost, you also start to lose the integrity of the plantain after it's blended and cooked. Overripe plantains have far more sugar content and less starch, so the final bread product is very sweet, mushy, and doesn't hold up well. The bread or pancake will still taste great, but you'll be left with a bread product that feels as if it's saturated with moisture.

Using plantains also means that you may have to organize some shopping and cooking around the ripeness of the fruit. If this feels too challenging, simply purchase plantains well in advance and freeze them when they reach their ideal ripeness. The frozen plantains can then be thawed and used in any of these recipes as needed. The same is true for bananas. If your plantains are overripe, simply pair them with underripe bananas or plantains to balance out the starch and sugar content.

These instructions may initially appear to be complicated, but I give you my word that learning to use plantains is worth the minimal effort. You can view instructions for how to peel plantains at deeprooted wellness.com/grainfree.

plantain blender pancakes

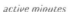

active minutes   total time   small pancakes   days   month

Let's be honest, I rarely make pancakes for my family since it requires that I stand at the stove for nearly 30 minutes first thing in the morning. I instead use this recipe on special holidays or weekends when time restraints are nonexistent. These pancakes are so good that they don't require a single topping; they can truly stand alone! Notice that this recipe closely resembles the Plantain Muffins recipe.

½ cup (75 g) raw sunflower seeds

2 teaspoons cinnamon

1 teaspoon baking powder

½ teaspoon baking soda

¼ teaspoon salt

2 ripe plantains (see *A Note about Plantains*, page 93), peeled and sliced in 2-inch (5 cm) pieces

2 eggs

¼ cup (60 ml) water

⅓ cup (65 g) coconut oil, for cooking, divided

Grind the sunflower seeds into a flour in a high-powered blender or food processor. Do not overblend or the seeds will start to turn into a seed butter. If using a high-powered blender, 5–8 seconds of blending should be adequate, but it will take closer to 30 seconds in a food processor. The flour will have the texture of almond flour. Scrape down the sides and corners after blending to free any lodged flour.

Add the remaining ingredients, except the coconut oil, to the blender or food processor in the order listed and blend just long enough to form a smooth batter.

Heat a large frying pan over medium-low heat and add approximately 2 tablespoons of the coconut oil to the pan. Using a ¼-cup (80 ml) measuring cup, pour batter into the pan to form pancakes. You can usually cook four pancakes at a time, but this depends on the size of your pan.

Cook each pancake for approximately 3 minutes or until the edges begin to brown, flip, and cook for an additional 2–3 minutes.

Continue cooking pancakes, being sure to add 1–2 tablespoons of coconut oil before each consecutive batch to prevent sticking.

Serve pancakes with fresh fruit or simply by themselves.

Batch Cooking and Leftovers: Freeze pancakes on a waxed paper–lined baking sheet, then transfer after frozen to Ziploc bags.

The batter is nearly identical to Plantain Muffins, so do a double batch of batter and make muffins with the other half (see the note on muffin batch prepping on page 93).

Make It a Meal: Serve topped with chopped fruit and a side of scrambled eggs or Vegetable Egg Scramble with Avocado and Salsa.

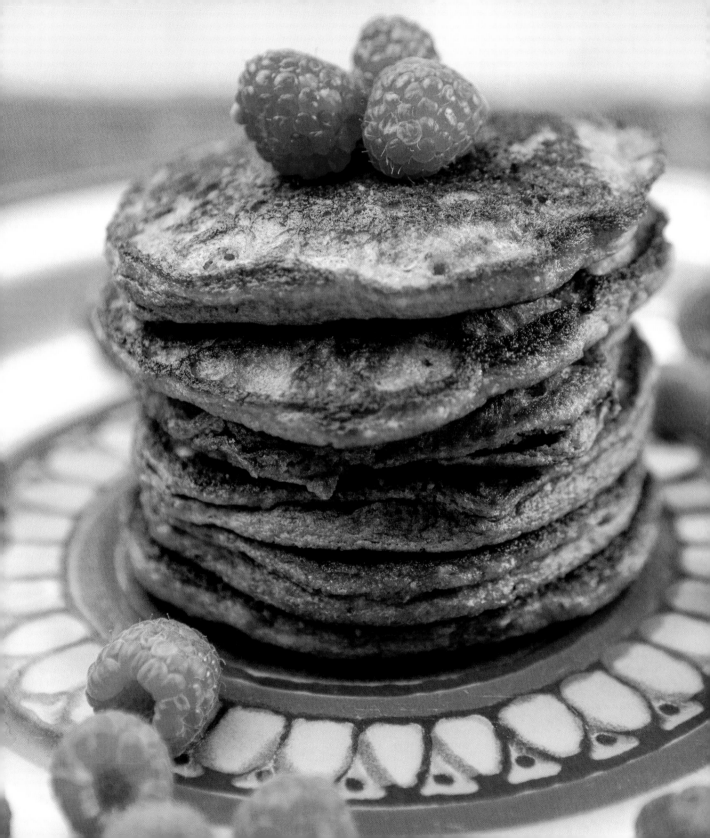

banana nut bread

active minutes   total time   loaves   days   month

This grain-free version of banana nut bread is so delicious (and nutritious) that you'll quickly move on from the sugar-laden version you've grown accustomed to. It's perfectly sweet and has just the right amount of crunch from the walnuts. I often buy bags of overripe bananas when they go on sale and then store them in the freezer for future use as banana bread. Buying walnuts and almond flour in bulk helps make this recipe far more economical. Shown on page 69.

6 overripe bananas
1½ cups (145 g) almond flour
4 eggs
½ cup (120 ml) water
½ cup (100 g) coconut oil,
   more for greasing
1 tablespoon vanilla extract
2 teaspoons baking powder
1 teaspoon baking soda
1 tablespoon cinnamon
1 teaspoon nutmeg
½ teaspoon salt
1 cup (115 g) chopped walnuts

Preheat the oven to 350°F (177°C).

Blend all the ingredients except the chopped walnuts in a high-powered blender or food processor until a smooth batter forms.

Mix the chopped nuts into the batter and divide the batter between two greased bread pans.

Bake the bread for 55 minutes.

Allow the bread to cool for about 5 minutes before turning the pans over onto a cooling rack, releasing the bread from the pans where it will remain till completely cool.

Batch Cooking and Leftovers: Double the recipe and freeze a few loaves for use at a later date.

Make It a Meal: Pack into a lunch box along with Hard-Boiled Eggs and Roasted Non-Starchy Vegetables for a simple yet filling lunch.

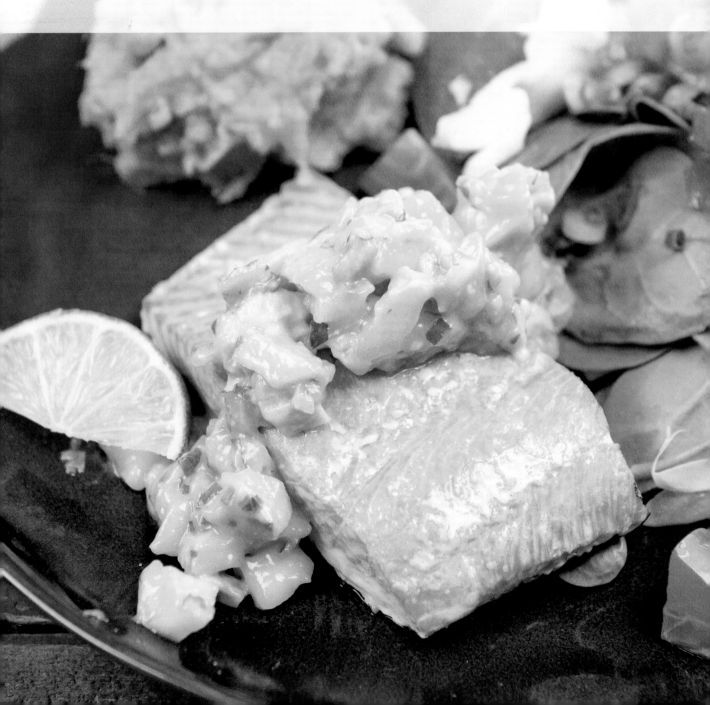

main courses

baked salmon with avocado-mango salsa

active minutes   *total time*   *servings*   *days*

People are often intimidated when it comes to preparing fish, but there's no reason to shy away from cooking this nutritious protein. My foolproof preparation provides you with an easy main course to flavor with a terrific salsa. I always serve this Baked Salmon with Avocado-Mango Salsa, but you could instead use Chimichurri Sauce, Pico de Gallo, or any other sauce of your choice. No time to make a sauce? Just add a squeeze of lemon and enjoy! Shown on page 97.

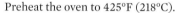

1½ pounds (680 g) wild-caught
   Alaskan salmon, cut into
    6 equal fillets
1½ tablespoons cooking oil
   (avocado or olive oil preferred)
Salt, to taste
Pepper, to taste
Avocado-Mango Salsa

Preheat the oven to 425°F (218°C).

Evenly coat each salmon fillet with oil and place the fish, skin-side down, on a baking sheet, leaving about 2 inches (5 cm) of space around each fillet. Sprinkle the fish with salt and pepper, and bake for 8–10 minutes or until the salmon appears just ever so slightly rare in the center. The salmon will continue to cook as it cools, yielding a fillet that is cooked through. Reduce your cooking time by about 2 minutes if you like your fish more rare.

Allow the salmon to rest for 2 minutes before topping it with salsa and serving immediately.

Batch Cooking and Leftovers: Try repurposing it into a salmon salad, much like The Tuna Salad Upgrade.

Make It a Meal: Add Coconut Lime Cauliflower Rice or Coconut and Cinnamon Sweet Potato Mash, include a small Everyday Salad for a well-rounded dinner.

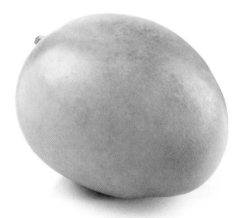

shrimp and mixed vegetable green curry

active minutes *total time* *servings* *days*

Serve this delectable shrimp curry over Simple Spaghetti Squash or Coconut Lime Cauliflower Rice and you'll have a meal with some incredible depths of flavor. Your kitchen will be smelling like Thai cuisine fit for a king, and you'll have a family that's excited about eating all of the vegetables hidden among the sweetness of creamy coconut! I use Thai Kitchen brand green curry paste. I'm sure you can find curry paste recipes to make on your own, but this paste does not contain questionable ingredients and it has a long shelf life when stored in the refrigerator after opening.

2 tablespoons coconut oil

1 onion, diced

2 carrots, diced

1 bunch of kale, chopped into bite-sized pieces (ribs intact)

1 red pepper, diced

3 cloves garlic, minced

1 can (13.5 ounces [398 ml]) unsweetened full-fat coconut milk

2 tablespoons Thai Kitchen green curry paste

1½ teaspoons lemon zest

2 tablespoons thinly sliced fresh basil leaves

¾ teaspoon salt

1 pound (455 g) shrimp, peeled and deveined

Heat a large frying pan on medium heat, add the coconut oil, and sauté the onion for about 3 minutes. Add the carrots, sauté for an additional 3 minutes, and then add the kale, red pepper, and garlic and sauté for 3 minutes more.

Reduce the heat to low, pour in the coconut milk, and add the curry paste, lemon zest, basil, and salt. Stir to dissolve the curry paste into the coconut milk.

Bring the coconut-and-vegetable mix to a low simmer, add the shrimp, and simmer for an additional 5 minutes, stirring the shrimp for even cooking.

Serve immediately.

Make It a Meal: Serve over a Simple Spaghetti Squash or Coconut Lime Cauliflower Rice.

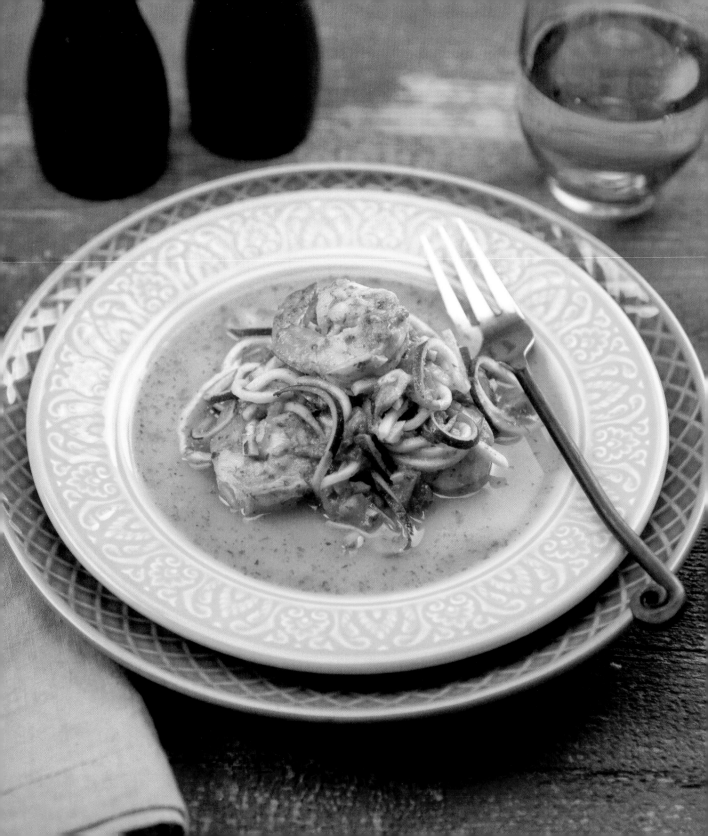

shrimp scampi with tomatoes and zoodles

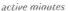 active minutes

 total time

 servings

 days

This dish was created by chance, but it is definitely one of my finer kitchen "accidents." Finding whole-food recipes that take less than 30 minutes from start to finish can feel like an impossible task, but this healthy version of shrimp scampi fits the bill. Not only is it quick, it's also packed full of deliciously bright flavors that are sure to please most any palate. Zoodles (zucchini noodles) are created using a vegetable spiralizer (countertop versions work the best) or with a julienne peeler if a spiralizer is not available.

¼ cup (60 ml) cooking oil (avocado or olive oil preferred)

5 cloves garlic, minced

½ cup (120 ml) dry white wine

1 tablespoon lemon juice

½ pound (225 g) Roma tomatoes, diced

2 tablespoons dried parsley

1 teaspoon dried oregano

Pinch of red pepper flakes

1 teaspoon salt

1 pound (455 g) shrimp, peeled and deveined

2 medium zucchinis, spiralized (see note above)

Heat the cooking oil in a large pan over medium heat and sauté the garlic in the oil for about 2 minutes or until fragrant.

Add the white wine, lemon juice, tomatoes, parsley, oregano, red pepper, and salt, and continue to cook for an additional 5 minutes or until the liquid is reduced to a thick sauce.

Add in the shrimp and cook for another 2–4 minutes or until the shrimp is solid in color and pink. Remove the scampi from the heat.

Cut the zucchini noodles in pieces 4–5 inches (10–12.5 cm) long and stir into the hot scampi. The noodles will lightly steam from the heat.

Serve immediately.

Make It a Meal: Add bulk by serving over a bed of Simple Spaghetti Squash. A side of Everyday Salad with Red Wine Lemon Vinaigrette rounds out the meal.

simple whole roasted chicken

active minutes	total time	servings	days	months
10	1h 30m	8	5	2

A classic whole chicken is always a safe bet when you're looking for an economical crowd pleaser. I find myself relying on whole chickens often since it's difficult to find a local farm that's willing to part with just the chicken breasts or thighs. This simple preparation boasts a perfectly crispy skin covered in just the right amount of herbs and salt. Cooking two whole chickens simultaneously is a great time-saver; in fact, I never cook just one. Use a pan large enough to hold both chickens in order to save space in the oven. You can remove the meat from the cooked chicken and freeze the meat in freezer bags, or you can simply freeze the entire cooked whole chicken. Both of these techniques work great for making less work down the road. If you have enough freezer space, you could even cook six to eight chickens at one time and store them all in the freezer.

1 whole chicken, approximately
   4 pounds (1.8 kg)
1½ tablespoons cooking oil
   (olive or avocado oil preferable)
1 teaspoon garlic powder
1 teaspoon dried sage
1 teaspoon dried thyme
1 teaspoon salt

Preheat the oven to 425°F (218°C).

Remove the giblets and neck from the chicken cavity, if present. Store these parts in the freezer to use for making stock at a later date.

Evenly coat the entire chicken with oil. Mix together the garlic powder, sage, thyme, and salt and evenly sprinkle the mixture over the entire chicken, sprinkling any excess into the chicken cavity.

Bake the chicken for 15 minutes and then reduce the heat to 375°F (191°C) and bake for another 45–65 minutes or until the juices run clear. Exact bake time depends on the size of the chicken. In general, it takes about 20 minutes of cooking time per pound of chicken.

Allow the chicken to cool for 10 minutes before serving.

Batch Cooking and Leftovers: Reserve the chicken carcass and freeze for later use.

Use extra chicken in Grilled Chicken Salad with Fresh Vegetables and Chicken and Vegetable Coconut Curry Soup.

Make It a Meal: Serve with Grain-Free Gravy, Apple Butternut Soup, and Garlicky Greens.

pulled mojo chicken

active minutes

total time

servings

days

months

This is one of my family's absolute favorite recipes! Pulled Mojo Chicken scores perfectly in all categories—taste, ease of preparation, versatility, and freezer storage. This brightly flavored chicken can be served in salads, on sandwiches, over Plantain Tortillas, or all of the above.

2½–3 pounds (1.1–1.4 kg) boneless chicken breasts

2–2½ pounds (910 g–1.1 kg) boneless chicken thighs, excess fat trimmed

1 tablespoon onion powder

1 tablespoon garlic powder

2 teaspoons dried oregano

1 teaspoon cumin powder

1 teaspoon salt

¼ cup (60 ml) lime juice

1 orange, juiced

Place the chicken into an electric pressure cooker or into an oven-safe baking dish if you don't own a pressure cooker. Mix together the spices, lime juice, and orange juice, and pour the mixture evenly over the chicken.

Secure the pressure cooker lid and cook on high pressure for 30 minutes. Release the pressure when done. If using an oven, cover the dish with aluminum foil and bake the chicken in a preheated oven at 375°F (190°C) for 35 minutes. Use a slotted spoon to transfer the chicken to a large bowl and allow it to rest for about 5 minutes or until it can be handled.

Using clean hands or two forks, shred the chicken. Pour a small amount of cooking liquid into the shredded chicken and toss before serving.

Serve hot.

Batch Cooking and Leftovers: Freeze at least half of this recipe after it has been prepared since it is so big. (Include liquid; it helps to preserve and enhance the flavor of the chicken after it's thawed.)

Make It a Meal: Serve with Plantain Tortillas, Garlicky Guacamole, Chimichurri Sauce, and Pico de Gallo for grain-free taco night.

grilled chicken breasts with basil and thyme

15	30m	16	6	2
active minutes	total time	servings	days	months

Herbed grilled chicken breasts are a summertime favorite for my family. Grilling outside means that we get to enjoy beautiful weather while also preparing a nutritious and simple meal that's refreshing, light, and easily served or repurposed for multiple meals. I always make an extremely large amount of grilled chicken because it can be easily added to most any meal or repurposed into Chicken Salad with Fresh Vegetables or "Pasta" Bowls. Grilled chicken along with olives and diced avocado are some of my favorite additions to a filling Everyday Salad. Preparing a few sauces in advance (or pulling them from the freezer), such as Sun-Dried Tomato Tapenade, Simple Vegan Pesto, Homemade Mayonnaise, or Fresh Basil and Garlic Balsamic Vinaigrette, makes grilled chicken a versatile addition to most any meal. Simply freeze any leftovers for a quick meal later in the month. Although this recipe calls for 5 pounds (2.3 kg) of chicken, you can prepare even more for freezing.

5 pounds (2.3 kg)
  boneless chicken breasts
  (I prefer thinly sliced)
2 tablespoons cooking oil
  (olive or avocado oil preferred)
1 tablespoon garlic powder
1 tablespoon onion powder
2 teaspoons dried thyme
2 teaspoons dried basil
2 teaspoons salt

Preheat the grill to high heat.

Evenly coat each chicken breast with oil and place on a large baking sheet in a single layer.

Lightly sprinkle the garlic and onion powders, thyme, basil, and salt on one side of the chicken breasts, flip, and repeat. Place the chicken on the grill for 8–12 minutes (8 minutes for thinly sliced breasts, 12 or more for full sized) until the edges are cooked through. Cooking time varies depending on size of the chicken breasts and temperature of the grill. Flip the chicken and cook for another 5–8 minutes (5 minutes for thinly sliced breasts, 8 or more for full sized), or until juices run clear when cut through the thickest part of the meat.

Allow the chicken to cool for 5 minutes before serving.

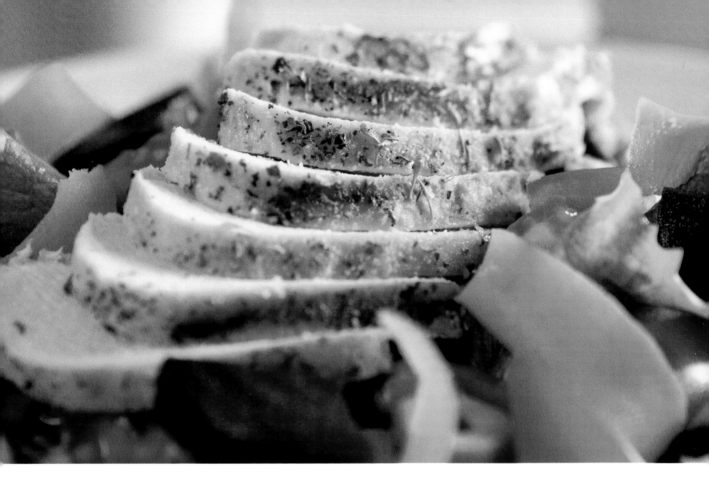

Note: Chicken breasts can be prepared in the oven or on the stovetop if you don't have a grill. For the oven, place the entire baking sheet of breasts into a preheated oven at 400°F (204°C) and bake the chicken for 15–20 minutes. If using the stovetop, place the chicken breasts into a large frying pan over medium heat (add 1–2 tablespoons of olive or avocado oil to the pan first). Flip the breasts after about 10 minutes, allowing the other side to cook for an additional 7 minutes. Exact cooking time will vary depending on the size of the breasts.

Batch Cooking and Leftovers: For freezing: Spread the individual breasts onto a waxed paper–lined baking sheet, then place the baking sheet into the freezer. Once the breasts are frozen, transfer to a freezer bag for storage.

Add Homemade Mayonnaise and some vegetables to create Grilled Chicken Salad with Fresh Vegetables, or use on top of an Everyday Salad or "Pasta" Bowl.

Make It a Meal: Serve with Grilled Zucchini and Yellow Squash, Dilly Sweet Potato Salad, and sliced cucumbers.

homemade mayonnaise

5 active minutes   **5m** total time*   **1** cup   **10** days

You can make mayonnaise by hand—my preferred method—as indicated in the recipe instructions. But be prepared for a *lot* of whisking. An immersion blender makes this process easier, but it's not necessary and takes a bit of practice to get it right. In fact, I have only been successful preparing mayonnaise by hand. Whatever method you choose, you will be shocked by the perfectly creamy, tangy, and rich consistency of the homemade mayo you make! After the mayo is prepared you can try adding different spice combinations or minced raw garlic for added flavor. You can also use lime in the place of lemon for a fun variation.

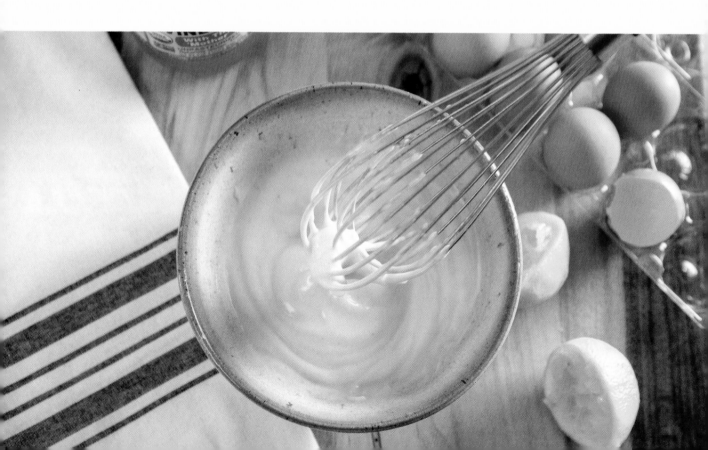

1 large egg yolk

1 tablespoon lemon juice

1 tablespoon raw apple cider vinegar

½ teaspoon Dijon mustard

½ teaspoon salt, plus more to taste

¾ cup (175 ml) avocado oil (or olive oil), divided

* If blending by hand, it will take about 15 minutes.

WHISKING BY HAND INSTRUCTIONS

Combine the egg yolk, lemon juice, vinegar, mustard, and salt in a medium bowl. Whisk until blended, slightly frothy, and bright yellow, about 30 seconds.

Whisking vigorously and constantly, slowly add ¼ cup (60 ml) of the oil to the yolk mixture a few drops at a time, to form an emulsion. This will take about 6 minutes, so be patient. Using a ⅛-teaspoon measuring spoon will help prevent adding too much oil at a time. If you hurry this step, your mayo will not form and your ingredients will be wasted.

Gradually add the remaining ½ cup (120 ml) oil in a very slow, thin stream, whisking constantly until the mayonnaise is thick, about 5 minutes (the mayonnaise will be light in color, but the exact color depends on the color of your oil).

Mayonnaise is best if chilled about an hour before use, but can be used immediately.

IMMERSION BLENDER INSTRUCTIONS

I suggest watching a YouTube instructional video before attempting this method.

Combine all ingredients in a slender glass or jar in the order listed.

Place the immersion blender on the bottom of the glass, start to blend, but do not move the blender from the bottom of the glass until the mixture begins to thicken, about 5–10 seconds.

Slowly move the immersion blender up and down in the glass until the remaining oil is combined and you reach your desired consistency, 10–15 seconds.

Mayonnaise is best if chilled about an hour before use, but can be used immediately.

Batch Cooking and Leftovers: Double the batch if you want to prepare Summer Potato Salad, The Tuna Salad Upgrade, and Simple Egg Salad all in one week, but plan to eat it all that week.

Make It a Meal: Use the mayo to prepare Summer Potato Salad to serve alongside Grilled Chicken Breasts with Basil and Thyme and Grilled Zucchini and Yellow Squash.

grilled chicken salad with fresh vegetables

active minutes

total time

servings

days

If your child isn't particularly keen on eating vegetables, this recipe just might change their mind. Rich mayo, herbs from grilled chicken, and lots of fresh vegetables make this a wonderfully nutritious (and diverse) meal for any age group. This recipe is a great way to repurpose leftover chicken into a new meal. The tastiest way to make this salad is by using leftover Grilled Chicken Breasts with Basil and Thyme, but you can use a Simple Whole Roasted Chicken, Pulled Mojo Chicken, or any other leftover chicken you have on hand. You can also substitute any of the vegetables for ones that your family enjoys. Don't have red pepper? Just add extra cucumber and carrot. No celery? Try peas. (Don't forget that fermented vegetables like Dilly Beans or others using the Basic Brine are great options, too!) This is not meant to be a complicated recipe, so just use whatever vegetables your family enjoys.

2½ pounds (4–5 cups [1.1 kg]) Grilled Chicken Breasts with Basil and Thyme, diced

1 red pepper, finely diced

1 medium carrot, grated

½ medium cucumber, finely diced

3 stalks celery, finely diced

Homemade Mayonnaise, about 1 cup (115 g)

2 tablespoons Dijon mustard

1 teaspoon onion powder

1 teaspoon garlic powder

½–1 teaspoon salt

Pepper, to taste

Mix the chicken, red pepper, carrot, cucumber, and celery in a large bowl.

In a small bowl, mix together the mayonnaise, mustard, onion powder, garlic powder, salt, and pepper and pour the mayo mixture over the chicken and vegetables. Mix until evenly coated.

Batch Cooking and Leftovers: Freeze cubed chicken to assemble the dish in the future, stored with a label stating: "Chicken Salad; add 1 grated carrot, ½ diced cucumber, etc." (see *Freezing Meals Before They're Actually Cooked* on page 61). Labeling is especially helpful when using for a vacation or weeknight meal.

Stores longer than 4 days in the refrigerator if you don't dress it immediately, so wait to dress the salad till you're ready to eat it.

Make It a Meal: Serve with Summer Cucumber and Tomato Salad and Roasted Beet and Citrus Salad for a summertime meal that can be largely prepped in advance.

turmeric-ginger baked chicken

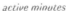

5 active minutes	35m total time	12–16 servings	6 days	2 months

I simply cannot imagine another dish that's so simple to prepare, yet packs so much depth of amazing flavors. There's virtually zero prep work involved, and the chicken cooks itself while you use that valuable time to prep for future meals. If you're like me, you'll quickly add this recipe to your repertoire of "emergency" meals. Start the meal by throwing a Simple Spaghetti Squash into the oven, next prepare the chicken, and finally throw in a tray of Roasted Non-Starchy Vegetables (I'd use broccoli). You'll have a piping-hot meal in about an hour that took minimal effort on your part. Use the baking time to hang with the kids after the school day or prepare a meal for later in the week. Chicken breasts can be used in the place of chicken thighs, but I prefer dark meat for this dish. Garnish the finished dish with fresh cilantro for an even more flavorful meal.

4–5 pounds (1.8–2.3 kg) boneless chicken thighs
1 teaspoon turmeric powder
1 teaspoon ginger powder
1½ teaspoons salt
1 can (13.5 ounces [398 ml]) unsweetened full-fat coconut milk

Preheat the oven to 350°F (177°C).

Arrange the chicken in a single layer in the bottom of a 10 × 15-inch (25 × 38 cm) baking dish. Evenly sprinkle turmeric, ginger powder, and salt on top of the chicken and pour coconut milk over the top.

Bake the chicken for 30 minutes. Allow it to cool for about 5 minutes before serving.

Batch Cooking and Leftovers: I often immediately freeze half since the dish yields such a large quantity of food. Freeze the chicken along with some of the sauce in a Ziploc freezer bag.

The recipe doubles well. Just divide the end yield into four evenly sized portions—one for eating and three for freezing.

Make It a Meal: Serve over spaghetti squash for a largely hands-off meal, or serve over Coconut Lime Cauliflower Rice using the coconut milk as a sauce. Steam or roast some broccoli—follow the recipe in Roasted Non-Starchy Vegetables for a quick and complete meal.

OMGrain-free chicken tenders

active minutes   total time   servings   days   months

My children (and husband) love these chicken tenders because they're a fun and delicious finger food. But I love them because they're so flippin' easy to make! The delicate undertones of coconut take this classic kid-friendly dish to the next level when it comes to taste and simplicity, and the shredded coconut makes the perfect grain-free breading. When shopping for ingredients, look for chicken tenders that are ready to be breaded. You can also use large chicken breasts (not thinly sliced) and cut the breasts into strips that are about 1½ (3.8 cm) inches thick. If you're looking for a perfectly golden chicken tender, you can transfer the pan to the top rack in the oven and broil the chicken for the last 2 minutes of the cooking time. Be sure to keep an eye on it so the chicken tenders don't burn. I only broil the tenders when I have someone to impress, which is almost never, but it's nice to have the option. Lightly frying the chicken tenders in a few tablespoons of avocado oil or lard on the stovetop is another great option, especially if you'd prefer not to use the oven on a hot day. The result is a healthy version of a classic comfort food. No one will even notice that you didn't use real breading.

3 eggs

1½ cups (170 g) unsweetened
   shredded coconut

1½ teaspoons salt

2 pounds (910 g)
   chicken tenders

Preheat the oven to 425°F (218°C).

   Beat the eggs together in a bowl. Set aside.

   Mix the unsweetened shredded coconut with salt in a wide, shallow bowl. You'll be covering the chicken tenders in this mixture, so it might be easier to use a plate if you don't have a bowl with a wide base.

   Dip each chicken tender and cover completely in egg, then immediately transfer into the coconut, turning the chicken until it's completely and evenly coated. Transfer the chicken onto a parchment paper–lined baking sheet.

   Bake the chicken tenders for 10 minutes, flip, and cook for another 7–10 minutes or until cooked through.

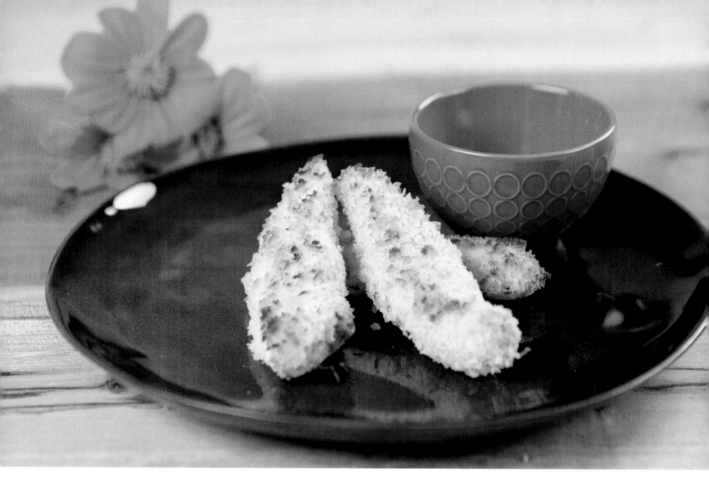

Batch Cooking and Leftovers: If you want a super-easy weeknight meal component, take an hour to prepare and cook as many chicken tenders in the oven as you can (you'll be limited by pan size and oven space). Cool, then transfer the pans to the freezer, and store the frozen tenders in a Ziploc freezer bag.

Reheat just like frozen store-bought chicken tenders: Bake at 425°F (218°C) for 10–12 minutes or until hot.

Make It a Meal: Serve with Crispy Sweet Potato Fries and a Summer Cucumber and Tomato Salad for a kid-friendly meal to share with your smallest of dinner guests.

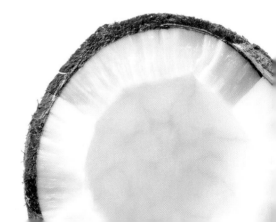

herb-encrusted drumsticks

active minutes   total time   drumsticks   days   months

Drumsticks are one of the most economical cuts of chicken, especially when you're buying organic. This recipe is packed full of flavor, is inexpensive, and has the added benefit of supplying you with bones to use for Chicken Stock. Use some caution when feeding this dish to kids: This is a particularly flavorful chicken, one that a picky eater may find overwhelming. (For a less adventurous eater, the drumsticks can simply be coated in oil and salt, and then baked as directed.) Removing the meat from the bone before serving can also encourage a picky kid to enjoy what might otherwise feel unfamiliar.

¼ cup cooking oil (avocado or olive oil preferred)

3 tablespoons garlic powder

3 tablespoons dried parsley

2 tablespoons onion powder

2 tablespoons dried thyme

1½ tablespoons dried sage

1 teaspoon smoked paprika powder

¼ teaspoon cayenne

1 teaspoon salt

12 chicken drumsticks (about 3 pounds [1.4 kg])

Preheat the oven to 400°F (204°C).

Pour the oil into a small bowl and set it aside. Mix the garlic powder, parsley, onion powder, thyme, sage, paprika, cayenne, and salt together in a small bowl and set it aside.

Evenly coat a piece of chicken with oil and then dredge the chicken through the herbs and pat the herbs onto the drumstick. Place the chicken onto a baking sheet or large Pyrex baking dish. Repeat this process until all drumsticks have been covered with oil and herbs.

Bake the drumsticks for 45 minutes, turning after 25 minutes. Allow the chicken to sit for about 5 minutes before serving.

Batch Cooking and Leftovers: Whole cooked drumsticks can be frozen on a parchment paper–lined baking sheet and then stored in a Ziploc freezer bag for later use.

If there are leftovers, remove the meat from the bone and use it for Grilled Chicken Salad with Fresh Vegetables, Chicken and Vegetable Coconut Curry Soup, or Chicken Noodle Soup. Always reserve bones for stock.

Make It a Meal: Serve with Black Bean and Vegetable Soup.

flavorful turkey burgers

15 active minutes   35m total time   10 burgers   5 days   2 months

The secret to a flavorful and moist turkey burger is the addition of egg. The egg makes the meat mixture a bit harder to work with (the burgers do not lend well to grilling), but the result is an amazing burger that is never dry. Add in an array of flavorful herbs and you have the perfect turkey burger. Ground turkey is often one of the most affordable ground meats available, making this an economical, simple, and delicious alternative to beef burgers.

2 pounds (910 g) ground turkey

2 eggs

2 teaspoons garlic powder

2 teaspoons onion powder

2 teaspoons dried basil

1 teaspoon dried sage

¾ teaspoon salt

Pepper, to taste

2 tablespoons cooking fat (preferably lard or reserved fats from cooked meats, but cooking oil will also work), divided

Combine all the ingredients in a bowl except the cooking fat and use your hands to mix everything together. Form 10 even balls to be formed into patties immediately before cooking. This mixture is harder to work with than ground beef for beef burgers, so it'll take a bit more finesse to create shapely burgers.

Preheat a large frying pan on medium-low heat, add 1 tablespoon of cooking fat, shape the preformed balls into patties, and carefully fill the pan with as many burgers as will fit. Cook the burgers for about 10 minutes, flip, and cook for an additional 10 minutes.

Repeat this process until all burgers have been cooked, adding more cooking fat to the pan before adding additional burgers.

Batch Cooking and Leftovers: Cooked burgers can be frozen for a quick meal, but note they'll be slightly dried out. Another option: Double the recipe and freeze half of the prepared meat mixture to cook at a later date.

Make It a Meal: Serve with Crispy Sweet Potato Fries and an Everyday Salad with Italian Dressing.

herbed beef burgers

active minutes   total time   burgers   days   months

When you're not eating burgers on a bun, the need for some herbs becomes apparent. Try wrapping this flavorful American classic with romaine lettuce or Plantain Tortillas for a healthy and filling meal. However, my family most often enjoys these delicious patties on their own, simply dipped in mustard. If you don't own a grill, you can instead panfry the burgers over medium heat. You'll need to increase your cooking time to 2–4 minutes longer than what is indicated for the grill preparation. Be sure to reserve any fat that remains in the pan (see *Saving Excess Fat from Cooked Meats*, page 71) after cooking. The instructions yield a medium-cooked burger; adjust the cooking time to reflect your own burger preference.

3 pounds (1.4 kg) ground beef
1 tablespoon onion powder
1 tablespoon garlic powder
1 tablespoon dried oregano
2 teaspoons dried rosemary
⅛ teaspoon crushed red
   pepper flakes
1½ teaspoons salt

Preheat the grill to high heat.

Place all the ingredients into a medium-sized bowl and use your hands to knead the herbs and spices into the meat. Once they are evenly distributed throughout, form 12–14 evenly sized balls and form each ball into a hamburger patty. I like to portion out the balls before forming even one patty to be sure that I've divided the meat correctly.

Place each hamburger on the hot grill and cook for 13 minutes, flipping after 7 minutes. Exact cooking time depends on the thickness of the burgers and the temperature of your grill. Transfer the cooked burgers to a plate and serve immediately.

Batch Cooking and Leftovers: Prep burgers in advance to make life easier: Double the recipe and freeze as many raw burgers as you'd like. (Remember to put parchment paper or waxed paper between the burgers to prevent them from freezing together.)

Burgers can be cooked frozen (increase cooking time by 4–5 minutes), or thawed in the refrigerator overnight. Note: Frozen cooked burgers will be slightly dry after being reheated.

Make It a Meal: Serve with Summer Potato Salad and an Everyday Salad with Fresh Basil and Garlic Balsamic Vinaigrette.

mexican shredded beef

active minutes — 20   *total time* — 2h   *servings* — 15   *days* — 6   *months* — 2

As one who grew up mostly vegetarian I'll be the first to admit that beef roasts posed a particular challenge to me when I was learning to cook meat. Thank goodness for a pressure cooker and some spices, because I'm guaranteed to serve up some restaurant-quality beef shredded into a taco-ready masterpiece! This recipe is a foolproof preparation for moist, fall-off-the-bone, flavorful beef. You can prepare this dish in the oven by placing the beef and all other ingredients into a large baking dish, covering the dish with aluminum foil, and baking it at 275° (135°C) for 4–5 hours. But, as you can see, using an electric pressure cooker produces the same dish in a fraction of the time.

4½–5 pounds (2–2.3 kg) beef roast or stew beef
2 teaspoons garlic powder
2 teaspoons onion powder
1 teaspoon chili powder
1 teaspoon cumin powder
½ teaspoon smoked paprika
1 teaspoon salt
5 cups (1.2 l) Beef Stock or enough to cover the roast

Evenly coat both sides of the beef roast with spices and salt, and place it in the bottom of an electric pressure cooker. Pour the stock over the roast and cook the roast on high pressure for 1 hour and 15 minutes.

Release the pressure when the cooking time is complete. Remove the beef from the liquid and allow it to cool for 5–10 minutes before pulling the meat apart with two forks. The beef will easily fall apart at this point and can even be shredded by hand (my preferred method) if allowed to cool long enough. Discard any large pieces of fat.

Pour a small amount of the cooking liquid back onto the shredded beef for added moisture, and serve hot.

Note: For extremely large batches use the oven method, because you're limited by the size of your pressure cooker.

Batch Cooking and Leftovers: Reserve the cooking liquid for use in future soups and stews with similar flavor profiles such as Not Quite Your Mama's Chili. (Or freeze the liquid until you're ready to use it.)

For freezing, add the desired amount of beef to a freezer-safe container or bag, and cover the beef in cooking liquid to maintain moisture and flavor.

Make It a Meal: Serve for taco night with Plantain Tortillas, Chimichurri Sauce, Garlicky Guacamole, Fermented Salsa Fresca, and shredded romaine lettuce.

garlic and cumin slow roast with napa cabbage

active minutes
15

total time
2h 30m

servings
8

days
5

months
2

Don't be deterred by the extended cooking time for this dish—the active time is minimal. The dish is largely unattended because it's left in the oven to cook, and it has the added advantage of being a one-pan meal. It's a wonderfully flavorful dish that's perfect for a Saturday at home with the kids. Start the roast, play outside, come in to chop some vegetables, switch out the meat, and voilà, dinner is served!

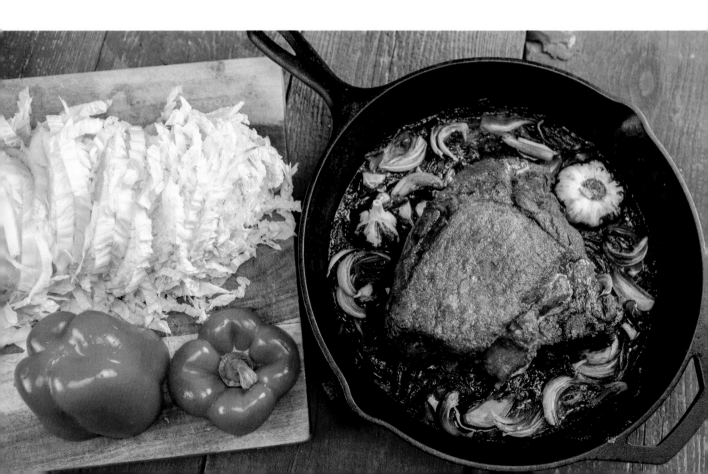

2½ pounds (1.1 kg) beef roast

½ teaspoon cumin powder

½ teaspoon onion powder

¾ teaspoon salt plus more
  if needed

1 head garlic

½ cup (120 ml) apple cider vinegar

½ cup (120 ml) water

1 onion, sliced

1 small head napa cabbage,
  shredded

1 red pepper, thinly sliced

3 tablespoons coconut aminos

Preheat the oven to 275°F (135°C).

Evenly sprinkle both sides of the roast with cumin powder, onion powder, and salt.

Heat a large cast-iron or other oven-safe pan over medium-high heat. Place the roast into the pan once it's hot, searing the roast for about 4 minutes on each side.

Place the head of garlic on its side and slice through the center, exposing the middle of the cloves. Pour the vinegar and water into the hot pan, add the onion, and place the garlic (clove-side down) into the pan. Place the roast in the oven for 2 hours and 15 minutes.

Remove the roast and the garlic from the pan, leaving behind the liquid and onion. Turn the oven up to 450°F (232°C).

Place the shredded cabbage, red pepper, and coconut aminos into the hot pan and toss. The pan will likely be very full but the cabbage will cook down. Return the pan to the oven and roast the vegetables for 10 minutes or until the cabbage reaches your desired consistency. Allow the roast to rest while the cabbage cooks.

Remove the cabbage-and-red-pepper mixture from the oven, stir, salt to taste, and serve sliced beef over the cabbag- and-red-pepper mix.

Batch Cooking and Leftovers: Cook two batches (one to eat and one to freeze), but only if you have two oven-safe pans. If preferred, place the vegetable mixture into the Ziploc freezer bag along with the beef for freezing, which will help to improve the flavor over time.

Make It a Meal: For a more filling meal, serve alongside Coconut and Cinnamon Sweet Potato Mash, or make it a roast beef and cabbage sandwich by preparing the Plantain Sandwich Bread.

cottage pie

35 active minutes

1h 45m total time*

12–15 servings

6 days

2 months

This upgraded, healthier version of the traditional Cottage Pie is a stand-alone meal that most any kid will enjoy. The warmth of mashed sweet potatoes smothering a bed of ground beef and mildly flavored, familiar vegetables makes it a great recipe to try when transitioning the family to a whole-food diet. However, Cottage Pie is not a dish to cook from start to finish in one day. I almost always prepare the sweet potatoes and stuffing and assemble the pie a day or two in advance, cover it with aluminum foil to store in the refrigerator, and bake it another night. I often put it in the oven before my family heads to the gym or soccer practice at 4:00 or 5:00 p.m. and use the Delayed Start feature on my oven so that it cooks while we're away. We come home hungry and dinner is ready to eat!

4 pounds (1.8 kg) sweet potatoes (about 7 large or 12 small)
2 pounds (910 g) ground beef
1 large onion, diced
1 bunch celery, chopped
5 medium carrots, chopped
1 bunch kale, finely chopped
6 cloves garlic, minced
1 pound (455 g) frozen peas
2 teaspoons dried basil
2 teaspoons dried thyme
2 teaspoons dried sage
2 teaspoons salt, divided

If you are baking the sweet potatoes in the oven, plan on the total cooking time to be 2 hours and 30 minutes.

Place the sweet potatoes into the electric pressure cooker on the steamer rack and add 1 cup (235 ml) water. Cook the potatoes on high pressure for 20 minutes for large potatoes or 15 minutes for small potatoes. Release the steam and remove the potatoes from the pressure cooker to cool. Alternatively, bake the sweet potatoes by placing them in an oven-safe dish covered in aluminum foil in a preheated oven at 400°F (204°C) for about an hour or till the potatoes can be easily pierced with a fork (exact cooking time depends on the size of the potatoes).

While the potatoes are cooking, heat a large frying pan over medium heat, place the ground beef into the pan, and break it apart as best you can using a metal spatula. Add in the onion, celery, and carrots and continue to sauté, breaking the ground beef apart, for about 10 minutes.

Add in the kale, garlic, peas, basil, thyme, sage, and 1½ teaspoons of the salt, and continue to sauté the beef-and-vegetable mixture for another 5 minutes. The vegetables (or meat, for that matter) don't have to be fully cooked since they'll be baked in the pie.

If you're planning to bake the Cottage Pie at this time, preheat the oven to 350°F (177°C); otherwise wait to preheat the oven till you're ready to cook the pie, but continue with the following steps.

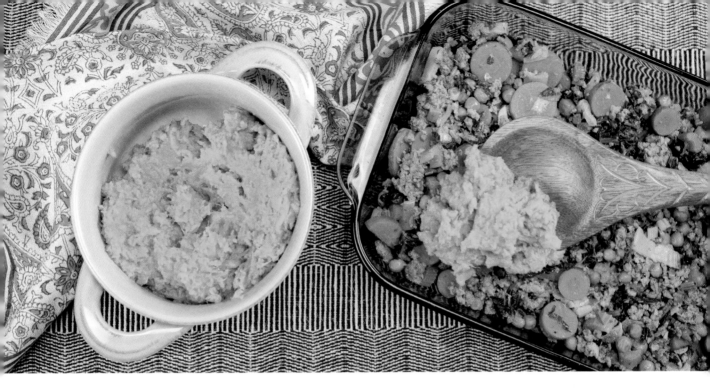

Evenly spread the vegetable-and-beef mixture into the bottom of an 11 × 15-inch (28 × 38 cm) baking dish.

Remove the skins of the sweet potatoes and return the flesh to the pressure cooker insert (dump out the cooking liquid before doing so and give it a quick rinse) or to the baking pan used to cook the sweet potatoes. Thoroughly mash the potatoes using a potato masher, stir in the remaining ½ teaspoon of salt, and evenly spoon the potatoes on top of the meat-and-vegetable mix. Smooth the potatoes flat using the back of a spoon. You can either store the pie in the refrigerator covered in aluminum foil at this point, or bake it uncovered for 1 hour.

Allow the Cottage Pie to cool for about 10 minutes before serving.

Batch Cooking and Leftovers: The entire dish can be prepared in advance and frozen whole, but I choose not to do this because I only own one pan large enough. I instead double the beef and vegetables recipe, assemble a pie to eat for the week using half, and place the other half into a Ziploc freezer bag to be frozen for use on a later date.

Make It a Meal: Serve with an Everyday Salad with Italian Dressing.

marinated grilled pork chops

active minutes

total time

servings

days

Simple marinades provide you with a flavor profile that will have people believing you spent hours in the kitchen, when the reality is that most of that time was hands-off. Take a few minutes to start this dish in the morning and you'll have a delicious protein for that evening's meal. You can start to marinate the pork chops as many as 24 hours before you plan to cook, but marinating past that point will start to change the muscle fibers in the meat, resulting in a stringy pork chop.

4 pork chops
½ cup (120 ml) Chicken Stock
   or water
¼ cup (60 ml) coconut aminos
¼ cup (60 ml) cooking oil
   (avocado or olive oil preferred)
2 cloves garlic, minced
Zest from ½ lemon
Salt, to taste

Combine the pork chops and all the ingredients except the salt in a shallow container with a lid or Ziploc bag. Be sure that the meat is submerged in the liquid, and store it in the refrigerator for 2–24 hours to marinate.

Preheat the grill to medium-high heat, salt the pork chops, and place them on the grill once it's hot. Alternatively, you can panfry the pork chops in 2 tablespoons of cooking oil over medium heat. Cook each side for 4–6 minutes or until the center is no longer pink. Exact cooking time depends on the thickness of the chops.

Allow the pork chops to rest for about 4 minutes, then serve immediately.

Batch Cooking and Leftovers: Best served immediately. If you want to eat pork chops for more than one meal in a week, double the marinade recipe and store it in the refrigerator until you're ready to marinate the meat (start marinating up to 24 hours in advance). You could even reuse the same marinade as long as an adequate amount remains.

Make It a Meal: Serve with Grain-Free Tabbouleh and Coconut and Cinnamon Sweet Potato Mash.

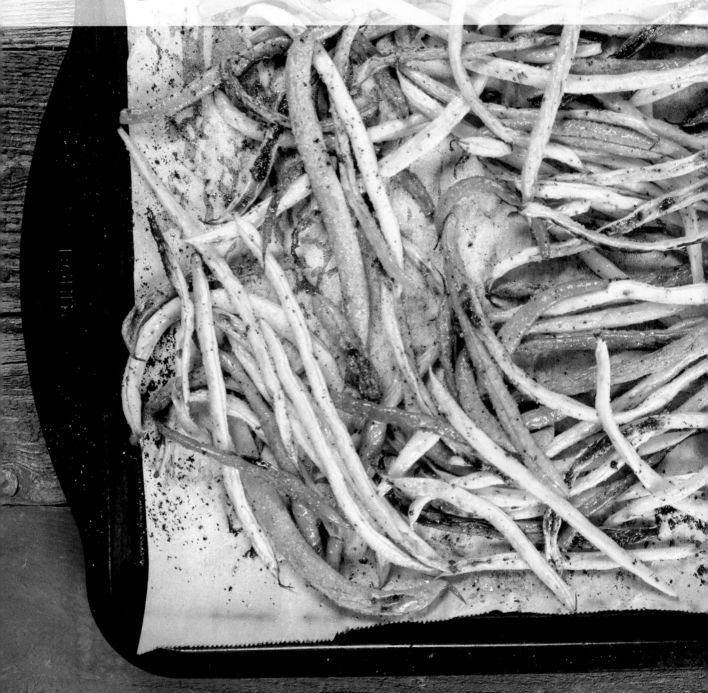

vegetable sides and salads

summer cucumber and tomato salad

active minutes · total time · servings · days

Mid-July marks the season to start preparing this summery salad on a regular basis. Fresh cucumbers and tomatoes from your home garden or local farmers market put any store-bought vegetable to shame. Using fresh ingredients is key in preparing simple yet delicious and satisfying salads. The crunch of watery cucumbers, the satisfaction of heirloom tomatoes, and the sweetness of fresh basil and balsamic are the perfect combination to serve on a hot, humid day. The speed at which this recipe can be prepared will have you coming back for more time and again!

1 pound (455 g) small cucumbers (about 5)

1 pound (455 g) mixed heirloom tomatoes (about 2 large or 8 small)

1 clove garlic, minced

¼ cup (60 ml) Fresh Basil and Garlic Balsamic Vinaigrette

Salt, to taste

Dice the cucumbers and tomatoes into bite-sized pieces and toss together with garlic, dressing, and salt (if desired).

Serve immediately.

Batch Prepping and Leftovers: Chop vegetables as early as 4 days in advance, but reserve dressing for when you plan to serve the salad. Only dress the portion of salad that will be eaten immediately. The salt in the dressing causes the tomatoes and cucumbers to lose their juices and the salad will become extremely watery over time.

Make It a Meal: Serve with grilled or boiled corn on the cob (see *But Isn't Corn a Grain?*, page 158) and Grilled Chicken Salad with Fresh Vegetables for a seasonal, light meal on a hot summer day.

grilled zucchini and yellow squash

10 active minutes   20m total time*   8 servings   5 days

This simple yet satisfying dish is one that I love especially during the summer when I have an abundance of zucchini in the garden. Marinating these gems with some coconut aminos and simple spices yields a quick, simple dish that most kids will love. Better yet, get the kids involved and let them practice their knife and measuring work! Be sure to buy organic versions of these vegetables, since conventionally grown zucchinis can be genetically modified (GM).

1 pound (455 g) zucchinis
   (about 3 medium zucchinis)
1 pound (455 g) yellow squash
   (about 4 small squash)
3 tablespoons coconut aminos
2 tablespoons cooking oil
2 teaspoons garlic powder
2 teaspoons onion powder
Salt, to taste

more for marinating (optional)

Preheat the grill to high heat. If no grill is available, prepare the recipe as follows, but bake the zucchinis and squash in a preheated oven at 425°F (218°C) for 15 minutes.

Cut the zucchinis and squash into lengthwise quarters or halves (depending on size) and place them in a bag or large mixing bowl (do this directly on the pan you plan to place in the oven if using the baking method).

Mix together the coconut aminos, cooking oil, garlic powder, and onion powder in a small bowl and pour the marinade over the top of the zucchinis and squash. Toss until all vegetables are evenly coated. You can allow this to marinate in the refrigerator for up to 6 hours or place the vegetables on the grill (or into the oven) immediately.

If quartered, cook zucchini and squash for 3 minutes on each of their 3 sides (9 minutes total). If halved, cook each side for 5 minutes (10 minutes total). Remove the vegetables from the grill and salt to taste.

Serve immediately.

Batch Cooking and Leftovers: Reduce your cooking load later in the week by chopping and adding leftovers to a Summer Cucumber and Tomato Salad or an Everyday Salad. The vegetables can be chopped and the marinade can be mixed as much as 5 days in advance. (Store the two components separately until you're ready to start marinating.)

Make It a Meal: Serve with Grilled Chicken Breasts with Basil and Thyme, Grain-Free Tabbouleh, and a pitcher of Hibiscus Zinger Iced Tea for a colorful and delicious meal.

everyday salad

active minutes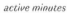

total time

servings

week

Making a large salad every week should become a habit, especially in the summer. This assures you have a quick, nutritious side to complete your meal plan for the week. You can use whatever ingredients you like, but don't skimp and don't make it boring! Salads taste best when created with varying greens, uniquely flavored vegetables, healthy fats, and delicious proteins. A correctly built salad has lively visual appeal, can easily stand alone as a filling meal, and doesn't leave you feeling hungry an hour later. Start by making a "base" salad of greens and vegetables, one large enough to last for an entire week (large enough to serve 20 people!). Add in varying proteins, fats, and dressings at different meals to mix and match, which prevents boredom from repetitive combinations.

**GREENS
(CHOOSE 1 OR MORE)**

Arugula

Baby bok choy

Baby kale

Baby leaf lettuce

Dandelion leaves (use
  sparingly)

Green leaf lettuce

Micro greens

Mixed greens

Napa cabbage

Romaine

Spinach

Watercress

**VEGETABLES (BETTER
WITH MORE VARIETY)**

Artichoke hearts, sliced

Banana peppers

Beets (cooked), peeled and
  sliced or diced

Beets (raw), grated or very
  thinly sliced

Bell peppers, slice or diced

Broccoli (cooked or raw),
  diced

Carrots, grated or very
  thinly sliced

Cucumbers, sliced

Fermented vegetables

Onion (red, yellow, white, or
  green), thinly sliced

Purple cabbage, shredded

Radishes, grated or
  thinly sliced

Sauerkraut

Sprouts

Tomatoes, diced

**FRESH HERBS
(CHOOSE 1 OR MORE)**

Basil

Chives

Dill

Fennel leaves

Onion tops

Parsley

Sage

Thyme

**PROTEINS
(CHOOSE 1–3)**

Bacon pieces

Beans

Bean sprouts

Chicken, tuna, or egg salad

Eggs (hard-boiled, fried,
  or scrambled)

Fiesta Sunflower Seed
  Hummus

Grilled meats

Hummus

Leftover meats

Nuts

Sardines

Seeds

**HEALTHY FATS
(CHOOSE 1 OR MORE)**

Avocados or Garlicky
  Guacamole

Nuts

Olives

Olive or avocado oil

Seeds

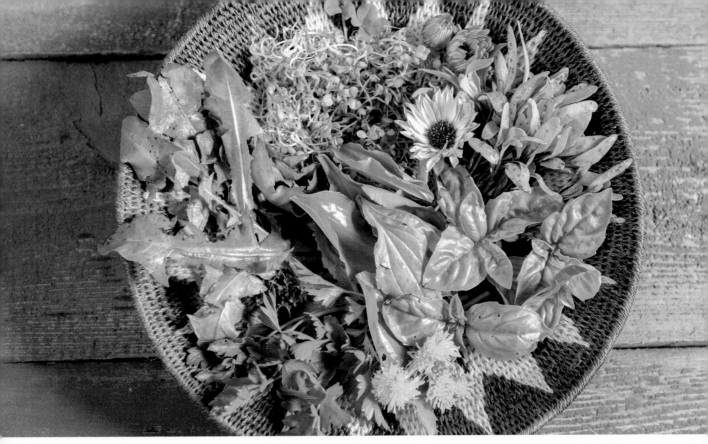

Salads can contain any number of ingredients including dandelion or wild plantain leaves, micro greens, edible flowers, or fresh herbs.

DRESSINGS

Chimichurri Sauce

Fresh Basil and Garlic
  Balsamic Vinaigrette

Italian Dressing

Pico de Gallo

Raw apple cider vinegar and
  olive oil

Red Wine Lemon
  Vinaigrette

Sun-Dried Tomato
  Tapenade

Tahini-Miso Sauce

Batch Cooking and Leftovers: A large salad will last for about 6–7 days in the refrigerator. Do *not* dress the entire salad! The dressing should be stored separately, and you should only dress the portion of salad that is placed on your plate at each meal.

I prepare the entire salad in one sitting, placing the washed and chopped greens in the bottom of a large stainless steel bowl with the other chopped vegetables layered on top. I then place a large dinner plate on top of the bowl and store the salad in the center rack of the refrigerator (my vegetables will start to freeze if I store it on the top shelf). A large food storage container can be used instead, but I don't own one large enough to accommodate such a large salad. I have found that Saran Wrap is unnecessary; the salad stays fresh enough by simply using a plate as a lid.

Make It a Meal: Serve repeatedly as a side dish for varying meals, but it can easily stand alone when topped with The Tuna Salad Upgrade, Fresh Basil and Garlic Balsamic Vinaigrette, sliced olives, roasted sunflower seeds, and diced avocado.

roasted non-starchy vegetables

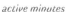

active minutes   total time   servings   days

Roasting is one of the easiest and tastiest vegetable preparations. This is a general recipe—you can plug in most any vegetable or combination of vegetables to create a quick and easy side that most kids will enjoy. Some of my family favorites include roasted multicolored green beans from the garden, red peppers with zucchini chunks, and broccoli with carrots. Try whatever's seasonal or on sale! Shown on page 121.

2 pounds (910 g) non-starchy vegetables

3–4 tablespoons cooking oil (avocado or olive oil) or melted cooking fat (bacon grease is preferable)

1 teaspoon garlic powder

1 teaspoon onion powder

Salt, to taste

Preheat the oven to 450°F (232°C).

Cut vegetables as desired. For example, cut broccoli into bite-sized florets, carrots into ½-inch (1.3 cm) slices, peppers into long strips, or leave vegetables like green beans and asparagus whole.

Pile the vegetables onto a parchment paper–lined 12 × 16-inch (30 × 40 cm) baking sheet. Evenly pour oil or cooking fat over the top, and toss the vegetables until evenly coated. Spread the vegetables into a single layer and evenly sprinkle garlic and onion powder on top. Bake for 20–25 minutes, stirring halfway through. Exact cooking time varies depending on the vegetable and how that vegetable was cut.

Remove the pan from the oven and evenly sprinkle your desired amount of salt on top of the vegetables. Toss and serve immediately.

Batch Cooking and Leftovers: Prep in advance by cutting the vegetables and storing them in the refrigerator for up to 5 days. If you don't like leftover roasted vegetables, bake only the amount of vegetables you plan to eat for that meal and reserve the rest for a second meal another night.

Make It a Meal: Serve with Roasted Beet and Citrus Salad and Marinated Grilled Pork Chops.

garlicky greens

15 active minutes   20m total time   10 servings   1 week   2 months

Garlicky Greens is a flavorful way to enjoy most any green. You can substitute an onion for the leek, and you can use any greens in the place of collards. Collards take longer to cook than most other greens, so you'll have to reduce your cooking time if using kale, chard, bok choy, or another green. For a more enhanced flavor, try topping the greens with your favorite sauce or dressing (see *Sauces, Dips, and Dressings*, page 193). Excess cooked greens can be easily frozen for future meals.

2 tablespoons cooking fat

4 small bunches of collards, chopped, ribs intact

1 leek, cleaned and chopped

⅓ cup (80 ml) Chicken Stock or water

4 cloves garlic, minced

1 teaspoon salt, or to taste

Melt the cooking fat in a large skillet or frying pan on medium heat. Add in the collards, leek, and stock, and sauté the mixture for about 15 minutes, stirring frequently.

Add in the garlic and sauté for another 5 minutes or until the greens reach your desired texture. Remove the greens from the heat, mix in the salt, and serve.

Batch Cooking and Leftovers: I often double this recipe since it's so easy to store in the freezer, but you'll be limited by the size of your pot. Greens will not expand in the freezer, so I store leftovers in freezer-safe glass jars.

Make It a Meal: Use as a base for fried eggs, diced fresh tomatoes, Fermented Salsa Fresca, and diced avocados for an easy breakfast dish that takes very little time to prepare and is packed full of nutrition!

grain-free tabbouleh

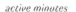

active minutes   total time   servings   days

Parsley, lemon, and garlic are the stars of the show when it comes to tabbouleh. Although the traditional recipe is made with bulgur wheat, you honestly don't need any grains when cauliflower acts as the perfect accompaniment. This flavorful, densely nutritious, low-carb, and brightly colored dish is the perfect side for most any protein. I use an English cucumber for this dish, which is a large cucumber, 12–14 inches (30–35 cm) in length. English cucumbers are my preferred store-bought cucumber since they are usually wrapped tightly in plastic and the peel has not been coated in a waxy substance like most other store-bought cucumbers. You can sub in three medium cucumbers if you have access to local, fresh ingredients. Also notice that the dish uses half of a head of cauliflower. Plan to prepare Cauliflower Hash Browns or Coconut Lime Cauliflower Rice in the same week to use up any leftovers. You can buy bagged, riced cauliflower at most grocery stores or make it yourself by roughly chopping a head of cauliflower and running it through the grater on your food processor. Rice all of your cauliflower for the week in one sitting and store excess in the refrigerator until it's ready to be used.

3–3½ cups (320–375 g) riced cauliflower, about ½ head

1 bunch parsley, chopped

1 large tomato, diced

1 English cucumber, diced (see note above)

⅓ cup (42 g) minced red onion, about ½ small onion

2 cloves garlic, minced

¼ cup (60 ml) olive oil

1 lemon, juiced

1½ teaspoons salt

Rice the raw cauliflower using the grater on a food processor, or you can buy bags of riced cauliflower at many grocery stores.

Combine all the ingredients in a large bowl and mix.

Serve immediately.

Batch Cooking and Leftovers: This dish holds up better than you would guess, but it quickly deteriorates after day 4. You can rice your cauliflower and chop the vegetables up to 4 days in advance, storing these in the refrigerator in airtight containers or bags. Simply wait to dress the tabbouleh until you're ready to eat it.

Make It a Meal: Serve with Herbed Beef Burgers and Coconut and Cinnamon Sweet Potato Mash.

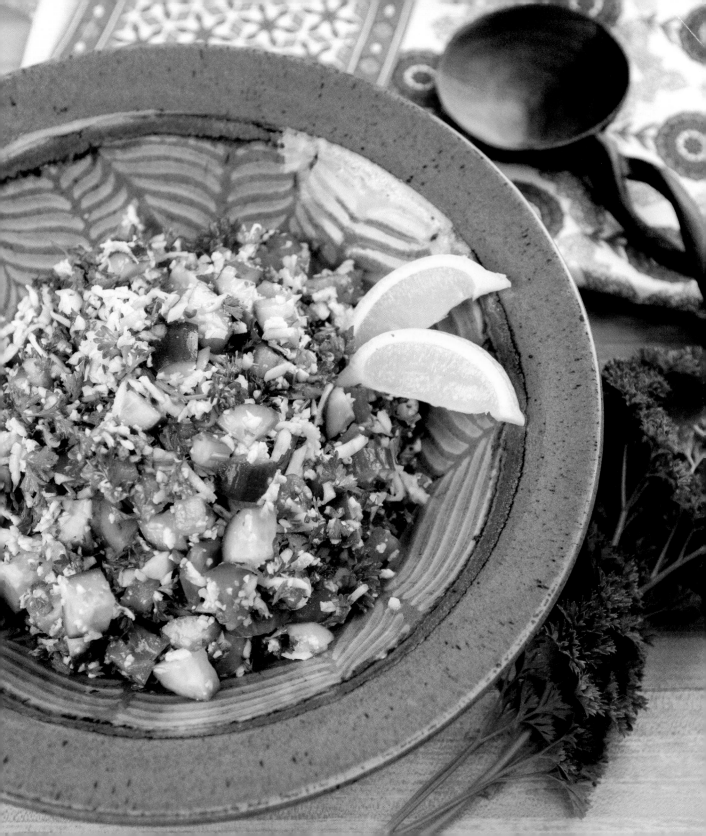

roasted brussels sprouts with bacon

15 *active minutes*

55m *total time*

8 *servings*

6 *days*

Your holiday guests will love the combination of toasty bacon, fragrant onions, and perfectly caramelized brussels sprouts—it doesn't get any better than that! This is a great dish for introducing brussels sprouts to the kids. If you happen to forget to pull the bacon from the freezer, don't worry: You can chop frozen bacon, though it will require a sharp knife and a bit of muscle.

2 pounds (910 g) brussels sprouts, trimmed and halved (about 7 cups)
1 large onion, thinly sliced
2 cloves garlic, minced
12 ounces (340 g) bacon

Preheat the oven to 425°F (218°C).

Place the brussels sprouts, onion, and garlic in a heaping pile on a 12 × 16-inch (30 × 40 cm) parchment paper–lined baking sheet.

Slice the bacon into 1 × 1-inch (2.5 × 2.5 cm) pieces by leaving the bacon in its original stack (straight from the package) and slicing every inch. Break the bacon apart as best you can until single pieces are formed. You don't have to spend too much time on this step since the bacon will break apart more as it's cooked and stirred.

Place the bacon pieces onto the brussels, onions, and garlic, and mix everything together. Spread the mixture into a single layer and bake for 40 minutes, stirring every 10 minutes. (This is especially important since it helps to coat the brussels sprouts and onions in bacon grease for even cooking.)

Serve immediately.

Batch Cooking and Leftovers: Prep all ingredients in advance and store together in a Ziploc bag in the refrigerator until you're ready to prepare the dish.

Make It a Meal: Serve as a delicious side to accompany a Simple Whole Roasted Chicken, Grain-Free Gravy, and Red and Yellow Rosemary Potatoes.

coconut lime cauliflower rice

active minutes   total time   servings   days

Missing white rice will be a thing of the past once you try this replacement that has far fewer carbs and much better flavor. The richness of coconut is perfectly complemented with tangy lime and cilantro. Cauliflower rice can easily become a main dish by simply adding leftover cooked chicken, beef, shrimp, or any other protein of your choice. For more information on how to rice cauliflower, see Grain-Free Tabbouleh, page 128.

2 tablespoons coconut oil
1 medium onion, diced
1 red pepper, diced
1 medium head cauliflower, riced
1 can (5.4 ounces [160 ml]) unsweetened coconut cream
Juice from 1 lime
½ bunch cilantro, minced
2 teaspoons salt, more to taste

Preheat a large frying pan over medium heat. Add the coconut oil and sauté the onion for about 5 minutes, stirring frequently. Add the red pepper and sauté for another 3 minutes.

Pour in the cauliflower and stir frequently for about 2–3 minutes, just until the cauliflower starts to change color. You don't want the cauliflower to become mushy or you'll lose the rice texture.

Pour in the can of coconut cream and mix the rice until the cream appears to be absorbed, about 2 minutes.

Remove the pan from the heat and stir in the lime, cilantro, and salt. Serve immediately.

Batch Cooking and Leftovers: You can rice the cauliflower and chop the vegetables up to 4 days in advance and store in the refrigerator. Simply wait to cook the rice until you're ready to eat it.

Make It a Meal: Serve topped with Shrimp and Mixed Vegetable Green Curry.

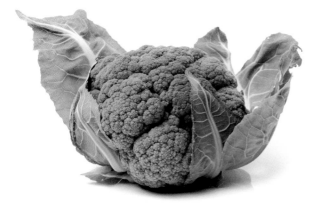

roasted cabbage wedges with tahini-miso sauce

active minutes

total time

servings

Roasted cabbage wedges are a striking dish that can act as an excellent conduit for your favorite dressing or sauce. I just so happen to love cabbage wedges with a thick and creamy Tahini-Miso Sauce, but the flavor possibilities are endless (see *Sauces, Dips, and Dressings*, page 193, for some options)! I use green cabbage, but red cabbage makes an excellent substitute, especially if you're trying to add vibrant color to a meal. Red cabbage has a sweeter, stronger flavor with a slightly tougher leaf, but the two can be used interchangeably here. You could even use both for a decorative effect.

1 head cabbage (about 3 pounds [1.4 kg])
2 tablespoons cooking oil (avocado or olive oil preferred)
¼ teaspoon coriander powder
Tahini-Miso Sauce

Preheat the oven to 425°F (218°C).

Cut the cabbage into 10 wedges by placing it on a cutting board with the core facing up. Slice straight through the cabbage on one side of the core to remove approximately one half of the cabbage. This half can be cut into four wedges. Continue removing wedges from the cabbage by cutting around the core and being careful to keep the cabbage wedges intact. See Dill Pickle Kraut (page 242) for a visual demonstration.

Place the wedges on a parchment paper–lined baking sheet and brush them with cooking oil. Turn the wedges over and repeat. Evenly sprinkle coriander over the wedges and bake for 25 minutes or until the edges are browned.

Serve cabbage wedges topped with Tahini-Miso Sauce or any dressing of your choice.

Batch Cooking and Leftovers: Cabbage wedges don't store particularly well. These become limp and lifeless in the refrigerator, and no one in my family is excited to eat them as leftovers. Better to cook only the desired amount, and then refrigerate the rest for a quick side dish later in the week.

Make It a Meal: Serve with Flavorful Turkey Burgers and Crispy Sweet Potato Fries.

bok choy and red peppers with thai peanut sauce

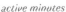

active minutes   *total time*   *servings*   *days*

I'm always looking for ways to use new and diverse greens such as bok choy—a wonderfully mild and crisp green that's most familiar as an ingredient in Asian-flavored vegetable preparations. Use the entire leaf, including the thick stem, for a mix of flavor, texture, and color. I love how the sweetness from the red peppers, carrots, and onions is accented by the creamy goodness of a delicious peanut sauce. Try serving these flavorful vegetables along with OMGrain-Free Chicken Tenders for a delightfully sweet and fragrant small meal.

2 tablespoons coconut oil

1 medium onion, halved and
   thinly sliced

2 medium carrots, thinly sliced
   in rounds

1 bunch bok choy, chopped

2 red peppers, thinly sliced in
   long strips

4 cloves garlic

1 teaspoon salt

Thai Peanut Sauce

Heat the coconut oil in a large pan over high heat. Add in the onion and carrots, and sauté the mixture for about 5 minutes. Add in the bok choy, red peppers, garlic, and salt, and continue to sauté for another 7 minutes.

Prepare the Thai Peanut Sauce while the vegetables cook.

You can either pour the sauce over the top of the vegetables and toss the mixture until the vegetables are evenly coated, or serve the sauce on the side.

Serve immediately.

Batch Cooking and Leftovers: Prepare in advance by chopping and bagging the vegetables and then storing them in the refrigerator until you're ready to cook. The Thai Peanut Sauce recipe can be doubled and frozen for use at a later date.

Make It a Meal: Serve over a bed of Simple Spaghetti Squash with leftover Simple Whole Roasted Chicken.

massaged kale salad with lentils

active minutes   *total time*   *servings*   *days*

I just love a good, hearty kale salad! This dish is sure to leave your taste buds feeling satisfied from all of the flavorful, crunchy, and creamy ingredients. Meanwhile, your belly will be in a state of nutritional bliss! Try preparing this salad in advance as a quick yet substantial lunch for busy workdays.

Kale is one of the simplest greens to grow, and like most cruciferous vegetables it offers a variety of unique health benefits. Crucifers boast high concentrations of calcium and have a cancer-fighting quality that is only reaped when the vegetable is eaten raw and chewed well. Enzymes that exist within the cell walls are released during mastication, which initiates a reaction that yields a cancer-fighting compound. Blending crucifers into smoothies is one way to achieve this benefit, as is massaging it to disrupt the cell walls.

SALAD

1 cup (210 g) dried French lentils
3 cups (710 ml) water or stock
1 bunch kale, stems removed and torn into bite-sized pieces
½ small red onion, finely diced
1 can (14 ounces [400 g]) hearts of palm (or artichoke hearts), thinly sliced
1 avocado, diced
1 pint grape tomatoes, diced
½ bunch parsley, minced
4 hard-boiled eggs, sliced

Combine the lentils and water in a small pot, bring the water to a boil, cover the pot, and simmer for 40 minutes or until the lentils are cooked.

Prepare the dressing and salad while the lentils cook. Combine all dressing ingredients in a small jar with a tight lid, shake vigorously, and set aside.

Place the kale into a large mixing bowl, pour half of the dressing over the kale, and massage with your hands for approximately 2 minutes or until the kale becomes soft and wilted.

Once the lentils have finished cooking, drain and rinse them with cool water until they reach room temperature.

Combine the kale, lentils, red onion, hearts of palm, avocado, tomatoes, parsley, and eggs in a large bowl, pour the remaining dressing on top, and toss. Serve immediately.

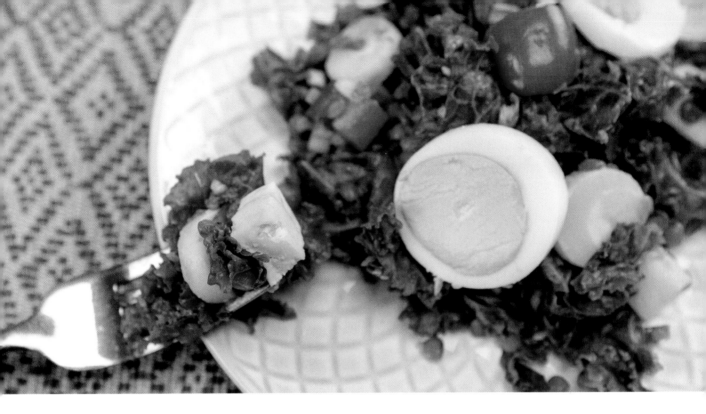

DRESSING

3 tablespoons red wine vinegar

2½ tablespoons olive oil

1 clove garlic, minced

1 tablespoon lemon juice

2 teaspoons Dijon mustard

¼ teaspoon cumin powder

⅛ teaspoon dried oregano

½ teaspoon sea salt

Pepper, to taste

Batch Cooking and Leftovers: Prepare the kale, chopped vegetables, lentils, eggs, and salad dressing separately up to 4 days in advance for extremely quick meal assembly on a busy weeknight. You could prepare a double batch of lentils and freeze the excess to prepare this salad again in the future, but be sure to label your freezer bag.

If you want to serve this salad over the course of 3–4 days as a lunch, leave out the egg and avocado and add when serving.

Make It a Meal: Serve with Coconut and Cinnamon Sweet Potato Mash and a warm cup of Winter Immunity Tea for a hearty wintertime salad meal.

coconut and cinnamon sweet potato mash

active minutes — 10

total time* — 40m

servings — 4–5

days — 6

months — 2

Who wants the diabetic coma that follows the consumption of marshmallow-covered sweet potato casserole so often found at the Thanksgiving buffet when you can just add coconut oil and cinnamon to achieve a sweet yet nutritious and guilt-less side? This fragrant and flavorful dish is good enough to serve for special occasions, yet it's simple enough for any old weeknight. I have even been known to use mashed sweet potatoes as a breakfast food to serve with Probiotic Pork and Vegetables. Although this may seem like a large amount of sweet potatoes, the final product is less than you would expect because you lose quite a bit of mass when you peel the cooked potatoes. I therefore almost always double (or even triple) this recipe, especially since it can be easily paired with so many other dishes.

3 pounds (1.4 kg) sweet potatoes, about 5 large or 9 small

1 cup water (for pressure cooker method)

¼ cup (50 g) coconut oil

¼ teaspoon cinnamon powder

¼ teaspoon salt

* If you are baking the sweet potatoes in the oven, plan on the total cooking time to be 1 hour and 10 minutes.

If using an electric pressure cooker, place the sweet potatoes on the rack, add water, and cook on high pressure for 20 minutes. Release the steam when done.

If using an oven, preheat the oven to 400°F (204°C). Place the sweet potatoes in a baking dish covered with tinfoil and bake for 50–60 minutes or until soft.

Carefully peel the sweet potatoes, discard the peels, and place the remaining flesh in a large bowl or pot (you can also use the baking dish or pressure cooker insert to cut down on dirty dishes).

Add the remaining ingredients and mash the sweet potatoes using a potato masher until they are creamy.

Serve immediately.

Batch Cooking and Leftovers: Leftovers work well alongside Grilled Chicken Breasts with Basil and Thyme. Use this recipe as a base for Garlicky Greens and your protein of choice, or even make it as a side dish for breakfasts like Probiotic Pork and Vegetables.

Make It a Meal: Serve as a simple breakfast with two fried eggs and a couple of pieces of Perfectly Baked Bacon.

red and yellow rosemary potatoes

| 10 active minutes | 1h total time | 8 servings | 6 days | 2 months |

Roasted potatoes are an easy and inexpensive side to pair with most any protein. I prefer the creaminess of yellow potatoes, but I most often mix in some red potatoes to make this an especially colorful dish. Choose whichever variety you'd prefer, but try to find organic potatoes if your budget allows since potatoes are listed as one of the Dirty Dozen (see *Is Organic Really Better?*, page 51, for more information). The recipe calls for dried rosemary, but you could instead use a couple of sprigs of fresh rosemary from the garden. Add the fresh rosemary halfway through the bake time to prevent burning. Be sure to toss it well with the potatoes and oil.

4 pounds (1.8 kg) red and
yellow potatoes, about 15 small
potatoes (any combination
of the two)
1 large onion, thinly sliced
4 cloves garlic, minced
1 tablespoon dried rosemary
4 tablespoons cooking oil
(avocado or olive oil)
Salt, to taste

Preheat the oven to 425°F (218°C).

Dice the potatoes into 1-inch (2.5 cm) cubes and heap them into a pile on a parchment paper–lined baking sheet along with the onion, garlic, and rosemary. Pour the oil evenly over the top of the potatoes and use your hands to mix until all ingredients are evenly coated. Spread the potato mix into a single layer.

Place the potatoes in the oven and bake for 45–55 minutes, stirring halfway through (add your fresh rosemary at this time, if applicable). Evenly sprinkle the potatoes with salt and toss to combine.

Serve immediately.

Batch Cooking and Leftovers: Best eaten fresh, but for leftovers reheat on the stovetop or in the oven for optimal flavor and texture. With that said, my kids don't seem to mind these reheated in the microwave.

The potatoes and onion can be chopped, bagged, and refrigerated up to 5 days in advance.

You can freeze this dish as indicated in *Batch Cooking and Leftovers* for the Roasted Roots, page 139. The only difference is that you'll reheat the rosemary potatoes at 425°F (218°C) rather than 450°F (232°C).

Make It a Meal: Serve alongside the Eat Your Greens Frittata for a made-ahead, hearty breakfast option.

roasted roots

10	1h	8	6	2
active minutes	total time	servings	days	months

When a chill is in the air it's time to pack the oven with some gorgeous fall-flavored vegetables that, fortunately, are readily available at your local farmers market. What better way to celebrate a colorful leaf display than with a local, colorful dish to match? Roasting root vegetables brings out their natural sweetness in a way that doesn't even require the addition of spices. Some great root vegetable choices include sweet potatoes, parsnips, carrots, beets, turnips, onions, and even leeks. Pick just one or two of the vegetables, or create a medley using whichever are in season.

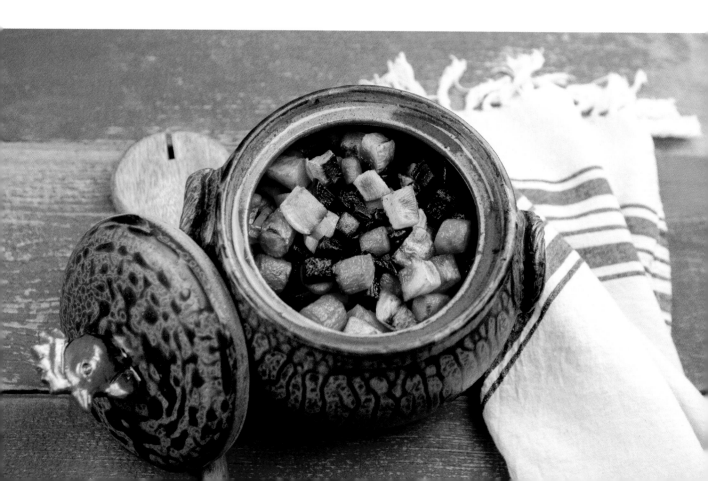

4 pounds (1.8 kg) mixed
 root vegetables
3 tablespoons cooking oil
 (avocado or olive oil preferred)
⅛ teaspoon salt, more to taste

Preheat the oven to 450°F (232°C).

Dice the vegetables to match cooking times. For example, beets take slightly longer to cook than carrots, so I cut the carrots into larger pieces than the beets.

Pile the diced roots onto a parchment paper–lined baking sheet, drizzle the oil over the top, and toss until all vegetables are evenly coated. Spread them into a single layer and bake for 45–55 minutes, stirring halfway through. Exact cooking time depends on the vegetables and size of your pieces.

Sprinkle salt over the top of the vegetables and lightly toss.

Serve immediately.

Batch Cooking and Leftovers: The vegetables can be chopped, bagged, and refrigerated up to 5 days in advance to make preparation easier when you're ready to cook the dish.

If time allows, reheat in the oven or a toaster oven to yield a better texture, but the stovetop or microwave will also work.

If prepping for later use, remove the portion you want to freeze 10 minutes before it has finished cooking. Freeze your desired portion on a parchment paper–lined baking sheet and then transfer the vegetables to a freezer bag for long-term storage.

Make It a Meal: Pair with frozen OMGrain-Free Chicken Tenders for an instant freezer meal, or serve with Creamy Cauliflower Soup topped with bacon bits made from Perfectly Baked Bacon. (Best to use leftover bacon, as the oven temperature for the bacon and vegetables is very different.)

crispy sweet potato fries

active minutes · *total time* · *servings*

You may have to prepare these fries a few times before you find your ideal cooking temperature, but this recipe is *so* worth it! My kids *love* sweet potato fries, and this quick and nutritious side takes minimal attention once the fries are cooking. I often chop enough fries for the week in one sitting, and then simply cook them when needed. When I'm finished using the lard, I leave it in the pan to use again and again until it's gone. You can make this recipe using unrefined coconut oil, but you have to reduce the heat since unrefined coconut oil has a lower smoke point than lard. (Refined coconut oil has a higher smoke point than unrefined, but you'll want to buy a brand like Nutiva that uses a steam-processing method for refining.) The fries will take closer to 30 minutes to cook when using unrefined coconut oil and they're not quite as crunchy, but they're still delicious. You can also sub in parsnips or carrots if you want to try using a different vegetable.

2 pounds (910 g) sweet potatoes, about 3 large or 5 small
1 cup (220 g) Homemade Lard or Tallow
Salt, to taste

Cut one slice, approximately ¼ inch (6 mm) thick, from the long side of the sweet potato, creating a flat side. Place the sweet potatoes flat-side down onto the cutting board to prevent them from rolling and continue cutting the potato into ¼-inch-thick slices. Next, cut each slice into ¼-inch-thick fries.

Preheat the lard to medium heat in a large frying pan. Once melted, the lard should be approximately ¼ inch (6 mm) deep. More or less is okay; it doesn't have to be exact, since you'll be stirring the fries. It's best to start preheating the lard when you're about halfway done cutting the fries.

Drop the fries into the hot lard and stir frequently, about every 3 minutes, until the fries are beginning to brown and appear crispy, about 25 minutes total. You can most likely fit all of the fries into the pan at once (not all of the fries will be submerged in the lard at one time, thus the need for frequent stirring), but you may have to work in batches depending on the size of your pan.

Remove the fries from the pan using a slotted spoon and place them on a paper towel– or napkin-lined plate. Sprinkle salt evenly over the fries and cool for 2 minutes before enjoying.

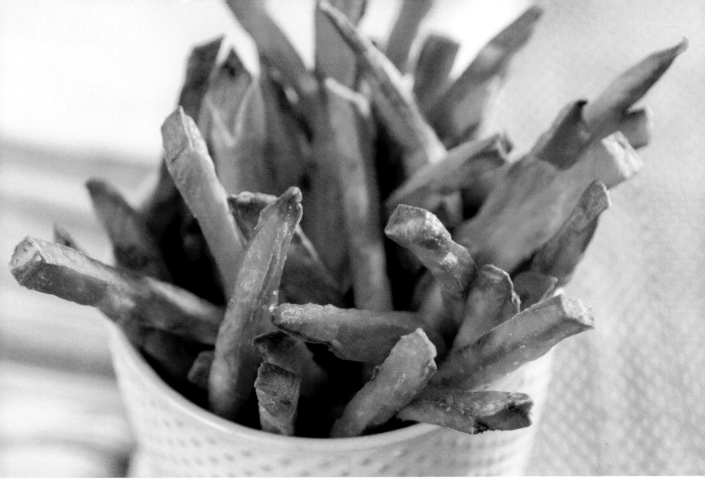

Batch Cooking and Leftovers: Best served fresh, but my kids will usually eat them as non-crunchy leftovers anyway.

I prep all of the fries in advance, storing them in a Ziploc bag in the refrigerator until they're ready to be cooked. The size of your pan will likely mean you will only be able to prepare four servings at a time. To make a larger batch, coat the fries in oil and bake at 400°F (204°C) for about 40 minutes (stirring halfway). The fries will be delicious, but they won't be crispy.

There is leftover lard in the pan after stovetop cooking, so I plan to serve this side at least two, sometimes three times in one week and reuse the lard until it's gone.

Make It a Meal: Serve with OMGrain-Free Chicken Tenders and broccoli prepared using the recipe found in Roasted Non-Starchy Vegetables for a classic kid-friendly meal.

homemade lard or tallow

active minutes   total time   pounds   months   months

Saturated fats are stable when heated (this prevents food oxidation) and are therefore a good choice as a healthy, nutrient-dense cooking fat. Tallow is made from beef, while lard is made from pork. Talk with your local farmers or butcher shops to find a good source of healthy fat to render into lard or tallow. Pastured animals that have access to fresh grass every day are always your best option. Cows should be eating nothing more than grass, and pigs and chickens should be fed organic or non-GMO feed. If you don't have a slow cooker you can instead render fat on the stovetop, heating a pan on low and letting the fat melt off the pieces. However, you'll need to tend to the fat in order to prevent burning. Rendering on the stovetop is a much more labor- and time-intensive process than using a slow cooker.

2–8 pounds (0.9–3.6 kg) beef or pork fat

Cut the fat into 2-inch (5 cm) cubes. This doesn't have to be done perfectly, but uniform sizes are best. (Note: It's easiest to work with cold fat.)

Place all the cubed fat into a pressure cooker with a slow-cook function, or into a Crock-Pot. Cook the fat on low temperature for 24 hours. The fat will render from the animal tissues and create a liquid in the pot.

Carefully (the fat is *hot!*) strain the liquid fat through a metal fine-mesh colander into glass jars for storage. The liquid will appear almost yellow in color, but will cool to a solid white. Lard that appears darker in color after cooling has been slightly overcooked—but don't worry, it's still good to use.

If additional fat remains on the original 2-inch (5 cm) pieces, return those pieces to the Crock-Pot or pressure cooker and continue to cook until you've rendered most of the usable fat. Don't cook it longer than 2 days, however,

as the fat will start to overcook and it will become brown in color, indicating oxidation.

As the liquid cools you may notice a very small amount of water in the bottom of a jar. If this happens, you will need to store your rendered fat in the refrigerator as this liquid can go bad sitting on the countertop. This usually only happens with the last jar to be poured, since fat floats on top of water and the fat is therefore the first liquid to be poured from the vessel, making the last jar the recipient of the water. Store all other jars either in the freezer for long-term storage or on the countertop for up to 2 months.

Batch Cooking and Leftovers: I make extremely large batches (1½–7 pounds [0.7–3.2 kg]) of lard or tallow in order to save time in the long run. Rendered fat stores indefinitely in the freezer, so there's no reason to have to repeat this process more often than once a year, especially if you're supplementing with reserved fats from cooked meats.

dilly sweet potato salad

active minutes — total time — servings — days

Nothing says "potluck" quite like a huge bowl of this Dilly Sweet Potato Salad. The sweetness of the potatoes is accentuated by zesty vinaigrette, and the addition of dill gives it visual and culinary appeal. The unique flavors of this dish may be challenging for a young child transitioning to a whole-food diet. Consider setting a small portion of the sweet potatoes aside to remain undressed until you feel that your child will be more agreeable to such strong flavors.

SALAD

3 pounds (1.4 kg) sweet potatoes, diced into ¾-inch (1.9 cm) cubes

2 tablespoons cooking oil (avocado or olive oil)

¼ cup (13 g) lightly packed minced dill

DRESSING

¼ cup (60 ml) olive oil

2 tablespoons red wine vinegar

1 clove garlic, finely minced

1 lemon, juiced

1 teaspoon Dijon mustard

½ teaspoon salt

Preheat the oven to 425°F (218°C).

Pile the potatoes onto a 12 × 16-inch (30 × 40 cm) parchment paper–lined baking sheet, and pour the cooking oil over the top. Toss until the sweet potatoes are evenly coated with oil and spread them into a single layer. Bake the potatoes for 45 minutes, stirring after 25 minutes.

Prepare the dressing while the sweet potatoes cook. Combine all dressing ingredients in a small jar with a lid, secure the lid, and shake until well combined. Set aside.

Place the cooked sweet potatoes into a bowl, pour your desired quantity of dressing over the top (start with half and adjust to taste), and add the dill. Stir the salad until well combined and evenly coated.

Dilly Sweet Potato Salad can be served at room temperature or chilled.

Batch Cooking and Leftovers: The dressing recipe yields ½ cup (120 ml). I typically use about ⅓ cup (80 ml) for the sweet potato salad and reserve the rest for use on Roasted Non-Starchy Vegetables or an Everyday Salad. It can be stored on the countertop for up to 3 weeks or 2 months in the refrigerator.

Tasks that can be performed in advance to complete this dish include chopping, bagging, and refrigerating the sweet potatoes until you're ready to cook the meal, mincing the dill (storing it in the refrigerator in an airtight container), and preparing the dressing.

Make It a Meal: Serve with a chilled Summer Cucumber and Tomato Salad and Herb-Encrusted Drumsticks.

summer potato salad

20	45m	12	4	
active minutes	*total time*	*servings*	*days*	

Potato salad offers you a unique opportunity to increase your vegetable intake in an inconspicuous manner. Adding a multitude of vegetables increases the salad's bulk and contributes subtle textures and colors to a creamy, savory dish. Traditional potato salad is often considered to be unhealthy, but I would argue that it's actually quite the opposite when quality ingredients are used. The ingredients for this salad are available starting in mid-summer from local farms and gardens, and preparing your own mayo ensures the use of quality fats. Potato salad is a family favorite that is frequently consumed (in large quantities) throughout the summer and into the early fall when fresh vegetables abound and easy sides are in high demand. Having a prepared dish that's ready to serve just waiting in the refrigerator makes a busy summer day feel easier. I most often prepare this dish using yellow potatoes, but red or russet potatoes work as well. Most potato salad recipes use celery, but I prefer cucumbers since I always have such an overabundance in the summer. Feel free to sub in celery if you'd like.

3½–4 pounds (1.6–1.8 kg)
  potatoes
Water, for cooking
  (see instructions)
1 red pepper, finely diced
1 medium cucumber, finely diced
1 bunch green onions, chopped
½ cup (36 g) minced dill
6 Hard-Boiled Eggs, diced
1½ cups (340 g) Homemade
  Mayonnaise (prepare a double
  batch and you'll have leftovers)
1 tablespoon raw apple
  cider vinegar
1½ teaspoons salt

Place clean potatoes on the rack in the pressure cooker along with 1 cup (235 ml) of water. Cook the potatoes on high heat for 15 minutes and release the steam when done. Remove the lid and allow the potatoes to cool. If a pressure cooker is not available, place the potatoes in a large pot completely covered with water, bring the water to a boil, and allow the potatoes to cook for about 30 minutes or until easily pierced with a fork. Strain off the water and allow the potatoes to cool.

Once the potatoes are cool enough to handle, dice them into bite-sized pieces and combine the potatoes with all of the other ingredients in a large mixing bowl. Gently mix the potato salad until the ingredients are evenly dispersed and coated with mayo.

Serve potato salad immediately or transfer to the refrigerator to completely cool before serving.

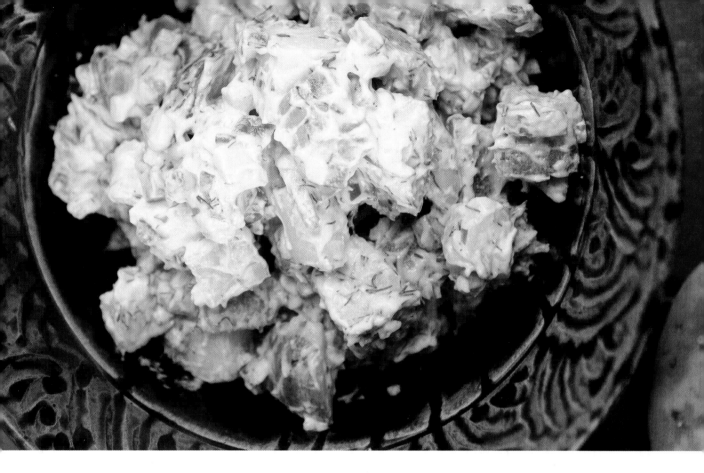

Batch Cooking and Leftovers: The recipe yields quite a bit of food, so I don't recommend doubling it unless you plan to serve it to guests.

I try to cook the potatoes in advance since they can often take quite a bit of time to cool. Prep your potatoes, chop your vegetables, and prepare the mayo the night before you plan to serve the dish.

Undressed potato salad can be stored in the refrigerator for up to 6 days, which makes it a good choice for pre-prepping and taking on vacation. Simply add your mayo, mustard, vinegar, and salt immediately before you plan to serve. Once the salad is dressed, you can store it in the refrigerator for up to 4 days.

Make It a Meal: Serve with Grilled Chicken Breasts with Basil and Thyme, Summer Cucumber and Tomato Salad, and Grilled Zucchini and Yellow Squash on a hot summer day.

kobocha casserole with pecans

| 20 active minutes | 2h 10m total time | 12 servings | 1 week | 1 month |

Kobocha squash is one of the superstars of the winter squashes, yet it's a variety that people often ignore. With a sweet, dry flesh, kobochas can be easily incorporated into casseroles without the need for added sugar. This dish is so sweet, in fact, that you may even be able to trick your kids into believing that they're actually eating dessert! Unlike a butternut, the flesh of a kobocha is extremely dry, which produces a firm texture that complements the light crunch of the chopped pecans. Flavors from cinnamon with coconut undertones make this a truly wonderful dish. Make sure to cook the squash a day or two in advance of serving, otherwise this dish is far too time consuming for an average weekday.

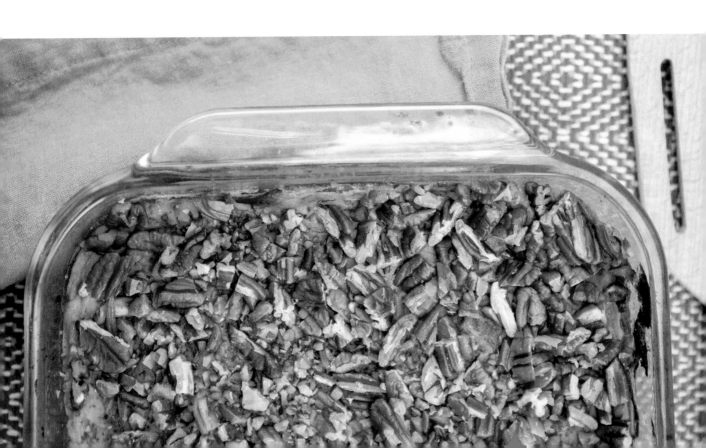

1 kobocha squash, about
  4½–5 pounds (2–2.3 kg)
4 eggs
2 cans (5.4 ounces [160 ml]
  each) unsweetened
  coconut cream
2 teaspoons cinnamon powder
1 teaspoon salt
2 tablespoons coconut oil,
  for greasing
1½ cups (180 g) pecans, chopped

Preheat the oven to 400°F (204°C).

Cut the kobocha squash into two even halves, remove the seeds, and place them facedown on a parchment paper–lined baking sheet. Bake the squash for 40–50 minutes or until it's easily pierced with a fork. Reduce the heat on the oven to 350°F (177°C). (Note: Kobochas do not hold together if cooked in the pressure cooker. I use this method for spaghetti and butternut squash, but I'm left with a crumbly mess that's nearly impossible to work with when using it for kobocha.)

Using a large spoon, remove the flesh of the squash from the peel and place it in the blender or food processor with eggs, coconut cream, cinnamon, and salt. You may have to work in batches for this. First blend half of the squash with half of the other ingredients and then repeat with the remaining squash.

Pour the squash mixture into a greased 10 × 15-inch (30 × 40 cm) baking dish. Sprinkle the pecans evenly on top of the squash and bake the casserole for 1 hour at 350°F (177°C).

Serve hot.

Batch Cooking and Leftovers: If you want an immediate, ready-to-serve meal, plan to bake the squash on Day 1, prepare and bake the casserole on Day 2, and serve it on Day 3.

If this casserole is too large for your family, simply halve the recipe and freeze the other half of the cooked squash to use for a second casserole later in the month.

Alternatively, prepare two casseroles in separate dishes and freeze one by covering it in Saran Wrap and then aluminum foil.

Make It a Meal: Serve with local link sausages made from pasture-raised pork and an Everyday Salad with Italian Dressing.

roasted beet and citrus salad

active minutes	*total time*	*servings*	*week*	
15	1h	10	1	

This salad is a refreshingly delicious twist on my favorite earthy vegetable. If you're new to the wonderful world of beets, start here with this tangy, sweet, and vibrantly colored salad, and you won't be disappointed! Beets contain unique pigments, betalains, that are particularly effective at supporting the liver in detoxification. Some of these pigments are destroyed during cooking, which is why I often reserve a small beet for grating raw into the prepared salad.

DRESSING

¼ cup (60 ml) cooking oil
   (avocado or olive oil)
¼ cup (60 ml) balsamic vinegar
1 tablespoon mandarin
   orange juice
1 tablespoon lemon juice
1 teaspoon lemon zest
½ teaspoon mandarin
   orange zest
1 teaspoon salt

SALAD

3 pounds (1.4 kg) beets,
   diced into 1-inch (2.5 cm) cubes
1 pound (455 g) mandarin
   oranges, peeled and diced into
   ½-inch (1.3 cm) cubes

Preheat the oven to 400°F (204°C).

Prepare the dressing by combining all ingredients in a small jar with a leakproof lid. Shake to combine and set aside.

Pile the diced beets onto a 12 × 16-inch (30 × 40 cm) parchment paper–lined baking sheet. Shake the dressing again before evenly pouring half of it over the beets. Reserve the other half of the dressing for after the beets have cooked. Toss the beets with the salad dressing, spread them into a single layer on the baking sheet, and bake for 45 minutes, stirring halfway through.

Remove the beets from the oven and allow them to cool for about 5 minutes before pouring them into a large bowl with the mandarin oranges. Pour the remaining dressing on top and mix everything together.

This salad can be served warm or chilled.

Batch Prepping and Leftovers: Simply serve any leftovers on top of a bed of baby spinach with a piece of grilled chicken for a quick and delicious lunch on the go. The beets can be chopped, bagged, and refrigerated up to 5 days in advance. You can also prepare the oranges and dressing in advance, but these are easiest to prepare while you wait for the beets to cook.

Make It a Meal: Serve with an Everyday Salad topped with Fresh Basil and Garlic Balsamic Vinaigrette and Turmeric-Ginger Baked Chicken.

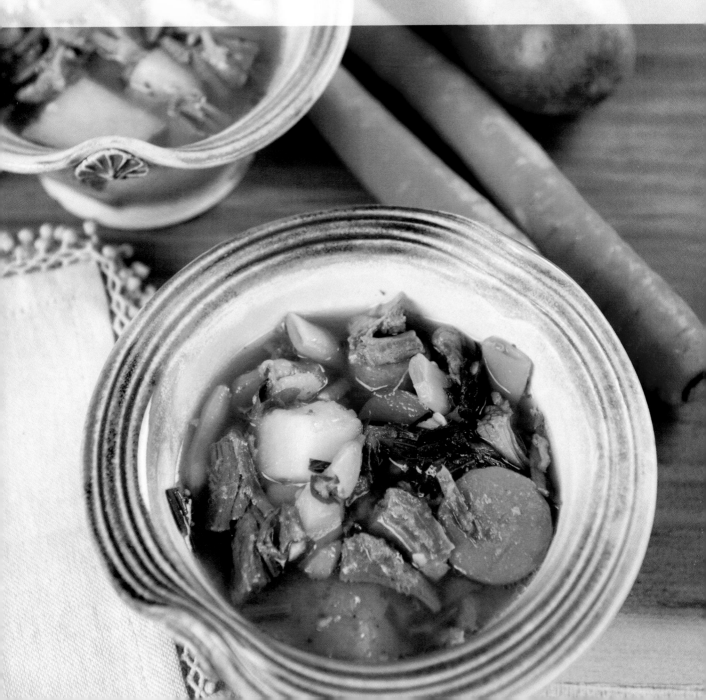

soups and stews

creamy cauliflower soup

active minutes   *total time*   *servings*   *days*   *months*

This is a thick, creamy, and savory soup that's *so* simple to prepare. Try topping each bowl of soup with a hefty serving of homemade bacon bits made from Perfectly Baked Bacon. You can use 1 pound (455 g) of frozen cauliflower in the place of one fresh head, which is often a more economical choice. I often prepare this soup as a double batch since it can easily accompany many of the main courses featured in this book including Grilled Chicken Breasts with Basil and Thyme, Simple Whole Roasted Chicken, Mexican Shredded Beef, and Garlic and Cumin Slow Roast with Napa Cabbage. Added bonus: This soup is a great way to get your kids to consume bone broth during the winter months when you're trying to boost and maintain their immunity. Stovetop preparation is possible if you don't have a pressure cooker. Simply sauté the onions and garlic as indicated, add the cauliflower and stock, bring the soup to a boil, and simmer for about 30 minutes or until the cauliflower is soft and falls apart easily. Proceed with the remainder of the preparation as directed.

1 tablespoon cooking fat (lard or reserved fat from cooking meats preferred)

1 large yellow onion, sliced

4 cloves garlic

1 large head cauliflower, roughly chopped

3–4 cups (710–945 ml) Chicken Stock (exact quantity depends on the size of your cauliflower and desired soup consistency)

1 can (5.4 ounces [160 ml]) unsweetened coconut cream

2 teaspoons salt

Pepper, to taste

Using the sauté function in an electric pressure cooker (see the note above for stovetop instructions), melt the cooking fat and sauté the onion for about 5 minutes, add the garlic, and sauté until the onion is caramelized and brown, about 7 minutes total.

Add in the cauliflower and 3 cups (710 ml) stock, and cook on high pressure for 10 minutes.

Release the steam when done, add the coconut cream, salt, and pepper, and blend the soup with an immersion blender or in batches using a blender or food processor. Adjust the soup thickness using the remaining stock.

Serve immediately.

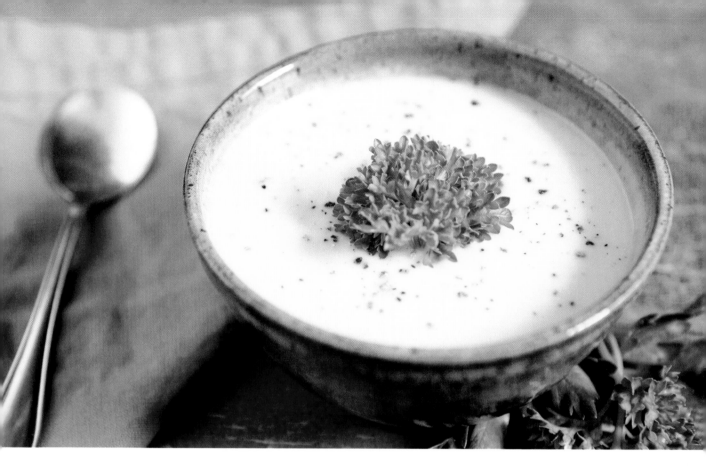

Batch Cooking and Leftovers: Use as a base for varying protein leftovers such as Pulled Mojo Chicken, Herb-Encrusted Drumsticks, Garlicky Greens, Roasted Roots, or Red and Yellow Rosemary Potatoes. Or chop leftover meat and vegetables into bite-sized pieces, and add them to the soup. See *Prepping for Soups and Stews* (page 152) for more information.

I often double this recipe since it can serve as a versatile side for busy weeknight meals or be frozen for a later date in Ziploc freezer bags.

Make It a Meal: Top with bacon bits made from Perfectly Baked Bacon, and serve with Roasted Roots and an Everyday Salad with Fresh Basil and Garlic Balsamic Vinaigrette.

Prepping for Soups and Stews

Soups and stews are some of my favorite wintertime meals. They're simple to prepare, highly nutritious, and yield large quantities of food that can be easily frozen for use on a later date. Put simply, they're the quintessential meal for the techniques I discuss throughout the book. However, these simple meals can become extremely time intensive when trying to prepare the meal from start to finish in one cooking session since there are often multiple steps involved. Chicken Stock and Beef Stock should always be prepped in advance. I keep stock on hand throughout the winter since I know that it will always be used in one way or another. You can prep the stock as far in advance as two weeks, or as late as the morning before you plan to make a soup or stew (for a pressure cooker method only; the stovetop takes 24 hours). Stocks can even be frozen in Ziploc freezer bags, but this requires a good bit of freezer space.

Preparing the other components for soups and stews in advance will also make for lighter work on the nights you plan to cook. For example, Chicken and Vegetable Coconut Curry Soup requires that you cook a whole chicken, a task that requires very little active time. Cook the chicken the night before while you eat dinner, or cook it or during one of your prep days, and you'll have one of the main soup components ready to go. Vegetables for soups and stews can also be chopped in advance. If you find that you have an extra 10 minutes while waiting for dinner to finish cooking, start chopping and bagging the vegetables to be used in the soup the following night.

Some of the soup recipes require the use of dried beans, which is another component that should be prepped in advance. Soaking beans, preparing stock, and then cooking the soaked beans in the stock is a multistep process that is actually largely hands-off and quite simple, *unless* you're trying to do it all in one day. Please note that stocks should *not* be salted before cooking dried beans. I'm not sure why, but salted liquid prevents the beans from cooking. Soups will quickly become your go-to wintertime meal once you implement a bit of organization and forethought in the kitchen.

Storing and Using Fresh Ginger

You'll need to keep ginger on hand if you plan to make Creamy Carrot Ginger Soup often (which you should). Store fresh ginger in the freezer. You can store the entire rhizome (the lateral root produced by a ginger plant) in the freezer or cut it into one- or two-inch pieces so that you have meal-sized portions readily available. The easiest way to peel ginger is by using the side of a spoon. Be sure to view a demonstration video online if you're not already familiar with this simple trick. Frozen ginger can be cut with a sharp knife and some effort, but use caution so as not to accidentally cut your hand. Alternatively, frozen ginger can be grated, which is a safer method.

creamy carrot ginger soup

active minutes

total time

servings

week

months

I just love the refreshing, tangy flavor of ginger in a creamy soup. It instantly brightens my mood on a cold winter night. The whimsical color of this soup brings me back to warmer summer months when Mexican sunflowers (*Tithonia rotundifolia*) are exploding in the garden and I gather the burning orange blossoms to brighten every corner of my home. Frozen carrots can replace fresh carrots. A stovetop preparation is possible if you don't have a pressure cooker. Simply sauté the vegetables as indicated, add the stock, bring the soup to a boil, and simmer the soup for about 30 minutes or until the carrots are soft and fall apart easily. Proceed with the remainder of the preparation as directed.

2 tablespoons coconut oil

1 onion, sliced

2 pounds (910 g) carrots, roughly chopped

2 cloves garlic, roughly chopped

1-inch (1.3 cm) piece of fresh ginger, peeled and chopped

5 cups Chicken Stock

1 can (13.5 ounces [398 ml]) unsweetened full-fat coconut milk

1 teaspoon salt

Using the sauté function in an electric pressure cooker (see the note above for stovetop instructions), melt the coconut oil and sauté the onion for about 5 minutes, add the carrots, garlic, and ginger, and sauté until the onions are caramelized and brown, about 7 minutes total.

Add in the Chicken Stock, and cook on high pressure for 10 minutes.

Release the steam when done, add the coconut milk and salt, and blend the soup with an immersion blender or in batches using a blender or food processor.

Serve immediately.

Batch Cooking and Leftovers: I often prepare a double batch of soup, eat half, and freeze the remaining half for a later date. See *Prepping for Soups and Stews* for more information.

Make It a Meal: Serve with OMGrain-Free Chicken Tenders and Bok Choy and Red Peppers with Thai Peanut Sauce.

AN EVERYDAY BASIC

chicken stock

active minutes   total time   quarts (1.9 l)   weeks   months

This simple and affordable preparation is a must for every home cook. Home-made chicken stock is one of the simplest ways to improve the flavor and nutritional value of numerous dishes. The dissolved amino acids in homemade stocks are beneficial for repairing tissues within the colon and joints. Stock by itself is an excellent beverage for the treatment or prevention of cold and flu. Using chicken parts such as feet, necks, and backs (which are some of the least expensive bones) will yield a stock that is higher in dissolved amino acids and is sure to "gel" when cooled. This gelling characteristic is indicative of high gelatin content, but the stock will become liquid again when heated.

1 whole chicken carcass
  (about 1 pound [455 g]
  of bones)
5 stalks celery, roughly chopped
3 carrots, roughly chopped
1 onion, quartered with
  peel intact
5 cloves garlic, halved
2 quarts (1.9 l) water
1 bay leaf
1½ teaspoons vinegar

Combine all the ingredients in an electric pressure cooker and cook on high for 2 hours (see the accompanying note for stovetop instructions). Allow the stock to cool for 15–20 minutes before releasing the steam.

Remove the bones and vegetables, and strain the liquid through a fine-mesh strainer into jars or directly into the dish you're preparing. I often pour the stock through the strainer into a large bowl before transferring it to jars, a method that results in less mess.

Store Chicken Stock in the refrigerator or freezer.

Note: Stock can be made on the stovetop, but doing so will require additional water because it needs to be simmered for at least 24 hours (some chefs recommend 48 hours) to fully extract the therapeutic and nutritive benefits from the bones.

Batch Cooking and Leftovers: Batch sizes will be limited by the size of your pot or pressure cooker. (I prefer to store the frozen bones and use them as needed since they require less freezer space.)

If storing in the fridge, leave the layer of fat on top; this helps seal and preserve the stock. (Some people say that stock can even store for months in the refrigerator as long as the layer of fat stays intact, although I've never tried it.)

beef stock

10	2h 45m	4	2	4
active minutes	*total time*	*quarts (3.8 l)*	*weeks*	*months*

The benefits of homemade stocks are endless, and the flavor profile is far better than most any product you can buy in the store. See the Chicken Stock recipe, page 154, for more details on nutrition and consistency. Homemade Beef Stock often yields a decent amount of fat that can be reserved for cooking. You can easily collect the fat from the stock once it has chilled—a solid layer of fat forms on top, which can be removed and stored in the refrigerator for cooking. Many people roast beef bones for about 15 minutes at 350°F (177°C) before preparing the stock in order to improve overall flavor.

3 pounds (1.4 kg) beef bones

6 stalks celery, roughly chopped

4 carrots, roughly chopped

1 onion, quartered with
   peel intact

8 cloves garlic, halved

4 quarts (3.8 l) water

3 bay leaves

1 tablespoon vinegar

Combine all the ingredients in an electric pressure cooker and cook on high for 2 hours. (See the note in Chicken Stock for stovetop instructions.) Allow the stock to cool for 15–20 minutes before releasing the steam.

Remove the bones and vegetables, and strain the liquid through a fine-mesh strainer into jars or directly into the dish you're preparing. I often pour the stock through the strainer into a large bowl before transferring it to jars, a method that results in less mess.

Store Beef Stock in the refrigerator or freezer.

Batch Cooking and Leftovers: You can often make two batches of beef stock using the same bones as long as connective tissue remains on the bones after the initial cook is complete (this cannot be done with chicken or poultry bones since they're much smaller and have less tissue). I've even made three batches of broth from the same bones by slightly reducing the amount of liquid with each consecutive cook. Assuming you have ample freezer space, freeze each consecutive batch after it has cooled in Ziploc freezer bags for up to 4 months. If not, refreeze the bones and be sure to label the bag with how many times they've been cooked. If storing in fridge, leave the layer of fat on top.

apple butternut soup

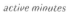

active minutes   total time   servings   week   months

The seasonal fall flavor of butternut squash and the tart yet slightly sweet flavor of Granny Smith apples truly welcome the changing of the seasons. This naturally sweet and creamy soup is one that most any kid would enjoy. I often prepare this recipe along with Apple Walnut Crisp Cereal in the fall when apple season is at its peak. Preparing the butternut squash in an electric pressure cooker while the apples bake makes this an even quicker meal to prepare. Halve and deseed the squash, and then place it on the rack in the pressure cooker with 1 cup of water and cook on high pressure for 10 minutes.

1 butternut squash, about 3 pounds (1.4 kg)

3 Granny Smith apples, peeled, cored, and diced

2 tablespoons melted coconut oil

1 tablespoon cinnamon powder

1 teaspoon ginger powder

½ teaspoon salt

2 cans (13.5 ounces [398 ml] each) unsweetened full-fat coconut milk

1 cup (235 ml) water or stock to adjust thickness

Preheat the oven to 400°F (204°C).

Remove the stem of the butternut squash, stand the squash on its end, and cut it into two even halves lengthwise. Remove the seeds and place the squash facedown on a parchment paper–lined baking sheet. Bake the squash for 45–55 minutes or until it's easily pierced with a fork.

Once the squash is in the oven, heap the apples onto a baking sheet. Pour the coconut oil on top and toss the apples until evenly coated with oil. Spread the apples into a single layer, place them into the oven along with the squash, and bake for 25 minutes or until soft.

Using a large spoon, scoop the flesh of the squash from the peel and place it in a large pot with the apples, cinnamon, ginger powder, salt, and coconut milk. Use an immersion blender to purée the soup until it's completely creamy. Adjust the thickness by adding the desired amount of water. Work in batches in a blender if you don't have an immersion blender.

Heat the soup to your desired temperature and serve.

Batch Cooking and Leftovers: Save time by prebaking the squash and apples. This way on the day of the meal, all you will have to do is throw everything in a pot, blend, and heat. A recipe that could take you over an hour turns into a 15-minute meal.

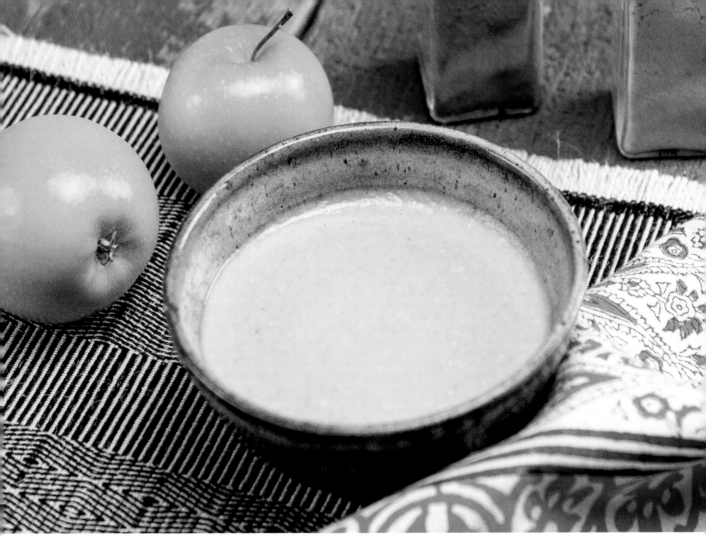

I often double the recipe and divide it into thirds—one-third for eating now and two-thirds for the freezer. See *Prepping for Soups and Stews* (page 152) for more information.

Make It a Meal: Serve with a Simple Whole Roasted Chicken and an Everyday Salad with Red Wine Lemon Vinaigrette. If baking both the soup ingredients and the chicken simultaneously, set the oven temperature to meet the requirements of the chicken, and then extend the squash cooking time by about 10 minutes.

black bean and vegetable soup

40 *active minutes*   1h *total time**   16–20 *servings*   1 *week*   3 *months*

Black bean soup brings me back to my early childhood when vegetarian stews were the norm in a household that rarely ate meat. My diet has drastically changed since that time, but my love for a bold yet simple bean soup has not diminished. Black beans and vegetables flavored with Mexican spices offer a soup that boasts powerful flavors similar to that of a hearty chili, but in a lighter way. Please note the yield for this soup and be sure to use an adequately sized pot (at least 9 liters, or 2½ gallons). Halve the recipe if your pot is not large enough. Beans are a food that can be as difficult to digest as a grain if not prepared correctly. Be sure to soak your beans for a minimum of 12 hours before preparing this delightfully nutritious soup (see *Soaking Seeds and Beans*, page 14, for more information). Do not use salted stock, as this prevents the beans from cooking. Beans should always be salted *after* being cooked. If you simply don't have the time or desire to prepare dried beans, you can replace them with canned beans: 1 pound (455 g) of dried beans is equal to approximately four 15-ounce (425 g) cans of beans. Drain and rinse the canned beans before adding them to the soup, and reduce the amount of stock by about 2 cups (475 ml).

But Isn't Corn a Grain?

You'll notice that I've added fresh and frozen corn to a handful of recipes in this cookbook even though corn is one of the most commonly eaten grains worldwide. The difference is that fresh corn—corn on the cob—is eaten before the seed is fully mature and is therefore considered a starchy vegetable. If you allow corn to continue to mature, the seed will fully develop. The corn is then dried and ground into a flour. It is at this point that corn becomes a true grain. I select organic corn, since otherwise, this crop relies heavily on pesticides and the use of genetically modified (GM) seed. Buying frozen organic corn is often your best option except for when fresh organic corn is available at your local farmers market. However, even with following all of these precautions, there are still individuals who cannot tolerate corn even in its immature starchy vegetable state. These individuals should, unfortunately, avoid corn altogether.

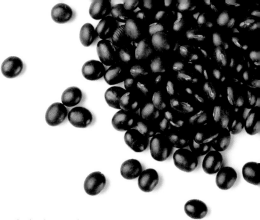

1 pound (455 g) dry black beans, soaked overnight

10 cups (2.4 l) Chicken Stock or Beef Stock

2 tablespoons cooking fat (lard or reserved fat from cooking meats preferable)

2 large onions, diced

1 bunch celery, sliced

4 medium carrots, sliced

2 red peppers, diced

3 medium zucchinis, diced

1 pound (455 g) frozen corn or 2 ears of fresh corn, kernels removed

1 head garlic, peeled and minced

1 tablespoon chili powder

1 tablespoon cumin powder

1 teaspoon smoked paprika

1½ tablespoons salt, or to taste

1 can (28 ounces [830 ml]) diced tomatoes

* plus 12–24 hours for soaking

Submerge the black beans in water and soak the beans for 12–24 hours (longer is better, but 12 hours is the absolute minimum; see *Soaking Seeds and Beans*, page 14).

Strain and rinse the black beans. Place the beans and stock into an electric pressure cooker, secure the lid, and cook on high for 30 minutes, releasing the pressure when complete. Prepare the rest of the soup while the beans cook. Soaked beans can be prepared on the stovetop, requiring approximately 2 hours to simmer. Watch your cooking liquid, adding more as necessary.

Preheat the cooking fat in a large pot on the stovetop and sauté the onions, celery, and carrots for about 5 minutes. Add in the red peppers, zucchinis (add corn at this time if using fresh), garlic, chili powder, cumin powder, paprika, and salt and continue to sauté until all vegetables are soft, about 10 minutes. Add in the corn (if using frozen) and tomatoes, and bring the soup to a low simmer.

Pour in the beans and stock, bring the soup to a simmer, and serve immediately. The flavors improve over time.

Batch Cooking and Leftovers: Divide the recipe in half: Eat one half and freeze the other.

Prepare the beans a day or two before you cook the soup to drastically reduce your total cooking time the day of serving. You can chop and bag the vegetables in advance for an even quicker meal. See *Prepping for Soups and Stews* (page 152) for more information.

Make It a Meal: Serve with leftover Pulled Mojo Chicken and a dollop of Garlicky Guacamole on top. You can even prepare a batch of Plantain Tortillas for a more filling meal.

not quite your mama's chili

 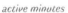

30	45m	8	1	2
active minutes	total time*	servings	week	months

This chili recipe incorporates all of the traditional ingredients required to create a flavorful, hearty bowl of steamy chili, but I've lightened it up ever so slightly with the addition of kale. I'm always looking for convenient (and undetectable) ways to incorporate more greens into our diet and this recipe fits the bill. This chili also lacks the heat that so many children dislike. Feel free to add in a few red pepper flakes or a chopped jalapeño if you're seeking a spicier option. You can use ground turkey or pork in the place of ground beef if desired—I often use half beef and half pork. Refer to Black Bean and Vegetable Soup (page 158) for information on subbing canned beans for dried. Also see *But Isn't Corn a Grain?* (page 158) for a brief explanation as to why I think fresh corn is an acceptable ingredient despite its use as a grain.

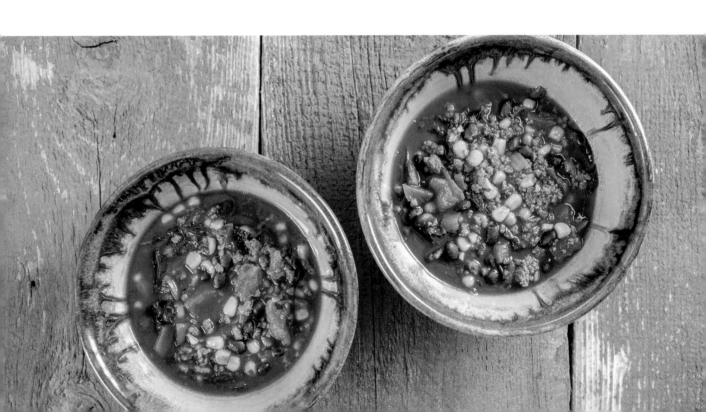

½ pound (225 g) dried
black beans

8 cups (1.9 l) Chicken Stock
or Beef Stock

2 pounds (910 g) ground beef

2 tablespoons cooking fat
(lard or reserved fat from
cooking meats preferable)

2 large onions, diced

1 green pepper, diced

6 cloves garlic, minced

1 bunch of kale, chopped
(ribs intact)

1 can (14.5 ounces [410 g])
diced tomatoes

1 can (6 ounces [170 g])
tomato paste

1 pound (455 g) frozen corn
or 2 ears of fresh corn,
kernels removed

1 tablespoon chili powder

1½ teaspoons cumin powder

¾ teaspoon smoked paprika

½ teaspoon dried oregano

1 tablespoon salt

plus 12–24 hours for soaking

Submerge the black beans in water and soak the beans for 12–24 hours (longer is better, but 12 hours is the absolute minimum; see *Soaking Seeds and Beans*, page 14).

Strain and rinse the soaked black beans. Place the beans and stock into an electric pressure cooker, secure the lid, and cook on high for 30 minutes, releasing the pressure when complete. Prepare the rest of the chili while the beans cook. Soaked beans can be prepared on the stovetop, requiring approximately 2 hours to simmer. Watch your cooking liquid, adding more as necessary.

Preheat a large pot and brown the ground beef for about 10 minutes. To do this, stir the beef frequently, breaking it apart as you go. Transfer the beef into a bowl and set aside.

Using the same pot, melt the cooking fat and sauté the onions for approximately 5 minutes; add the pepper and garlic, and sauté for another 5 minutes.

Add in the remaining ingredients and cook for an additional 5 minutes. Return the beef to the pot, and remove the beef-and-vegetable mixture from the heat until the beans are finished cooking.

Once the beans are done, pour the entire contents into the pot with the beef and vegetables. Bring the soup to a simmer and cook on low for about 30 minutes (optional).

Serve immediately.

Batch Cooking and Leftovers: I highly recommend doubling this recipe and freezing half for a later date, but this will require the use of a very large pot (about 10 liters, or nearly 3 gallons). See *Prepping for Soups and Stews* (page 152) for more information.

Make It a Meal: Serve with Plantain Tortillas and Pico de Gallo, or with an Everyday Salad and Italian Dressing.

white bean, fennel, and sausage stew

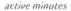

active minutes   total time*   servings   days   months

This is the perfect dish to serve when you're hosting guests. This stunning, fragrant, and all-around deliciously flavorful stew takes just an hour to prepare and it yields enough to feed most any size dinner party (see the accompanying *Make It a Meal* section for a complete meal suggestion). This is another stew recipe that will require the use of an adequately sized pot (at least 9 liters, or almost 2½ gallons). Working with two separate pots is always an option, but this will require cleaning both vessels when finished. You can substitute four 15-ounce (425 g) cans of white beans (strained and rinsed) for the dried beans. If doing so, reduce the amount of chicken stock by about 2 cups (475 ml).

1 pound (910 g) dried white beans

12 cups (2.8 l) Chicken Stock

2 pounds (910 g) sausage links

2 tablespoons cooking fat
(lard or reserved fat from
cooking meats preferred)

2 large onions, diced

1 large fennel bulb, halved and
thinly sliced, tops chopped

1 bunch celery, sliced

8 cloves garlic, minced

2 red peppers, diced

1 cup (235 ml) dry white wine

2 cans (14.5 ounces [411 g] each)
diced fire-roasted tomatoes

1½ tablespoons dried rosemary

1 teaspoon smoked paprika

1 bunch parsley, minced

1 tablespoon salt

* plus 12–24 hours for soaking

Submerge the white beans in water and soak the beans for 12–24 hours (longer is better, but 12 hours is the absolute minimum; see *Soaking Seeds and Beans*, page 14).

Strain and rinse the soaked beans. Place the beans and stock into an electric pressure cooker, secure the lid, and cook on high for 30 minutes, releasing the pressure when complete. Prepare the rest of the stew while the beans cook. Soaked beans can be prepared on the stovetop, requiring approximately 2 hours to simmer. Watch your cooking liquid, adding more as necessary.

Preheat the grill to high heat and cook the sausage links while you prepare the vegetables. Cook the links for about 10 minutes, flip, and cook for another 6 minutes until cooked through. Links can also be baked at 400°F (204°C) for about 15 minutes, flipping halfway through. Set the sausages aside until cool enough to handle.

Preheat a large pot over medium-high heat, melt the cooking fat, and sauté the onions, fennel, and celery for about 7 minutes, stirring frequently. Add in the garlic and peppers, and sauté for another 5 minutes.

Add the wine, tomatoes, rosemary, smoked paprika, and parsley. Bring the stew to a simmer and allow it to simmer for about 15 minutes.

Slice the sausage into bite-sized pieces and add it to the simmering stew.

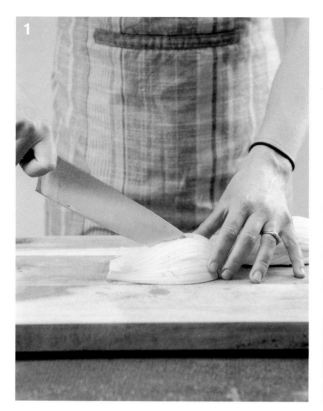

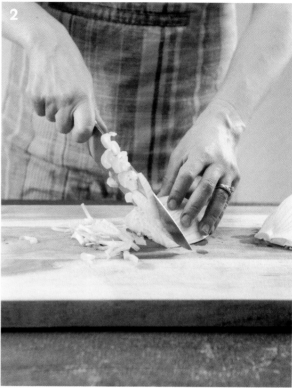

Step 1. Cut the fennel bulb in half, place it on the cutting board cut-side down, and slice the entire bulb similar to an onion, leaving more space between cuts. I usually only slice the bulb three times from the outside of the bulb toward the center. **Step 2.** Thinly slice the bulb perpendicularly to the cuts you just made.

The beans should be done at this point. Pour the entire contents of the pressure cooker into the vegetable-and-sausage mixture, add salt, stir, and allow the stew to simmer until ready to serve.

Batch Cooking and Leftovers: Prepare twice as many sausages and freeze the leftovers for later use. See *Prepping for Soups and Stews* (page 152) for more information.

Make It a Meal: Serve to dinner guests after first enjoying a plate of raw mixed vegetables with Fiesta Sunflower Seed Hummus as an appetizer, then with Roasted Beet and Citrus Salad and a stunning Everyday Salad with Fresh Basil and Garlic Balsamic Vinaigrette. End the evening with a slice of Apple Spice Bundt Cake.

chicken and vegetable coconut curry soup

40	1h	10	6	2
active minutes	total time	servings	days	months

This Thai-inspired soup boasts a beautifully layered flavor profile with the tang of citrus, creaminess of coconut, sweetness of red peppers, and accents of cilantro and curry paste. In addition to its delightful flavor, this soup is fragrant and colorful—all excellent qualities for a warming soup on a cold winter day. If you don't have any red curry paste, you can use instead 1–2 tablespoons of curry powder. The two have different flavors, but both work well for this recipe. Be sure to reserve and freeze the chicken carcass for making Chicken Stock in the future.

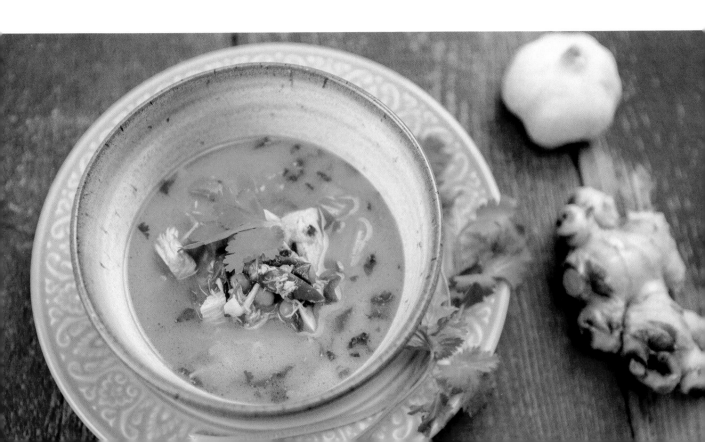

1 whole chicken, about 4 pounds (1.8 kg)

6 cups (1.4 l) Chicken Stock, divided

2 tablespoons cooking fat (lard, reserved fat from cooked meats, or coconut oil)

1 large onion, diced

2 medium carrots, sliced

1 red pepper, diced

1 bunch bok choy, chopped

1 tablespoon peeled, grated ginger

8 cloves garlic, minced

½ pound (225 g) frozen peas

2½ tablespoons Thai Kitchen red curry paste

Zest from 1 lemon

2–3 teaspoons salt

1 can (13.5 ounces [398 ml]) unsweetened full-fat coconut milk

1 bunch fresh cilantro, finely chopped

Place the whole chicken onto the rack in an electric pressure cooker, add 1 cup (235 ml) Chicken Stock, secure the lid, and cook on high pressure for 35 minutes. Release the steam and remove the lid to allow the chicken to cool. The chicken can also be prepared in the oven by following the instructions for Simple Whole Roasted Chicken. Prepare the chicken as instructed, but only coat it in oil; do not add the spices. Prepare the rest of the soup while the chicken cooks.

Preheat a large pot over medium-high heat, melt the cooking fat, and sauté the onion and carrots for about 5 minutes or until the onion becomes translucent. Add in the red pepper, bok choy, ginger, and garlic, and sauté for another 5 minutes or until the vegetables are soft.

Add in the frozen peas, red curry paste, lemon, salt, remaining stock, coconut milk, and any liquid from the pressure cooker. Bring the soup to a simmer.

Remove the chicken meat from the bone and chop the chicken into bite-sized pieces. Place the meat into the soup and reserve the bones for making stock. You can go ahead and prepare a batch of Chicken Stock at this time, or reserve the carcass in the freezer for a later date.

Stir in the cilantro and remove the soup from the heat.

Serve immediately.

Batch Cooking and Leftovers: Doubling this recipe is great, but you'll need a large pot (10 liters or 3 gallons), and you'll have to prepare the whole chickens in the oven because two chickens will not fit into the pressure cooker. You *could* pressure-cook them one after another, but this will actually take more time. See *Prepping for Soups and Stews* (page 152) for more information.

Make It a Meal: I like serving this soup with Crispy Sweet Potato Fries. The sweetness from the fries nicely complements the flavors of the soup.

chicken noodle soup

40 active minutes	1h total time	10 servings	5 days	2 months

Who says you can't eat soul-warming Chicken Noodle Soup when you don't eat grains? Turnip "noodles" are surprisingly delicious and give this soup a unique-ness that will be appreciated by everyone in the family! Turnips are one of the easier vegetables to grow, but I'm never quite sure what to do with them since neither my kids nor I particularly like the flavor of them when roasted. This soup has come to the rescue more times than you'll know when fall turnips are pouring out of the garden. You'll need a decent spiralizer to make a soup that's visually identical to the real deal; use a countertop version if you have one. If you're just not convinced that turnip "noodles" will be your thing, then simply leave them out and enjoy a delicious bowl of chicken and vegetable soup. A noodle-less ver-sion is the healing meal that I prepare as a nourishing gift to my kids or friends when someone is feeling unwell.

1 whole chicken, about 4 pounds (1.8 kg)

8 cups (1.9 l) Chicken Stock, divided

2 tablespoons cooking fat (lard or reserved fat from cooking meats preferred)

1 large onion, diced

3 medium carrots, sliced

1 bunch celery, sliced

1 pound (455 g) turnips (about 3 medium), spiralized

10 cloves garlic, minced

1½ tablespoons salt

1 bunch fresh parsley, finely chopped

Place the whole chicken onto the steam rack in an electric pressure cooker, add 1 cup (235 ml) Chicken Stock, secure the lid, and cook on high pressure for 35 minutes. Release the steam and remove the lid to allow the chicken to cool when done. The chicken can also be prepared in the oven by following the instructions for Simple Whole Roasted Chicken. Prepare the chicken as instructed, but only coat it in oil; do not add the spices. Prepare the rest of the soup while the chicken cooks.

Preheat a large pot over medium-high heat, melt the cooking fat, and sauté the onion, carrots, and celery for 8 minutes or until they begin to caramelize.

Cut the spiralized turnips into pieces about 3–5 inches (7.5–12.5 cm) in length. Add the garlic and turnips to the pot, and sauté for another 3 minutes. Don't overcook the turnips or they'll lose their texture.

Pour in the remaining stock and liquid from the electric pressure cooker, and bring the soup to a simmer. Add in the salt and parsley, and remove the soup from the heat to prevent overcooking the turnip noodles.

Chop the chicken into bite-sized pieces and stir into the soup.

Serve immediately.

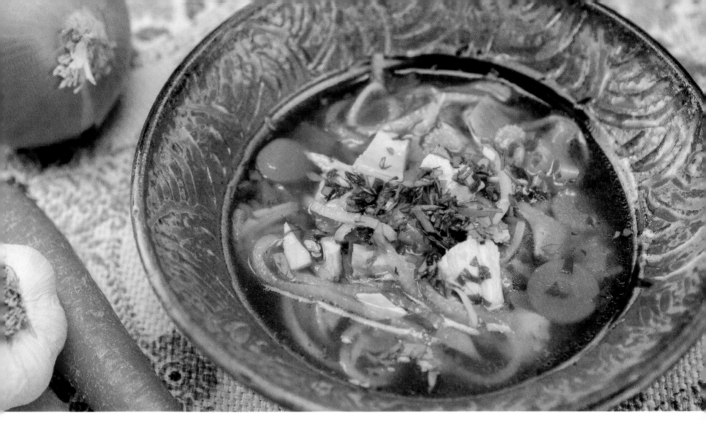

Batch Cooking and Leftovers: This soup doesn't freeze particularly well because of the turnip noodles. However, it can be easily frozen without the noodles. The noodles can instead be sautéed the day of serving and added after the soup has thawed and been reheated. See *Prepping for Soups and Stews* (page 152) for more information.

Make It a Meal: Serve as a stand-alone meal and add Apple Spice Bundt Cake for dessert.

40-minute beef stew

active minutes   total time   servings   days   months

Most beef stew recipes require a minimum of eight hours of cooking with the use of a slow cooker, but the preparation with an electric pressure cooker accomplishes the same thing in a fraction of the time. You can still use a slow cooker for this recipe: Simply combine all ingredients and cook on low heat for eight hours. If using this method, I recommend preparing the ingredients the night before. In the morning, simply throw everything into the slow cooker. I love that this beef stew is rich, flavorful, hearty, and can be easily served as a one-pot meal. I've also found this to be a good recipe for finicky eaters since it contains a number of subtly flavored and familiar ingredients. Shown on page 149.

2 pounds (910 g) stew beef, cubed

2 pounds (910 g) yellow potatoes, diced into 1-inch (2.5 cm) cubes

2 onions, diced

5 carrots, thinly sliced in rounds

1 bunch celery, sliced

1 pound (450 g) fresh green beans, cut into 1-inch pieces, or cut frozen green beans

1 head garlic, peeled and minced

8 cups (1.9 l) Beef Stock

1 teaspoon dried tarragon

2 bay leaves

Pepper, to taste

1 tablespoon salt, more to taste

Combine all the ingredients in an 8-quart electric pressure cooker. You may have to slightly reduce the amount of vegetables and stock if using a 6-quart version. Secure the lid and cook the soup on high for 20 minutes. If preparing on the stovetop, place all the ingredients into a large pot and allow the soup to simmer, covered, for about 2 hours or till the beef is easily pulled apart.

Allow the pressure cooker to sit for 10 minutes before releasing the steam. Remove the lid, add your desired amount of salt, mix, and serve.

Batch Cooking and Leftovers: If you want extra stew for freezing, simply prepare the ingredients to make a second batch of stew while the first batch is cooking. Empty the pressure cooker of its contents when the first batch is complete and start the second batch while you enjoy the first. See *Prepping for Soups and Stews* (page 152) for more information.

Make It a Meal: Serve with Plantain Sandwich Bread for dipping, or with an Everyday Salad with Red Wine Lemon Vinaigrette for a lower-carb option.

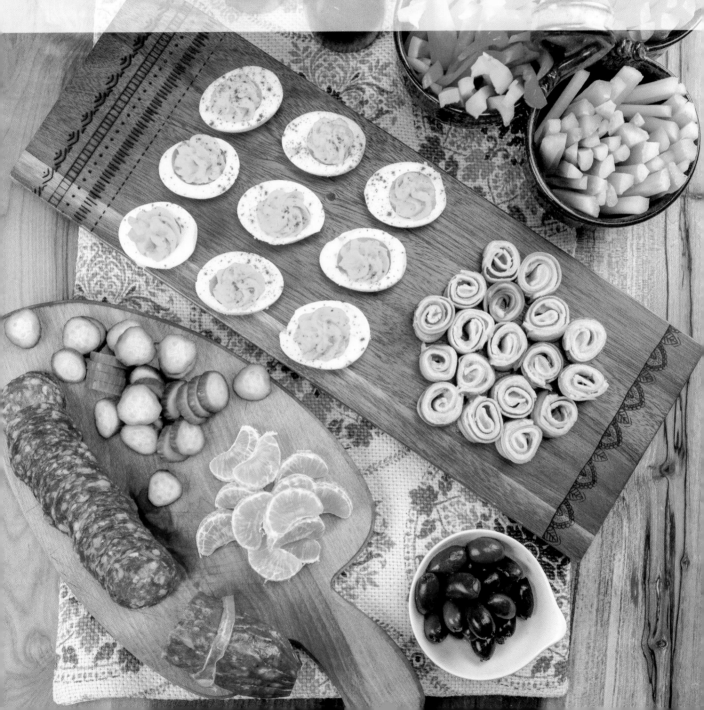

Quick and Easy Snacks

Some of the items on this list are recipes from the book, but many are quick snack foods that you can throw together in a matter of minutes. I believe that snacks should be small, uncomplicated morsels that can tide the kids over between meals. If they fill up on snacks (or calorie-rich beverages like juice or milk), then you can't possibly expect them to have an appetite for the wonderfully nutritious lunch or dinner that you prepare. I've included a handful of packaged snacks with recommendations for store-bought foods that I buy for my own family.

Apple slices with nut or
  seed butter
Banana Nut Bread
Carrot Cake Applesauce Muffins
Coconut Cream Goji Bites
Cold-Pack Dill Pickles
Fruit
Fruit kebabs

100 percent grass-fed beef sticks
Hard-Boiled Eggs
Homemade (Fiesta Sunflower
  Seed Hummus) or
  store-bought hummus
Organic grain-free chips
Plantain Blender Pancakes
  (leftovers)

Olives
Plantain Muffins
Roasted and Salted Walnuts
  (or seeds)
Superfoods Trail Mix
Smoothies
Turkey Cucumber Rolls
Raw vegetables, sliced

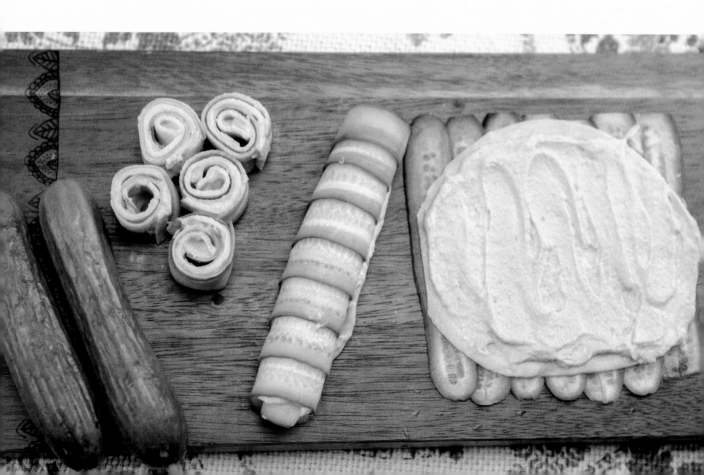

turkey cucumber rolls

active minutes   total time   rolls   days

You can prepare a number of these protein-packed bites as an appetizer for guests or as a delightfully savory snack that can go in your kids' school lunches. You can string them on a skewer or individual toothpicks to guarantee that they won't come unrolled en route to school. I've tried slicing the cucumber using a mandoline, but the slices came out too thick, even on the thinnest setting. You really need a vegetable peeler. I buy deli meats that are free of hormones and antibiotics, and from animals that are certified humanely raised. For hummus, I buy a variety of brands, but closely check the ingredients list. You can also prepare Fiesta Sunflower Seed Hummus for a homemade, bean-free version.

1 large or 2 small cucumbers

4 slices turkey breast
  (see note above)

4 tablespoons hummus
  (see note above)

Use a vegetable peeler to cut the cucumbers into thin slices, lengthwise. Form a "sheet" of cucumbers by lining up the thin slices lengthwise with a small amount of overlap between each one. Make the sheet as wide as the slice of turkey. You'll make 4 sheets in total, one for each piece of turkey.

Place one piece of turkey on top of each sheet of cucumbers and evenly spread 1 tablespoon of hummus across the turkey.

Carefully roll the cucumber into what looks like a sushi roll. You can serve it as is or slice the roll into pieces resembling sushi.

Serve immediately.

Batch Cooking and Leftovers: If packing in a school lunch, pack the lunch box with an ice pack.

Make It a Meal: Serve 2 turkey rolls with apple slices and peanut butter (or Apple Slice Monsters, if you're feeling ambitious), and raw sliced vegetables to dip in Garlicky Guacamole for a kid-friendly packed lunch.

superfoods trail mix

active minutes	total time	cups (565 g)	months	year
5	5m	5	6	1

Finally, a chocolaty trail mix you can feel good about serving to your kids! The sweetness of the mulberries and goji berries combined with the crunch from the cacao nibs makes for a sweet and crunchy snack minus the refined sugar found in most store-bought trail mixes. Notice that this is a nut-free recipe that can be taken into your child's nut-free school zone! Try subbing in your favorite nuts or seeds for a personalized mix.

2 cups (120 g) coconut flakes
1 cup (150 g) hemp hearts
1 cup (130 g) cacao nibs
1 cup (110 g) dried mulberries
½ cup (55 g) dried goji berries
½ teaspoon salt

Combine all the ingredients in a large jar, cover the jar with a lid, and shake until the ingredients are evenly mixed.

Batch Cooking and Leftovers: This recipe takes very little effort and yields a good amount. If it turns out to be a family favorite, you can always double the recipe and freeze half.

Make It a Meal: Serve ¼ cup of the trail mix along with Turkey Cucumber Rolls, Summer Cucumber and Tomato Salad, and Dilly Sweet Potato Salad for a packed lunch for the kids.

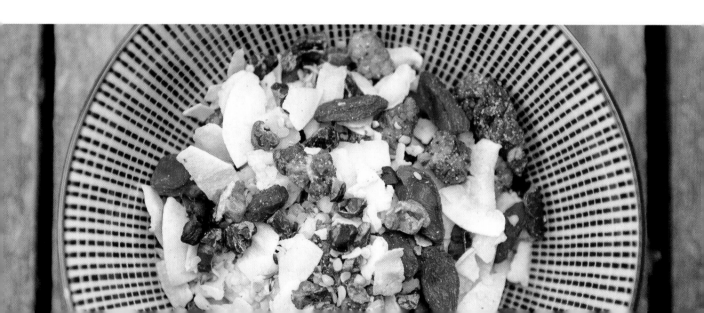

roasted and salted walnuts

active minutes   *total time**   *servings*   *weeks*   *months*

10   1h 10m   16   3   6

Much like grains, nuts contain compounds like phytic acid and enzyme inhibitors that are difficult to digest or prevent the absorption of nutrients. Soaking nuts in warm salt water for 12–24 hours helps to increase nutrient availability, improve digestibility, and degrade compounds that are less than desirable for consumption. This extra step takes very little active time, but makes a huge difference in the digestibility, health benefits, and flavor of nuts. And soaking nuts results in a creamy texture. I use walnuts in this recipe, but you can use any nut or seed of your choice. When cooking small seeds like sunflower seeds, reduce the baking time. The nuts and seeds need to be cooked until they're crispy and dry so that they no longer contain any water.

1 tablespoon plus ¼ teaspoon salt, divided

4 cups (945 ml) warm water

4 cups (510 g) raw walnuts

* plus 12–24 hours for soaking

Dissolve 1 tablespoon of salt into the water using a bowl or jar large enough to hold the entire volume of nuts and water combined. Once the salt is dissolved, add the walnuts to the bowl or jar and allow the nuts to soak at room temperature for 12–24 hours.

After soaking is complete, preheat the oven to 250°F (121°C).

Strain the walnuts through a colander and rinse well to remove any salt water. Pour them onto a clean towel and toss them around to remove any excess water.

Spread the walnuts in a single layer on a baking sheet and sprinkle with the remaining salt. Bake the walnuts for 1 hour, stirring every 20 minutes.

Allow the nuts to completely cool before placing them in an airtight container.

Batch Cooking and Leftovers: This recipe can be easily doubled or even tripled. The ease of preparation and the long freezer storage time make them an excellent choice for large batches, and they don't need to be thawed before eating.

cold-pack dill pickles

active minutes

total time

pickle spears

months

Homemade pickles are a snack staple in our house! These crispy dill pickles are easy to make and retain all the nutrients that would be lost if they were heated at high temperatures for canning. Preparing your own pickles takes very little time, and it's a tremendous upgrade from store-bought varieties that can contain food dyes. You can add ingredients like red pepper flakes, jalapeño peppers, or peppercorns for a spicier version.

2¼ cups (530 ml) warm water

2 pounds (910 g) pickling cucumbers, quartered into spears

½ large bunch of dill

3 cloves garlic, smashed

1 teaspoon whole mustard seed

1 tablespoon salt

1¾ cups (415 ml) apple cider vinegar

Heat the water while you cut and pack your cucumbers. The water just has to be warm enough to easily dissolve salt.

Place the dill, garlic, and mustard seed into a ½-gallon-sized glass jar or divide ingredients among three quart-sized jars. Lean the jar on its side while placing the cucumber spears upright into the jar, packing them as tightly as you can without damaging the cucumbers. Pack a second tier of cucumbers if using a ½-gallon-sized jar.

Place the salt in a separate 1-quart-sized jar and pour the water over the top. Stir to dissolve. Pour the vinegar into the salt water and mix.

Pour the water-and-vinegar mixture over the top of your cucumbers and place a lid on the jar. Refrigerate the jar, allowing a minimum of 2 days before eating.

Batch Cooking and Leftovers: Pickles make a great addition to salads, such as The Tuna Salad Upgrade or Simple Egg Salad, which means that a double batch is often in order. However, you will be limited by space in your refrigerator, so plan accordingly.

strawberry santas

15	15m	12	3	
active minutes	*total time*	*santas**	*days*	

These adorable little treats are so much fun for the kids to make! Strawberry Santas are a delightful, easy, and nutritious treat for holiday parties. They also make for a fun indoor winter activity on a snowy day. The recipe for Coconut Whipped Cream makes more than you'll need. You can simply store excess in the refrigerator for up to 2 weeks. Just be sure to whip the cream again before serving it.

Coconut Whipped Cream
1 pound (455 g) strawberries
½ teaspoon flaxseeds

* depends on strawberry size

Place a small amount of whipped cream into the corner of a small plastic bag. Cut a small hole into the corner of the bag to create an icing pipe.

Remove the tops of the strawberries. Slice a round from the bottom of each strawberry and keep both the top and the bottom together as a set.

Place the strawberry round on a plate, pipe a circle of coconut cream on top of the round, place the top of the strawberry onto the whipped cream, and finish the hat with a small dab of whipped cream on top. Complete the Santa by placing two flaxseeds where the eyes should be.

Enjoy immediately.

Batch Cooking and Leftovers: Strawberries tend to go bad quickly, so I don't recommend you prepare a double batch unless you're certain your family will eat the Santas within 3 days.

Leftover whipped cream can be stored in the refrigerator for up to 2 weeks.

Make It a Meal: Serve with a variety of easy, light finger foods around the holidays when you're experiencing holiday-food burnout. Try pairing them with raw sliced vegetables dipped in Avocado-Mango Salsa and OMGrain-Free Chicken Tenders.

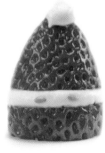

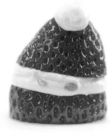

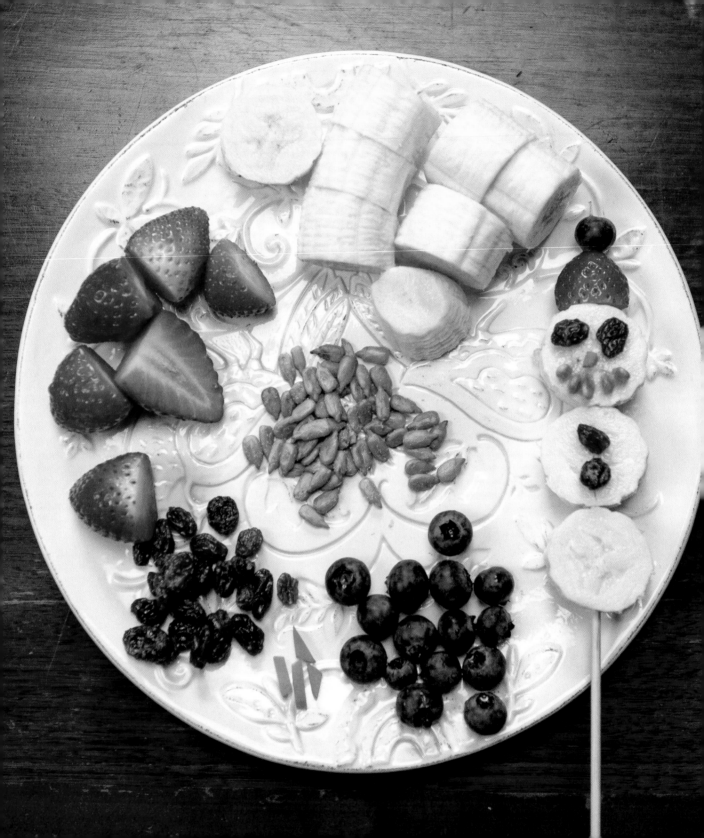

banana snowmen

active minutes
15

total time
15m

snowmen
10

days
2

Changing your diet doesn't mean that you have to miss out on fun food ideas for the holidays; it just means preparing something a little different. Your kids will love assembling these Banana Snowmen for the winter holidays and it's a treat-like snack you can actually feel good about eating! The ingredients list includes only enough to build the snowmen. I suggest having far more ingredients on hand if you're doing this project with kids, because they will surely munch on the ingredients during assembly.

3 bananas

5–10 strawberries

10 blueberries

¼ cup (37 g) raisins

3 small slices of carrot

1 tablespoon sunflower seeds

Cut the bananas into 1-inch-thick (2.5 cm) rounds. You can get about 10 rounds per banana. Place three banana rounds onto each skewer to form the snowman bodies.

Remove the tops of the strawberries and slice them in half lengthwise if using large strawberries. Keep them whole if using smaller strawberries. Place the strawberry on top of the bananas followed by one blueberry to form a hat.

Carefully cut the carrot slices into triangles to use as noses.

Decorate the snowmen using raisins, carrot triangles, and sunflower seeds. Serve immediately.

Batch Cooking and Leftovers: The bananas will start to brown after 2 days, so only prep as many snowmen as you plan to eat within that 2-day period.

Make It a Meal: My kids and I assemble the snowmen over the winter holidays along with Strawberry Santas, Lemon Coconut Date Balls, and Chocolate Walnut Brownies topped with Chocolate Icing. The kids are able to help, which has now become our tradition!

apple slice monsters

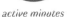

20
active minutes

20m
total time

8
monsters

2
days

These fun and healthy snacks are made from 100 percent whole-food ingredients. It's the perfect recipe for a Halloween gathering, as a unique school project, or on days when you're feeling like putting a bit of creativity into your child's snack. The ingredients only list what you'll need to make eight monsters. You'll likely want extra blueberries and strawberries if kids are helping, because they'll likely munch on these ingredients as you build. You can use any nut or seed butter to attach the tongue and eyes, but SunButter keeps the flavor consistent with the sunflower seed teeth. Assembling Apple Slice Monsters in a school setting would be a fun and manageable project to do with a large group of children, but be sure to avoid any SunButter that was processed on shared equipment with nuts or peanuts, if any students in the classroom have nut allergies.

2 green apples
2 tablespoons sunflower seeds
3 strawberries
2 tablespoons SunButter
10–16 blueberries

Quarter the apples and carefully remove the seeds, leaving as much of the apple flesh as possible. Cut a wedge out of the peel side of the apple, keeping the wedge slightly off center. This leaves more room for the eyes on the top, and less space for the mouth on the bottom.

Place approximately 10 sunflower seeds into the top of each mouth, poking the pointed side of the seed into the apple flesh.

Remove the tops of the strawberries and cut them into thin slices. Use a small dab of SunButter to adhere the strawberry into the mouth as a tongue.

Adhere the blueberry eyes with a small dab of SunButter. Each monster can have one, two, or even three eyes.

Repeat with the remaining apple quarters and enjoy.

Batch Cooking and Leftovers: If stored in the fridge, apples will start to brown over time. Better to prep 4–6 hours in advance and they won't lose any of their color. Spritz them with a lemon water mixture if you're trying to prevent them from browning.

Make It a Meal: Add to your child's lunch box as a playful treat along with an Herbed Beef Burger, Grain-Free Tabbouleh, and Coconut and Cinnamon Sweet Potato Mash.

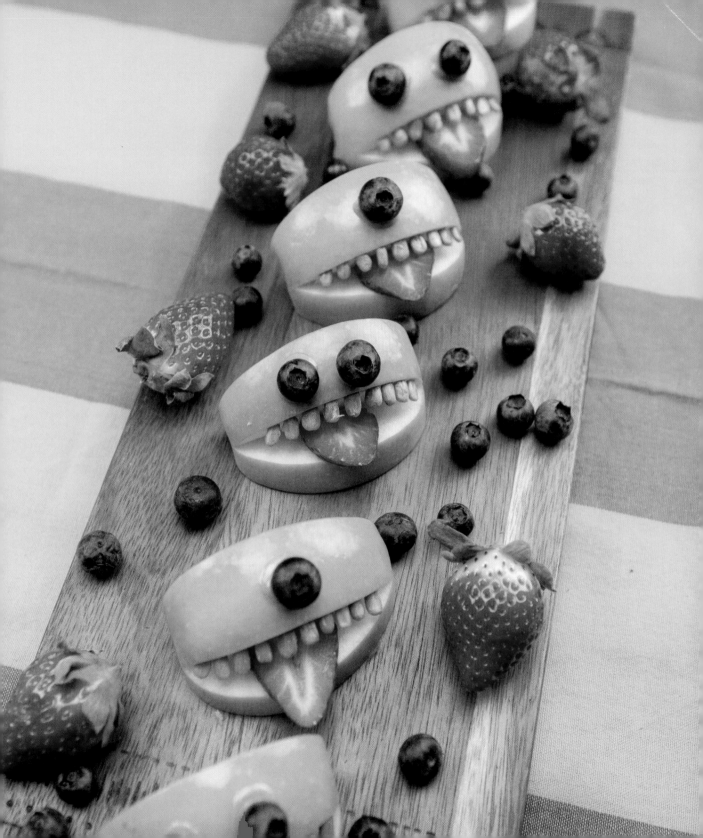

bacon-bundled green beans

active minutes   total time   bundles   days

I tested this recipe with varying vegetables, including asparagus, but green beans came out as the surprising winner. These savory little morsels are a hearty and nutritious finger food for any party. Not only are they delicious and visually stunning, but they're so easy to make! These beans store well in the refrigerator and make a great addition to a packed lunch.

1½ pounds (680 g) green beans, washed and trimmed
12 ounces (340 g) bacon

Preheat the oven to 350°F (177°C).

Using eight or nine green beans at a time, form a small bundle and tightly wrap the green beans in a piece of bacon from the top to the bottom.

Place the bundles on a baking sheet, allowing an inch (2.5 cm) of space between bundles. Bake the green beans for 1 hour, flipping halfway through.

Serve the green bean bundles immediately.

Batch Prepping and Leftovers: This is a recipe that can be easily doubled, so plan to use leftovers for snacks and meals throughout the week. Leftovers are delicious paired with soups such as Creamy Cauliflower Soup.

Make It a Meal: Pair with Apple Butternut Soup and a Massaged Kale Salad with Lentils for a hearty wintertime meal.

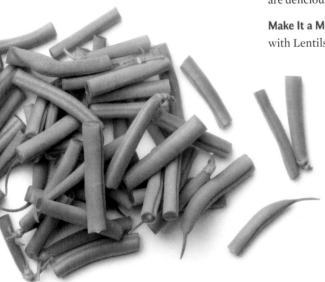

deviled eggs

active minutes   total time   servings   days

20   20m   6–12   5

Deviled eggs are one of my favorite prep-ahead proteins. Buying free-range eggs that come from hens fed a diet free of GMOs (seek out a local source and have them confirm this) guarantees that you're consuming one of the most nutrient-dense proteins in existence. Eggs from healthy chickens are loaded with protein, omega-3 fatty acids, HDL cholesterol (the good kind), and loads more vitamin E and A than store-bought eggs. Deviled eggs are creamy, savory, and delicious little morsels of nutrition! And they store and pack well. You can use a decorative icing pipe to fill each egg if you want a fancified dish for serving to guests. Using the pressure cooker method to prepare the hard-boiled eggs yields an egg that is much easier to peel, making it possible to complete this recipe in far less time than using the stovetop method. Shown on page 169.

12 Hard-Boiled Eggs

¼ cup (55 g) Homemade
   Mayonnaise

1½ teaspoons Dijon mustard

¼ teaspoon salt

⅛ teaspoon paprika

Peel the eggs and cut each egg in half.

Remove the yolks and place the yolks into a small bowl with the mayonnaise, mustard, and salt. Mash using a fork until the mixture is completely smooth.

Using a small spoon, evenly distribute the yolk mixture back into the egg whites. Place the finished eggs on a plate and evenly sprinkle paprika on top.

Batch Cooking and Leftovers: I always assume that we'll eat two eggs (four deviled eggs) per person for a meal or one egg (two deviled eggs) for a snack. Double the recipe if it's for a whole meal. Leftovers are quickly eaten in my household. We use them as the protein in salads or for a quick snack with a piece of fruit.

Prepare the Hard-Boiled Eggs up to 5 days in advance.

Make It a Meal: Serve with an Everyday Salad with Red Wine Lemon Vinaigrette and a fresh, local peach for a light packed lunch in the summer. Replace the peach with fresh corn on the cob when in season.

coconut cream goji bites

15	1h 15m	60	1	6
active minutes	*total time*	*squares*	*month*	*months*

These little treats seem to disappear almost as quickly as I can make them. They're wonderfully fatty little snacks for the kids, and I make them when I want something that's quick, easy, satisfying, and doesn't make a huge mess. Plus, I love all of the superfoods in them! These sweet and creamy morsels are a treat that both parents and kids can feel good about eating. They need to remain chilled or they'll melt, so send them with an ice pack if they're taken on the go.

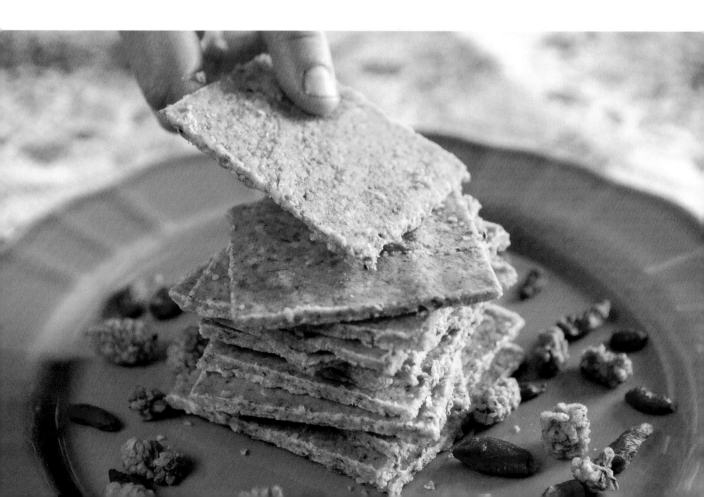

4 cups (450 g) unsweetened
  shredded coconut
1 tablespoon coconut oil
½ teaspoon salt
½ cup (55 g) dried goji berries
½ cup (55 g) dried mulberries
1 cup (150 g) hemp hearts

Combine the coconut, coconut oil, and salt in a high-powered blender and blend on high until the coconut becomes a liquid, about 6 minutes. You have to occasionally stop the blender to scrape the coconut down from the sides with a rubber spatula.

Add the goji berries and mulberries and blend on high for an additional minute.

Add the hemp hearts and blend just until combined, about 5 seconds.

Divide the mixture in half and place one half between two pieces of waxed or parchment paper. Using a rolling pin, smooth the mixture until it's as thin as a cracker, about ⅛ inch (3 mm) thick. Carefully slide the waxed paper onto a baking sheet. Repeat with the second half and refrigerate the mixture for 1 hour.

Once the mixture has completely hardened, remove it from the refrigerator and heavily score 2-inch (5 cm) squares with a knife or pizza cutter into the surface of the mixture. Break apart the squares, place them in an airtight container, and store them in the refrigerator. The squares will melt or become soft if stored at room temperature.

Batch Cooking and Leftovers: This is a great, calorie-dense snack to have on hand in the refrigerator or freezer.

If doubling the recipe, work in batches as the size of your blender will be a limiting factor. Prepare two batches, spread into thin layers, and then pile the sheets on top of each other. You can chill multiple sheets at a time this way.

Make It a Meal: Pack into your child's lunch box (don't forget the insulated sleeve and ice pack) along with Deviled Eggs, sliced raw vegetables, Fiesta Sunflower Seed Hummus (or a store-bought variety), olives, and a small handful of Roasted and Salted Walnuts.

collard wraps

active minutes   total time   servings

If you don't have a small garden or visit your local farmers market, it's time to start! These simple and delicious wraps are easy to prepare, and the collards adapt the wonderful flavors of whatever you put inside. However, it's hard to find a collard worth wrapping at the grocery store. Big, beautiful, fresh leaves are best found in your home garden or at the farmers market. I like to keep my wraps relatively small in diameter and increase the number of wraps I serve at one sitting, but you can overstuff Collard Wraps if you'd prefer to eat just one.

8 large collard leaves, stem removed at base of leaf

PROTEIN OPTIONS (CHOOSE ONE)

The Tuna Salad Upgrade

Simple Egg Salad

Fiesta Sunflower Seed Hummus

Grilled Chicken Breasts with Basil and Thyme (sliced)

Grilled Chicken Salad with Fresh Vegetables

Pulled Mojo Chicken

OTHER TOPPINGS (CHOOSE AS MANY AS YOU'D LIKE)

Chimichurri Sauce

Pecan Parmesan "Cheese"

Tomatoes, diced

Red onion, thinly sliced

Olives, sliced

Lettuce, shredded

Avocados, diced

Lay the collard leaves flat and distribute your protein of choice evenly among them along the mid-rib of the leaf, leaving the top of the leaf empty for folding downward. (Note: The side of the leaf with the thick stem will break when bent, so be sure to place the stuffing atop the thickest part of the stem, closest to the leaf base.) Distribute your other toppings on top of the protein.

Fold over one side of the collard, followed by the top of the leaf, and lastly roll the remaining side to form a wrap. Serve immediately.

Batch Cooking and Leftovers: Prepared collard wraps keep for only about 12 hours, so you'll need to prepare the wraps fresh each day. Simply prepare the stuffing ingredients and store these in the refrigerator till you're ready to assemble the wraps.

Make It a Meal: Pair with Summer Potato Salad or Dilly Sweet Potato Salad for a quick packed lunch or light dinner.

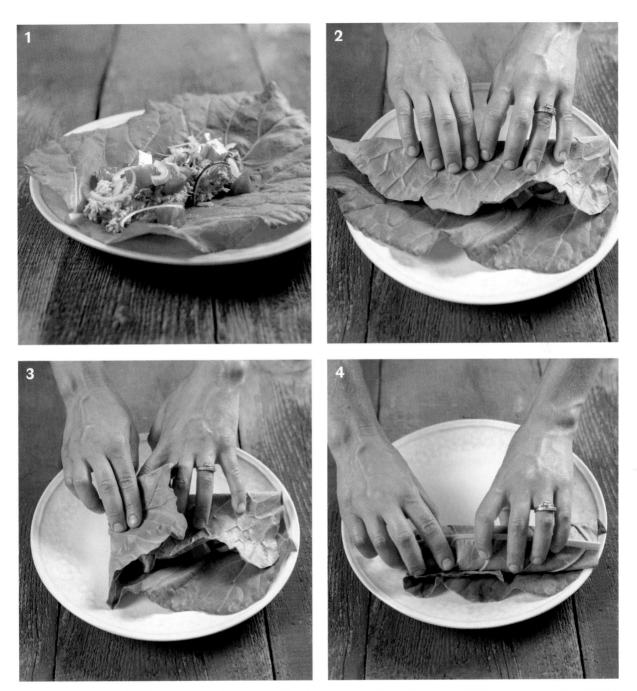

Step 1. Place the stuffing along the mid-rib of the leaf, leaving the top of the leaf empty for folding downward. **Step 2.** Fold over one of the sides of the collard. **Step 3.** Fold down the top of the leaf. **Step 4.** Roll up the remaining leaf to form a wrap.

"pasta" bowls

10
active minutes*

10m
total time*

6–8
servings

5
days

2
months

Creating varying flavor profiles atop a bed of a spaghetti squash can be an excellent way to use up leftovers. But don't underestimate these dishes! Serving any of the following flavor-packed options is a sure way to convince anyone that grain-free eating is creative, filling, and delicious!

"Pasta" Bowls make for a quick and easy weeknight dinner as long as the meal components have been made in advance. You can either prepare them in advance on Saturday and Sunday (prep days) or pull the components from the freezer (see the following *Batch Cooking and Leftovers* section).

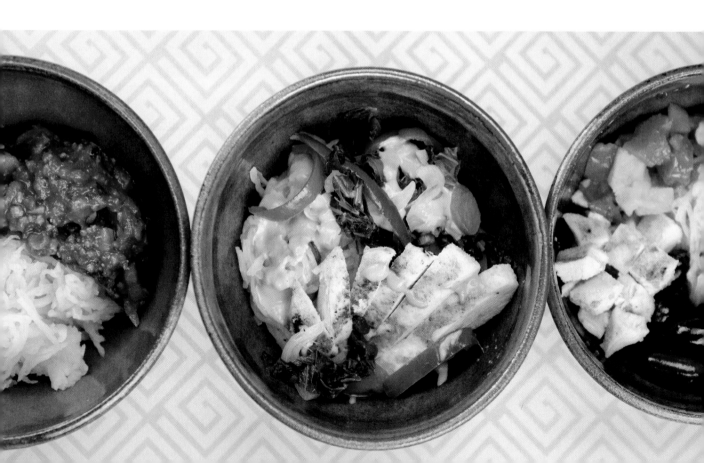

GREEK BOWL

1 Simple Spaghetti Squash
Grilled Chicken Breasts with
    Basil and Thyme†
Sun-Dried Tomato Tapenade†
Simple Vegan Pesto
1 jar (12.1 ounces [343 g])
    kalamata olives, sliced
2–3 handfuls spinach (optional)

MEXICAN FIESTA BOWL

1 Simple Spaghetti Squash
Pulled Mojo Chicken† or Mexican
    Shredded Beef†
Chimichurri Sauce†
Garlicky Guacamole
Fermented Salsa Fresca

THAI PEANUT BOWL

1 Simple Spaghetti Squash
Grilled Chicken Breasts with
    Basil and Thyme†
Bok Choy and Red Peppers with
    Thai Peanut Sauce

ITALIAN BOWL

1 Simple Spaghetti Squash
Hearty Meat Bolognese†
Pecan Parmesan "Cheese"

* after preparing meal components

*† Use half of the recipe. Freeze the
    other half if you don't plan to use
    it immediately.*

Determine your bowl of choice and combine the desired amount of each component into a bowl.

Serve "Pasta" Bowls warm.

Batch Cooking and Leftovers: Store each meal component in a separate storage container in the refrigerator for up to 5 days (components like Sun-Dried Tomato Tapenade can be stored much longer; refer to the individual recipes for more guidance). Assemble components immediately before serving.

Many of the recipes used to assemble "Pasta" Bowls can be pulled from the freezer if pre-prepared (refer to *Recipes That Freeze Well*, page 285, for a complete list).

For example, the Greek-style "Pasta" Bowl: Prep two spaghetti squashes (freeze one), one batch of Grilled Chicken Breasts with Basil and Thyme (freeze half), a single batch of Sun-Dried Tomato Tapenade (freeze half), and a double batch of Simple Vegan Pesto (freeze half). This means next week you have everything ready to thaw and eat! Just top with fresh kalamata olives and spinach and serve.

Make It a Meal: Serve your desired "Pasta" Bowl with a glass of Infused Water or Hibiscus Zinger Iced Tea for a 100 percent homemade meal, beverage and all!

pecan parmesan "cheese"

active minutes   *total time*   *servings*   *month*   *months*

This recipe originated when I was teaching raw foods cooking classes in my home. Participants were always shocked at how truly delicious this cheese substitute is. Its rich, nutty flavor will almost make you believe you're eating the real deal!

½ cup (60 g) pecan halves
1 tablespoon nutritional yeast
1 tablespoon olive oil
½ teaspoon salt

Place the pecan halves into a food processor and process until the pieces are approximately the size of peas.

Add in the nutritional yeast, olive oil, and salt. Process again until it's a coarse crumb. Avoid overprocessing, because you want to maintain texture and crunch to your "Parmesan."

Serve immediately.

Batch Cooking and Leftovers: This recipe freezes well. Make a large batch by spreading a single layer of it on a parchment paper–lined baking sheet, freezing it, and then pouring it into a freezer-safe container. The result will be a condiment that can be easily portioned out as needed.

If preparing in larger batches, keep an eye on the salt content to avoid an overly salted outcome.

the tuna salad upgrade

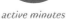

active minutes   total time   servings   days

Tuna salad is a relatively quick, easy, and nutritious food to prepare for busy weeknights or to have on hand for packed lunches. What I love about this salad is that it's actually quite bulky thanks to the addition of vegetables. It will be a nutritious way to fill your family's bellies! Skipjack tuna has less mercury compared with albacore (and it also happens to be less expensive), but neither should be eaten more than twice per week (refer to the Consumer Guide to Seafood from the Environmental Working Group, ewg.org). I purchase brands of canned, sustainably line-caught tuna to help protect the oceans from being overfished. You could also prepare the recipe using canned wild Alaskan salmon or sardines. Both have lower mercury content and are high in omega-3 fatty acids. Traditional tuna salad is often prepared with relish or pickles. I often use fermented vegetables such as green peppers, Dilly Beans, or radishes in the place of the celery in order to achieve this same flavor profile. You can use the Basic Brine to create your own unique ferments for use in tuna salad.

3 cans (5 ounces [142 g] each) tuna
½ cup (115 g) Homemade Mayonnaise
1 tablespoon Dijon mustard
4 stalks celery, finely diced
½ red pepper, finely diced
2 tablespoons finely diced red onion, about ⅛ onion
Salt, to taste
Pepper, to taste

Place the tuna in a medium-sized bowl and mash it with a fork until all of the pieces are broken apart. Stir in the mayonnaise and mustard until mixed well.

Add in all the remaining ingredients and mix until well combined. Serve immediately.

Batch Cooking and Leftovers: This recipe does not lend well to batch cooking unless you're serving the dish for a large group of people.

Make It a Meal: Perfect for school lunches with raw, sliced vegetables, Cold-Pack Dill Pickles, a Carrot Cake Applesauce Muffin, and a small handful of nuts.

simple egg salad

active minutes	*total time*	*servings*	*days*
15	15m	6	4

This egg salad appears on our table (and in the kids' lunch boxes) on occasions when I'm just too busy to pull anything else together. You can make this dish with any number of eggs to suit your specific needs at the time. Everyone is always happy with this simple yet flavorful and nutritious salad. You can add vegetables like grated carrots, pickles, onions, celery, or chopped ferments for a more flavorful dish.

12 Hard-Boiled Eggs, peeled
⅓ cup (75 g) Homemade
   Mayonnaise
1 tablespoon Dijon mustard
¼ teaspoon salt

Place the eggs into a medium-sized bowl and mash using a potato masher or fork.

Add the remaining ingredients and continue to mash and mix until you've achieved your desired consistency.

Serve immediately.

Make It a Meal: Serve on Plantain Sandwich Bread along with lettuce and tomato for a traditional sandwich, over an Everyday Salad with Fresh Basil and Garlic Balsamic Vinaigrette for a nutritious lunch, or simply as a dip for sliced cucumbers as a quick snack.

hard-boiled eggs

active minutes   *total time*   *week*

Fresh Hard-Boiled Eggs can be difficult to peel, but the pressure cooker method completely eliminates this problem. It's by far my preferred method! Hard-Boiled Eggs are great for snacks, in recipes like Deviled Eggs and Simple Egg Salad, or even for a quick on-the-go breakfast. They're quick, versatile, and packed with healthy fats, proteins, and other necessary nutrients. Finding a local source for fresh, pastured eggs is the absolute best choice since you can talk with the farmer about their methods to guarantee the chickens have not been fed GMO grains. Organic is always best, but I fervently avoid GMOs.

Desired number of eggs
(see *Batch Cooking and Leftovers* below)
Water, enough to cover the eggs, or 1 cup (235 ml) (pressure cooker method)

STOVETOP INSTRUCTIONS

Place the eggs in a pot and cover them completely with cool water. Place a lid on the pot and heat the pot on high. Bring the water to a boil, allow it to boil for 1 minute, turn off the heat, and allow the eggs to sit in the hot water for 10 minutes covered.

Transfer the eggs to a bowl fill with cold water. Allow the eggs to sit in the water to cool for about 5 minutes.

ELECTRIC PRESSURE COOKER INSTRUCTIONS

Pour 1 cup (235 ml) cool water into the bottom of the pressure cooker. Place the rack into the pressure cooker insert and gently line the rack with your desired number of eggs. Secure the lid and cook on high pressure for 5 minutes.

Release the pressure when the cooking time is complete and immediately transfer the eggs to a bowl filled with cold water. Allow the eggs to sit in the water to cool for about 5 minutes.

Batch Cooking and Leftovers: Works well in large batches—I prepare 12–18 Hard-Boiled Eggs at a time. Try peeling the eggs as soon as they're done cooking to make a grab-and-go salad topping or snack.

Eggs can be stored in their shells in the refrigerator for up to 10 days, or out of the shells for about 5 days.

bacon liver pâté

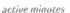

active minutes	total time	servings	days	months
20	20m	20	5	2

Organ meats are some of the most nutritious foods in existence, but their palatability can be a challenge. Liver has unmatched concentrations and bioavailability of iron, vitamin A, and various other nutrients that are important factors in building a healthy immune response. Bacon Liver Pâté was born from my dislike of yet strong desire to tolerate liver on a regular basis. My goal was to enhance my family's immune response, especially during cold and flu season. I've applied the "just add bacon" tactic to this pâté to produce a creamy spread that I can thankfully enjoy (and feed to my children) on a regular basis. If you don't like liver, but want to make it part of your diet, this recipe is for you. If you love liver, you're in luck because this recipe is also for you.

8 ounces (225 g) bacon, chopped

1 large onion, sliced

3 cloves garlic, roughly chopped

⅓ cup (80 ml) dry white wine

1 pound (445 g) grass-fed beef
  liver, roughly chopped

1 teaspoon dried rosemary

1 teaspoon tarragon

½ teaspoon salt

2–4 tablespoons water

Heat a large pan over medium heat and sauté the bacon along with the onion and garlic until the onion begins to turn translucent and the bacon has released most of its fat.

Pour in the white wine, bring the mixture back to a simmer, and add in the remaining ingredients except the water.

Continue to sauté the mixture until the liver is completely cooked through, 6–10 minutes depending on the size of your pieces.

Remove the pan from the heat and place the meat-and-onion mixture into a high-powered blender. Blend the mixture on high, pressing it down into the blades till a creamy consistency is reached. You may need to add water 1 tablespoon at a time till you reach a consistency that can be blended. Add as little water as possible.

Serve immediately.

Batch Cooking and Leftovers: The recipe yields a lot; I divide the pâté into four containers and freeze three, eating only one immediately.

Make It a Meal: This is one of the few instances in which I break out a box of acceptable grain-free crackers made from almond flour or cassava flour. I then add olives, sliced raw vegetables, and fresh fruit to make a small yet satisfying meal.

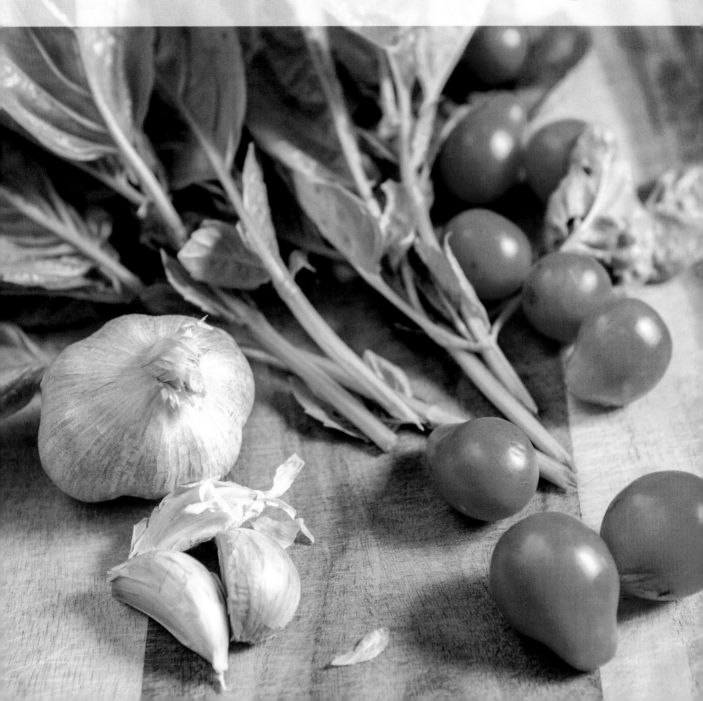

sauces, dips, and dressings

italian dressing

active minutes   *total time*   *cup (235 ml)*   *months*   *months*

Italian dressing is one of the easiest dressings to make, and your homemade version will boast flavors more delightful and refreshing than any store-bought brand. Use it as a marinade for vegetables before you throw them on the grill or in the oven, or use it as a simple topping for any salad. The oil will harden if stored in the refrigerator, which is why I store it on the countertop. If you do choose to store in the refrigerator (or even the freezer), it takes about an hour, sometimes more, at room temperature for the oil to liquefy again.

½ cup (120 ml) olive oil
¼ cup (60 ml) white vinegar
2 tablespoons apple
    cider vinegar
2 tablespoons water
1 tablespoon lemon juice
1 teaspoon garlic powder
1 teaspoon dried parsley
¾ teaspoon dried basil
½ teaspoon dried oregano
½ teaspoon salt

Combine all the ingredients in a jar that seals tight, and shake well to combine. Can be stored at room temperature for 2 weeks.

Batch Cooking and Leftovers: I almost always double (or triple) the recipe as prep for future meals. You could even make enough dressing for an entire year in one prep session using a number of small jars with lids, and store in the freezer.

Make It a Meal: Homemade dressings are what make an Everyday Salad truly tasty. Serve a dressed salad with The Tuna Salad Upgrade, Dilly Beans, and diced avocado.

From left to right: Red Wine Lemon Vinaigrette, Italian Dressing, and Fresh Basil and Garlic Balsamic Vinaigrette.

red wine lemon vinaigrette

active minutes   total time   cup (235 ml)   2 months   12 months

This simple salad dressing is as diverse as it is easy to prepare. The use of common ingredients ensures that you'll almost always be prepared to throw this together in a pinch. Pour this dressing over an Everyday Salad or your favorite Roasted Non-Starchy Vegetables. Try adding fresh herbs such as dill or parsley for additional flavor.

½ cup (120 ml) olive oil
¼ cup (60 ml) red wine vinegar
2 tablespoons fresh lemon juice
2 tablespoons raw apple
  cider vinegar
1 tablespoon coarse
  ground mustard
1 clove garlic, minced
½ teaspoon salt

Combine all the ingredients in a jar that seals tight, and shake well to combine. Can be stored at room temperature for 2 weeks.

Make It a Meal: Use this dressing to drizzle over Roasted Cabbage Wedges to replace the Tahini-Miso Sauce. Serve the dressed cabbage with Coconut and Cinnamon Sweet Potato Mash and Herb-Encrusted Drumsticks.

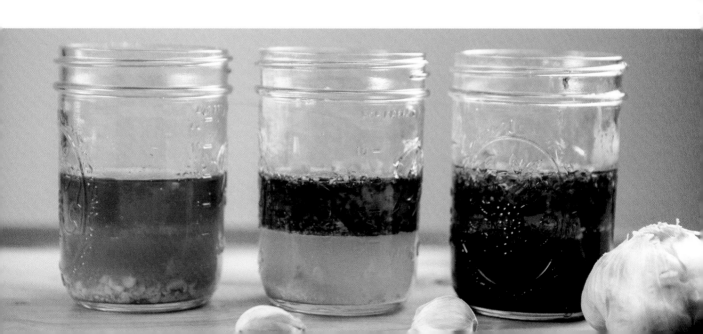

fresh basil and garlic balsamic vinaigrette

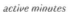
active minutes

total time

cup (235 ml)

months

months

Basil and balsamic create a rich and sweet addition to any salad. This is by far my kids' favorite salad dressing! I've used varying types of balsamic vinegar to create the dressing. I suggest a thicker vinegar, almost as if it has been reduced, because it results in a dressing that seems to smother and stick to whatever vegetables you've chosen to dress. Making large batches of this dressing in the summer when basil is readily available ensures that you're using quality ingredients. Dressings store well over the course of months, making them an excellent food to prep in bulk for freezing when fresh ingredients are in season.

½ cup (120 ml) balsamic vinegar (see note above)
½ cup (120 ml) organic olive oil
¼ cup (5 g) minced fresh basil
1 clove garlic, minced
½ teaspoon salt

Combine all the ingredients in a jar that seals tight, and shake to combine. Can be stored at room temperature for 2 weeks.

Make It a Meal: Use this dressing on an Everyday Salad made from shaved fennel, grated beets, and diced oranges for a unique summer salad. Serve it with Grilled Zucchini and Yellow Squash and Herbed Beef Burgers.

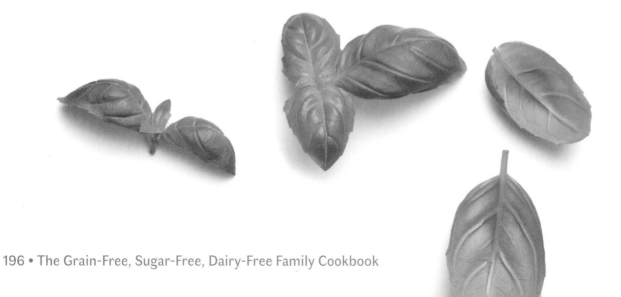

tahini-miso sauce

active minutes   total time   servings   months

This flavorful sauce really packs a punch and is perfect for dishes that might otherwise taste bland. This thick, creamy sauce adheres to most any food and is absolutely delicious paired with steamed or roasted vegetables. Miso is made from a variety of beans including black beans, soybeans, mung beans, and even garbanzo beans. This fermented condiment, which originates from Japan, can be found in the refrigerator section of your local co-op or health food store. The strong, pungent flavor of miso can be overpowering by itself, but small quantities mixed into sauces and soups add a distinct and delightful twist to everyday meals. You can use half a clove of minced fresh garlic in the place of garlic powder for a fresh flavor.

½ cup (130 g) tahini
2 tablespoons water
1½ tablespoons coconut aminos
1 tablespoon white vinegar
1 tablespoon miso
½ teaspoon garlic powder
¼ teaspoon salt

Combine all the ingredients in a bowl and whisk together using a fork or a whisk until completely smooth.

Serve the sauce over the top of most any dish (see *Batch Cooking and Leftovers* below for suggestions).

Batch Cooking and Leftovers: Consider preparing a double batch of Tahini-Miso Sauce for storage in the refrigerator as a quick condiment since the sauce keeps for such a long period of time. Roasted Cabbage Wedges are the suggested meal for serving with this sauce, but it could be used with any other dish that needs a flavor upgrade.

Make It a Meal: Prepare Turmeric-Ginger Baked Chicken with Garlicky Greens smothered in Tahini-Miso Sauce. Serve it with a side of Coconut Lime Cauliflower Rice or over a bed of Simple Spaghetti Squash.

chimichurri sauce

active minutes

total time

servings

week

months

Chimichurri is a light, yet densely flavored Argentinian sauce made primarily from fresh herbs and garlic. I adore this recipe over Mexican Shredded Beef or Pulled Mojo Chicken for its bright flavor and colorful accent. Be sure to use a quality organic olive oil when preparing this dish to enhance the nutrient (and flavor) profile. Herbs are a concentrated source of vitamins and minerals, which makes this sauce a nutritious topping for your favorite Mexican dish.

1 bunch flat-leaf parsley, roughly chopped

½ bunch cilantro, roughly chopped

½ cup (120 ml) olive oil

2 tablespoons (30 ml) raw apple cider vinegar or red wine vinegar

1 lemon, juiced

2 cloves garlic, roughly chopped

½ teaspoon cumin powder

½ teaspoon salt

Blend all the ingredients together in a blender or food processor until the herbs are mostly smooth and finely chopped.

Batch Cooking and Leftovers: I always prepare a double, sometimes triple batch of this sauce since it freezes so easily. You'll need to reduce the amount of lemon juice and garlic if quadrupling the recipe.

Tips on Freezing Leftovers: Use an ice cube tray to freeze the sauce in individual servings and transfer the frozen cubes to a Ziploc freezer bag for long-term storage, or put leftovers into a quart-sized freezer bag, place the bag on the counter, and use your hands to smooth the sauce flat, pushing out any air in the process. Freeze the bag flat because it will be easier to store this way. I opt for the flat-bag freezing method since I reuse the entire contents within a week.

Make It a Meal: Serve over Mexican Shredded Beef, Coconut Lime Cauliflower Rice, and a side of Plantain Tortillas.

From left to right: Pico de Gallo, Garlicky Guacamole, and Chimichurri Sauce.

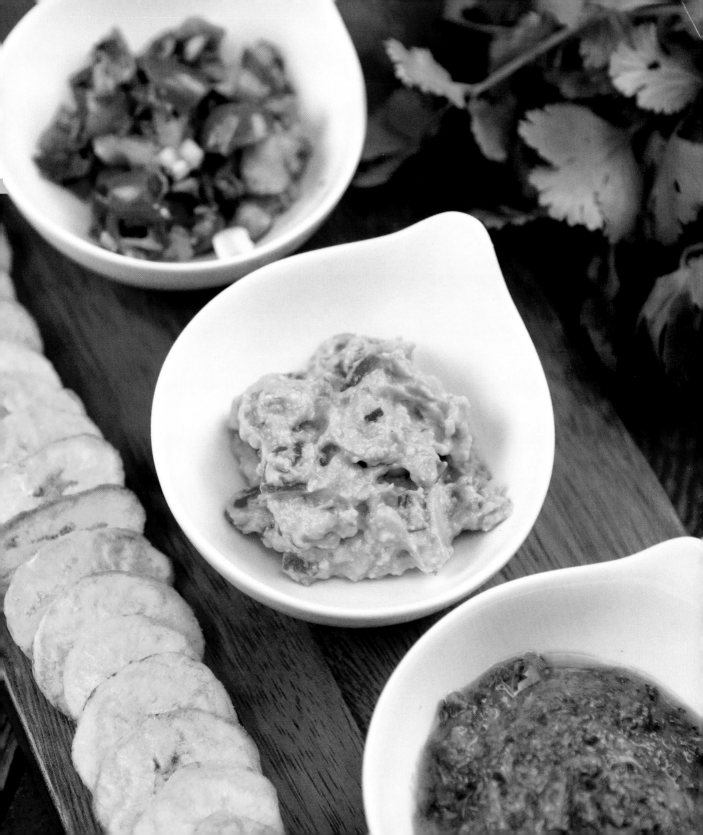

thai peanut sauce

| 10 active minutes | 10m total time | 8 servings | 2 weeks | 2 months |

Introducing this sweet sauce to a meal will make your eaters believe you have culinary skills beyond what is expected of a home cook. Most peanut sauce recipes use brown sugar or honey, but a similar effect is accomplished using naturally sweet coconut aminos. The sauce is creamy, sweet, and boasts vibrant undertones from garlic, lime, and ginger, making it an excellent choice when you're craving a sweet and savory dish. Peanuts are a crop that can be heavily sprayed with pesticides. I therefore recommend buying organic peanut butter with just two ingredients: peanuts and salt. Manufacturers squeeze all sorts of ingredients into peanut butter, especially sugar, so be sure you're buying a brand that's free of added sugar and oils.

½ cup (135 g) peanut butter
  (see note above)
⅓ cup (80 ml) water
2 tablespoons coconut aminos
1 lime, juiced
2 teaspoons grated ginger
1 clove garlic, minced
Salt, to taste

Combine all the ingredients in a shallow bowl and whisk together using a fork or a whisk until the sauce is thick and creamy.

Serve the sauce over most any dish (see *Batch Cooking and Leftovers* below for suggestions).

Batch Cooking and Leftovers: Leftover sauce can be stored in the refrigerator for up to 2 weeks or in the freezer for up to 2 months. Use leftovers to dress Simple Spaghetti Squash or Simple Whole Roasted Chicken, or use to add flavor to Coconut and Cinnamon Sweet Potato Mash or Coconut Lime Cauliflower Rice. If you enjoy the diversity and flavor of this sauce, you can prepare a double or even triple batch and store leftovers in the refrigerator or freezer for use at a later date.

Make It a Meal: This sauce is great with Bok Choy and Red Peppers and OMGrain-Free Chicken Tenders. You can pair these dishes with a bowl of Creamy Carrot Ginger Soup for a more filling meal.

simple vegan pesto

active minutes

total time

servings

days

months

Pesto is such a versatile sauce to have on hand since fresh basil and garlic instantly elevate most any dish—Vegetable Egg Scramble with Avocado and Salsa, Simple Spaghetti Squash, Roasted Non-Starchy Vegetables, or Grilled Chicken Breasts with Basil and Thyme. The simplicity of this sauce and its versatile nature make it an essential for every home cook! The early months of summer are a good time of year to consider prepping batches of fresh pesto to be frozen for use during the winter months. Fresh basil is an abundant and readily available ingredient from your home garden or local farmers market. Take advantage of this bounty!

1 cup (50 g) packed fresh
  basil leaves
¼ cup (32 g) pine nuts
¼ cup (60 ml) olive oil
1½–2 teaspoons fresh
  lemon juice
1 clove garlic, roughly chopped
¼ teaspoon salt

Combine all the ingredients in a food processor or blender and process until mostly smooth.

Batch Cooking and Leftovers: Leftover pesto will brown where exposed to air, but is fine to eat. Can be easily frozen into individual servings using an ice cube tray or quart-sized Ziploc bag (See the Chimichurri Sauce recipe for instructions.). You can easily double this recipe, but you'll need to reduce the amount of garlic if tripling or quadrupling.

Make It a Meal: Use to prepare Greek-style "Pasta" Bowls or as a topping for a fried egg with a tomato slice served over Hearty Almond Flour Bread for a high-fat, low-carb breakfast.

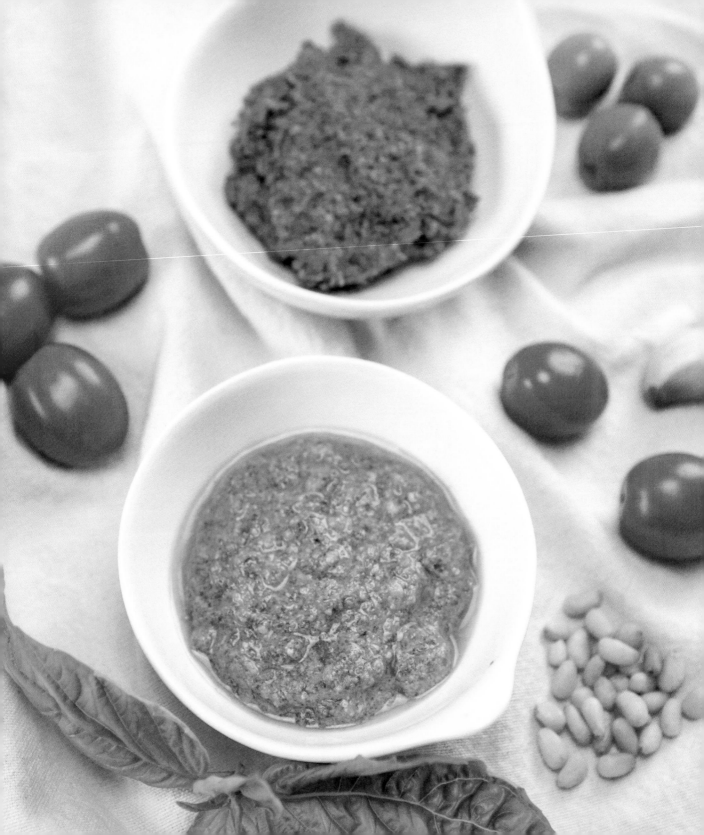

sun-dried tomato tapenade

active minutes	total time	servings	weeks	months
10	10m	12–15	2	6

If you enjoy olives then you will absolutely love this savory topping. The distinct sweetness of sun-dried tomatoes brings out the tart goodness of an assortment of olives and capers to create a topping that is both refreshing and bold. It's so good that I eat it by the spoonful! Tapenade is packed full of healthy fats that keep you feeling full longer, making it an excellent candidate for adding to breakfast foods like scrambled eggs or frittatas. Don't limit your use of tapenade to lunch and dinners, because it can be used in so many other ways! If you're not working with a good blender or food processor, you may need to soak the sun-dried tomatoes in water for a few hours before making this tapenade.

9 sun-dried tomato halves

½ cup (120 ml) olive oil

¾ cup (100 g) pitted and drained kalamata olives

½ cup (65 g) pitted and drained green olives

2 tablespoons capers

1 cup (50 g) roughly chopped parsley, packed

1 clove garlic, roughly chopped

Combine all the ingredients in a food processor or blender and process until you reach a consistency similar to a finely blended salsa. Some small chunks are to be expected, but all ingredients should be finely minced.

Batch Cooking and Leftovers: I suggest preparing a double batch of this recipe and dividing it among three separate jars—one for immediate use and two for freezing.

Leftovers can be repurposed to flavor many dishes including Greek-style "Pasta" Bowls, Eat Your Greens Frittata, Grilled Chicken Breasts with Basil and Thyme, on a sandwich made from Plantain Sandwich Bread, or as a topping for an Everyday Salad.

Make It a Meal: Prepare a Simple Spaghetti Squash and top it with Sun-Dried Tomato Tapenade, Simple Vegan Pesto, and leftover Simple Whole Roasted Chicken.

Sun-Dried Tomato Tapenade
and Simple Vegan Pesto.

fiesta sunflower seed hummus

      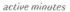

active minutes · total time* · servings · week

Not everyone can easily tolerate beans, which is why I've included this delicious hummus substitute made from 100 percent raw ingredients. This recipe is quick, easy, and makes more than enough hummus to serve on salads, as a dip, or simply by the spoonful! Cumin, garlic, and chili powder combine to create a flavor similar to your favorite taco seasoning, but without the added fillers. See *Soaking Seeds and Beans* (page 14) for information on the benefits of soaking for enhanced digestibility.

2 cups (290 g) raw sunflower
  seeds, soaked overnight
8 sun-dried tomato halves,
  soaked overnight
1 clove garlic, minced
2 tablespoons (30 ml) olive oil
⅓ yellow pepper, diced
⅛ white onion, diced
1 teaspoon chili powder
¾ teaspoon cumin powder
1¼ teaspoons salt
2 lemons, juiced
Water, to create desired
  consistency
¼ bunch fresh cilantro, minced

* plus 1 day for soaking

Soak the sunflower seeds and sun-dried tomatoes in separate jars overnight. (This prevents the sunflower seeds from taking on a burnt orange color from the tomatoes.) Strain both ingredients through a colander and rinse.

Place the sunflower seeds, sun-dried tomatoes, and garlic into a food processor or blender and process until the mixture is creamy, about 4 minutes. You may have to keep scraping down the sides with a rubber spatula to get a uniform texture or add your olive oil if it's simply too thick. Waiting to add the oil helps to better pulverize the sunflower seeds into a paste.

Add all the remaining ingredients except for the cilantro and process again until well combined and creamy, about 4 minutes more. Add the cilantro and process just long enough to mix the cilantro throughout. Do not overprocess or it will change the color and flavor of the hummus. You can even mix the cilantro in by hand if you're concerned about overprocessing.

The hummus is best if chilled for about an hour before serving, but can be served immediately.

Batch Cooking and Leftovers: Leftovers don't freeze well. Halve the recipe if hummus isn't a family favorite.

Make It a Meal: Serve for dipping with raw sliced cucumbers, carrot sticks, and red peppers.

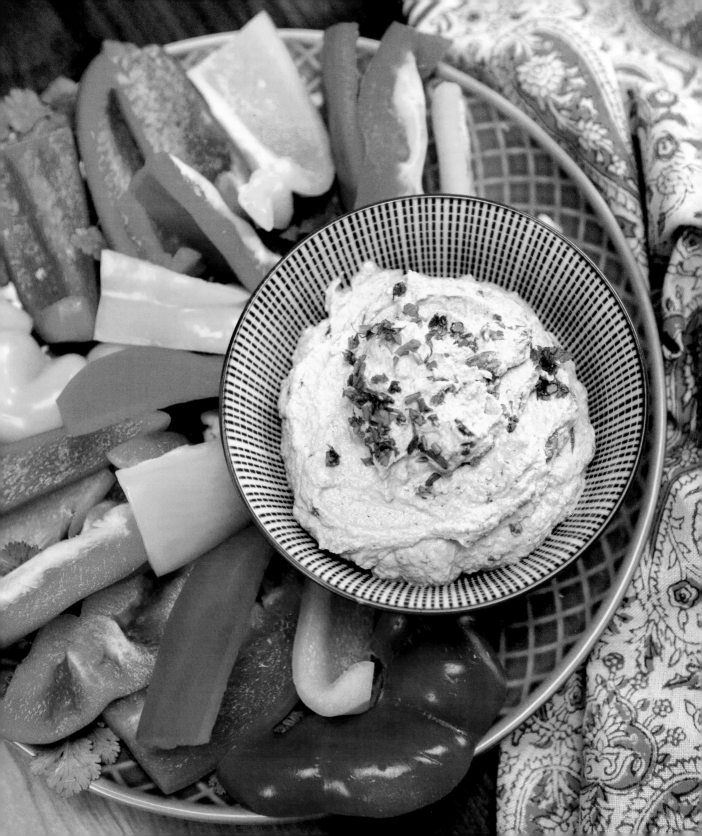

garlicky guacamole

active minutes · total time · servings · days

You can buy premade guacamole from a store, but the 10 minutes it takes to prepare homemade, fresh Garlicky Guacamole is totally worth the effort. Plus the flavor is leagues ahead of store-bought varieties. The creamy goodness of this guacamole makes it one of the tastiest and most versatile dips in existence! Try it on salads and proteins, as a dip for vegetables, or as a delicious and filling breakfast condiment. It's hard to go wrong with anything made from avocados. Try adding 2 tablespoons of minced cilantro for additional flavor.

2 ripe avocados
1 lemon, juiced
1 clove garlic, minced
½ cup (85 g) finely diced tomatoes
2 tablespoons finely diced red onion
¼–½ teaspoon salt

Combine the avocado and lemon juice in a bowl and mash it into a paste using a fork.

Add the remaining ingredients to the avocado paste and mix until all ingredients are evenly distributed throughout the guacamole.

Serve immediately.

Batch Cooking and Leftovers: Guacamole will oxidize and turn brown when in contact with air. To prevent browning, cover with Saran Wrap, store along with the pit, or squeeze lemon or lime juice on the surface.

Doubling, tripling, or even quadrupling this recipe for a party can be made easier with the use of a potato masher to work the avocados. Reduce the amount of garlic if quadrupling the recipe.

The tomatoes, garlic, and red onions can be prepped up to 3 days in advance.

Make It a Meal: Serve on an Herbed Beef Burger with Fermented Salsa Fresca and an Everyday Salad with Italian Dressing for a low-carb meal. Add in some Crispy Sweet Potato Fries for the kids or if carbs are not a concern.

pico de gallo

 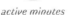

active minutes   *total time*   *servings*   *days*

This fresh salsa is far superior to any of the jarred salsas available in the grocery store. I often prepare this salsa in the summer when tomatoes are fresh off the vine and zingy, cool flavors are just what my body craves. Wait to salt this dish until you're ready to serve it. The salt causes the tomatoes to weep, and you'll have quite a bit of excess liquid if it sits too long. If you salt it earlier, you can just pour off the liquid before serving, if necessary.

2 cups (340 g) finely diced grape tomatoes (about 1 pint)
¼ green pepper, finely diced
¼ small red onion, finely diced
1 small jalapeño, seeds removed, minced
½ bunch cilantro, finely chopped
1 clove garlic, minced
1 lime, juiced
¼ teaspoon salt

Mix all the ingredients together in a medium-sized bowl and serve immediately.

Batch Cooking and Leftovers: This recipe can be easily doubled or tripled. Vegetables can be chopped and refrigerated up to 4 days in advance.

Make It a Meal: Enjoy grain-free taco night made from Plantain Tortillas, Pulled Mojo Chicken, Pico de Gallo, Chimichurri Sauce, and Garlicky Guacamole.

avocado-mango salsa

active minutes   total time   servings   days

Don't underestimate the powerful flavor profile of these simple ingredients. Sometimes less is more, and this salsa is a great example of how you can use a few limited ingredients to brighten up any boring meal. Creamy avocados, sweet mangoes, the ever so slightly pungent crunch of red onions, and the zippiness of lime come together in this tantalizing and colorful salsa.

1 ripe avocado, finely diced
1 mango, finely diced
1 tablespoon minced cilantro
1 tablespoon minced red onion
1 clove garlic, minced
Juice of ½ lime
Pinch of salt

Mix everything together in a medium-sized bowl. Serve immediately.

Batch Cooking and Leftovers: All ingredients (except for the avocado and salt) can be prepped up to 3 days in advance. Save time by preparing a double batch of this salsa to be used for multiple meals.

Make It a Meal: Serve with Coconut Lime Cauliflower Rice and a bowl of Creamy Carrot Ginger Soup.

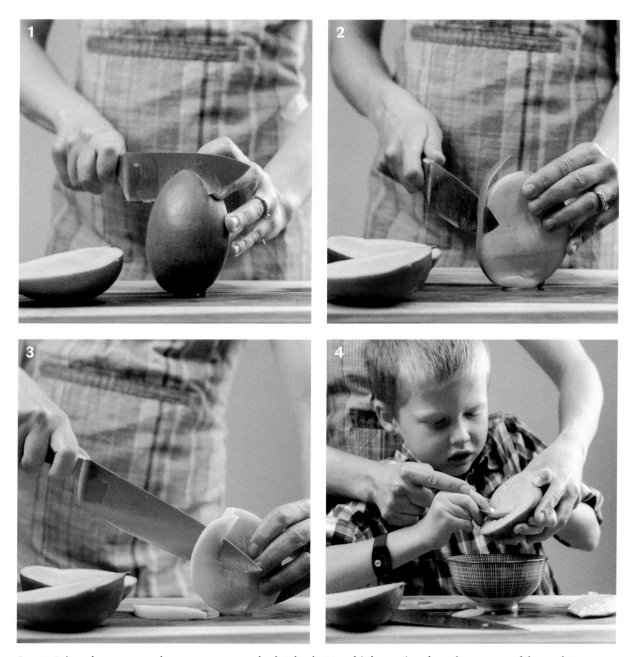

Step 1. Orient the mango so that you can remove both "cheeks." Do this by cutting along the contour of the seed. **Step 2.** Carefully remove the peel from the remaining portion of the mango. **Step 3.** Firmly holding the seed, carefully remove the remaining flesh from around the seed. **Step 4.** Score the mango "cheeks" in a checkerboard pattern, but do not cut through the peel. Scrape out the diced mango cubes with a large spoon.

hearty meat bolognese

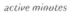

40 active minutes   50m total time   20 servings   1 week   3 months

Jarred or canned pasta sauce most often contains sugar, an addition that is entirely unnecessary. Rather than pay loads of money for organic sugar-free versions, make your own nutritious Bolognese using grass-fed beef from a local farm. You won't have to make this recipe often because it yields a huge quantity of deliciously hearty sauce that holds up well in the freezer. I also love that preparing my own sauce allows me the opportunity to add lots of fresh vegetables. Fresh herbs can be used in the place of dried herbs if you so choose. Fresh tomatoes can be used as well, but you'll need to first simmer and blend the tomatoes into a sauce-like consistency before adding the mixture to your Bolognese.

2 tablespoons cooking fat (lard, reserved fat from cooked meats, or olive oil)

2 onions, diced

1 pound (455 g) mushrooms, diced

3 carrots, diced

2 zucchinis, diced

1 head garlic, minced

2 cans (28 ounces [793 g] each) crushed tomatoes

2 cans (28 ounces [793 g] each) fire-roasted crushed tomatoes

2 tablespoons dried parsley

1½ tablespoons dried basil

1½ tablespoons dried oregano

½ tablespoon dried thyme

1 teaspoon salt, or to taste

2 pounds (910 g) ground beef

Preheat a large pot over medium-high heat, melt the cooking fat in the pot, and sauté the onions for 4–5 minutes. Add in the mushrooms and carrots, and sauté for another 5 minutes. Add in the zucchinis and garlic, and sauté until all the vegetables are soft, about 10 more minutes.

Pour in the canned tomatoes, herbs, and salt, and bring the sauce to a simmer. The amount of salt added depends on whether you're using salted or unsalted canned tomatoes.

Brown the beef in a separate pan while the sauce simmers. Add the cooked beef to the sauce and allow everything to simmer for 10 minutes.

Serve the sauce immediately.

Batch Cooking and Leftovers: This is a great recipe to freeze for future use, since it yields such a large amount. I often divide this recipe into thirds: Two-thirds are frozen in freezer-safe bags, and one-third is eaten immediately.

If you double the recipe for Pecan Parmesan "Cheese" and Simple Spaghetti Squash, it's possible to assemble Italian-style "Pasta" Bowls entirely from the freezer.

Make It a Meal: Serve over lightly sautéed zoodles (see notes in Shrimp Scampi with Tomatoes and Zoodles for instructions), and top the dish with Pecan Parmesan "Cheese." Serve with a side Everyday Salad and Italian Dressing.

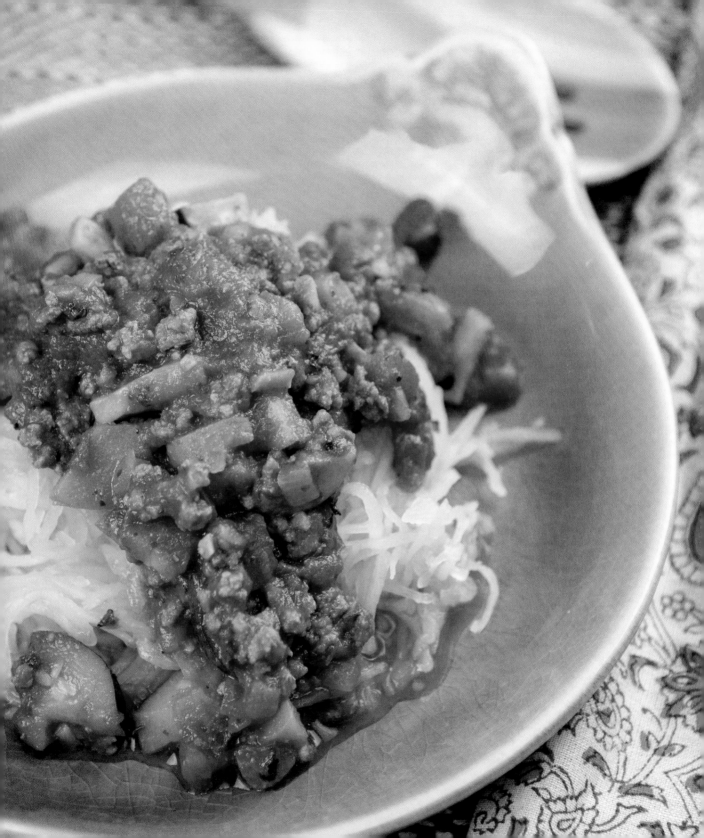

grain-free gravy

active minutes   total time   cups (940 ml)   days   months

I've tried this recipe with a variety of vegetables but none compare to the color and flavor achieved with onions, zucchinis, and celery. Grain-Free Gravy is such a simple and delicious upgrade for any weeknight or holiday meal. The thick, creamy goodness is a much healthier alternative to more traditional gravies made from cornstarch and other unhealthy thickeners.

Simple Whole Roasted Chicken
1 onion, diced
5 stalks celery, diced
2 medium zucchinis, sliced
4 cloves garlic, halved
1 tablespoon cooking oil
  (avocado or olive oil preferred)
1–2 teaspoons salt
½–2 cups (120–470 ml)
  Chicken Stock

Prepare the whole chicken as instructed in Simple Whole Roasted Chicken, and set it into a 9 × 13-inch (23 × 33 cm) baking pan. Set the uncooked chicken aside and prepare the gravy ingredients before placing the chicken into the oven.

Combine the onion, celery, zucchinis, and garlic in a bowl and toss with the oil until all vegetables are evenly coated.

Pack the vegetables into the baking dish alongside the chicken.

Cook the chicken as instructed in the Simple Whole Roasted Chicken recipe.

Remove the pan from the oven and transfer the cooked vegetables to a blender (or a vessel for use with an immersion blender). Carefully transfer the whole chicken to a large plate to cool, and pour the remaining drippings into the blender along with the vegetables. Add your desired amount of salt (start with a teaspoon and add more to adjust) and blend until smooth. Adjust the consistency of the gravy by adding warm Chicken Stock (the stock can be preheated on the stovetop in a small saucepan).

Serve the gravy immediately

Batch Cooking and Leftovers: This recipe makes enough gravy for two whole chickens, but can be used for other gravy-worthy dishes including Sage and Rosemary Sausage Patties.

Freeze leftovers. Be sure to blend the thawed, reheated gravy immediately before serving since some separation can occur after freezing.

Make It a Meal: Serve over a Simple Whole Roasted Chicken, Red and Yellow Rosemary Potatoes, and green beans prepared using the instructions for Roasted Non-Starchy Vegetables.

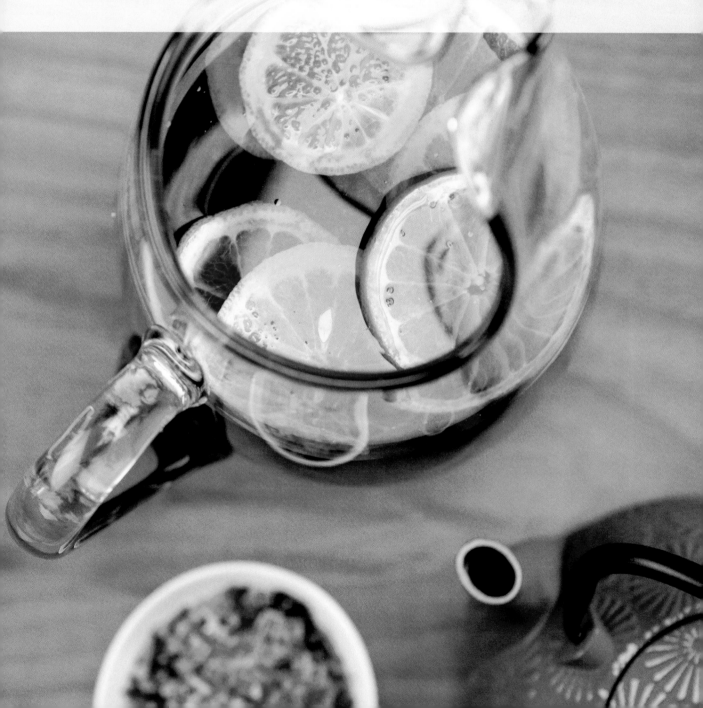

smoothies and other drinks

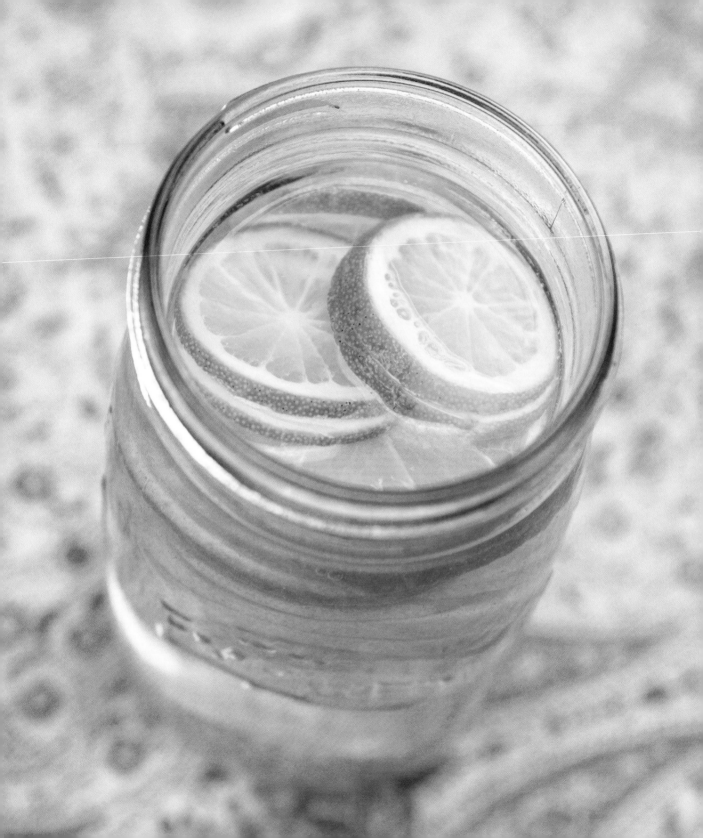

infused water

active minutes	total time	servings	days	
5	1h	4	6	

These refreshing beverages can be served over ice on a hot day as a healthy and refreshing upgrade when you're craving something a bit more flavorful than water. Even better, they can be enjoyed by guests at a party (making a large batch of Infused Water in a large clear glass vessel makes for colorful décor). Try other creative combinations such as rosemary-watermelon, mango-lime, or any other blend that suits your fancy!

CITRUS WATER

½ orange, sliced into thin rounds
½ lemon, sliced into thin rounds
½ lime, slice into thin rounds

RASPBERRY-LIME WATER

1 lime, sliced into thin rounds
1 cup (120 g), raspberries fresh or frozen

PINEAPPLE-MINT WATER

6-inch (15 cm) sprig of mint
1 cup (170 g) diced pineapple, fresh or frozen

BLACKBERRY-SAGE WATER

4 large sage leaves
1 cup (140 g) blackberries, fresh or frozen

IMMUNE-BOOSTING, ANTI-INFLAMMATORY WATER

½ lemon, sliced into thin rounds
1-inch (2.5 cm) piece ginger,
  sliced into thin rounds
1-inch (2.5 cm) piece turmeric,
  sliced intothin rounds

Choose any of the listed flavor combinations. Place the ingredients in the bottom of a ½-gallon-sized (or 2-liter) glass jar. Mash ingredients like berries if using fresh berries (this is not necessary for frozen, which seem to fall apart on their own). Fill the jar with water and allow the water to infuse for about an hour.

Batch Cooking and Leftovers: You can chop your ingredients up to 5 days in advance, which is a time-saver if you plan to heavily rely on flavored waters.

homemade almond milk

active minutes

total time*

cups†

week

months

Homemade almond milk is a quick and easy way to up your health game in the kitchen. Store-bought milk substitutes are full of ingredients including thickeners, flavorings, preservatives, and fortified vitamins and minerals that I'd prefer to avoid. This homemade, creamy goodness contains just two ingredients and takes just minutes to prepare. You can use this recipe to prepare other nut- and seed-based milks such as homemade hemp milk. Sub out the almonds for 1 cup (150 g) hemp hearts or any other nut or seed to achieve the perfect milk substitute.

1 cup (140 g) raw almonds, soaked overnight
2–4 cups (475–945 ml) water, more for soaking

* plus 12–24 hours for soaking
† 475–945 ml

Place the almonds in a jar and cover with water. Allow the almonds to soak overnight. Soaking is optional, but it helps to soften the almonds and improve digestibility. (See *Soaking Seeds and Beans*, page 14.)

Drain and rinse the almonds. (You can skip this step if you didn't soak your almonds.)

Combine the water and almonds in a blender and blend on high for 1–2 minutes or until the almonds become a fine meal. The amount of water you use will determine the thickness of the milk. I tend to try to stretch the almonds a bit further by using more water, but you should use less water if you want a thicker, creamier milk. You'll have to play with the recipe to achieve your preferred consistency.

Pour the contents into a nut milk bag while holding the bag over a large mixing bowl (see Homemade Coconut Milk, page 219). If you don't have a nut milk bag, line a fine-mesh strainer with cheesecloth (or an old, clean T-shirt), hold the strainer over a bowl, and carefully pour the mixture onto the cheesecloth.

Gather the nut milk bag (or four corners of the cheesecloth) and twist to form a ball. Using both hands, squeeze as much liquid from the almonds as possible. The leftover almond pulp can be spread into a thin layer and dried in a dehydrator or in the oven at 250°F (121°C) to make a flour. Alternatively, the wet pulp can be made into crackers.

Pour the milk into a jar and store it in the refrigerator. Contents will settle; shake before serving.

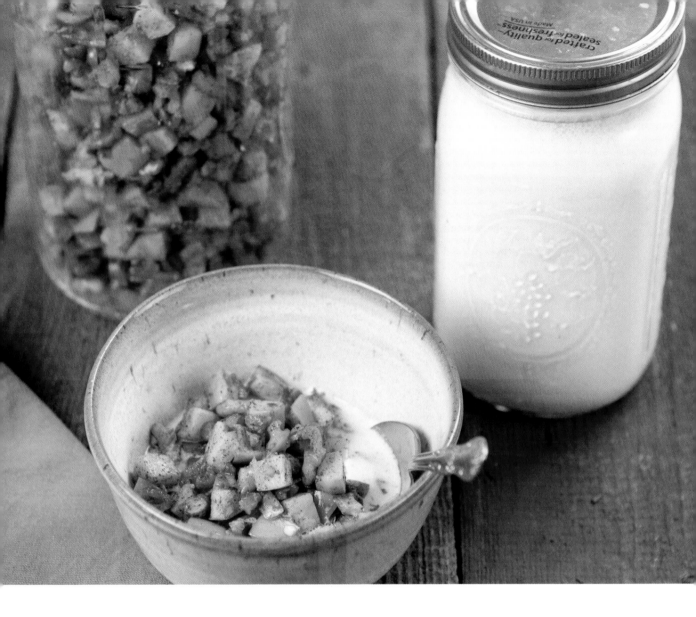

Above, Apple Walnut Crisp Cereal with Homemade Almond Milk.

Batch Cooking and Leftovers: While this freezes well, the amount of freezer space required to store almond milk isn't likely worth the time savings. I would just plan to make a fresh batch each week, unless preparing for a family vacation (where a block of frozen almond milk could help chill other items in your cooler).

You can easily double or even triple the recipe if your family uses a lot of almond milk, but you may have to work in batches since the size of your blender will be a limiting factor.

homemade coconut milk

active minutes

total time

cups (945 ml)

week

This nondairy milk is so delicious that you're going to have to hide it from your kids! It's good enough to drink on its own, but I most often use it for Apple Walnut Crisp Cereal, morning tea or coffee, or soups. It can also make for a delicious warm beverage for the kiddos on a cold or lazy afternoon. This milk is easy, creamy, flavorful, and will be adored by coconut lovers everywhere! Coconut milk is high in fat and will separate in the refrigerator. The effect is more pronounced the longer the milk is refrigerated; the milk can even form a solid layer of fat that floats above the liquid portion. If this happens, place the jar of milk in a warm-water bath till you can once again shake the contents back together.

4 cups (945 ml) warm water

2 cups (225 g) shredded unsweetened coconut

½ teaspoon vanilla extract (optional)

Heat the water on the stovetop until it's warm, but not boiling. Using warm water helps to release the fat from the coconut, creating a creamier milk.

Combine the warm water, coconut, and vanilla extract in a blender and blend for 1 to 2 minutes or until the coconut becomes a fine meal.

Pour the contents into a nut milk bag while holding the bag over a large mixing bowl. If you don't have a nut milk bag, line a fine-mesh strainer with cheesecloth (or an old, clean T-shirt), hold the strainer over a bowl, and carefully pour the mixture onto the cheesecloth.

Gather the nut milk bag (or four corners of the cheesecloth) and twist to form a ball. Using both hands, squeeze as much liquid from the coconut as possible. The leftover coconut pulp can be spread into a thin layer and dried in a dehydrator or in the oven at 250°F (121°C) to make a flour. Alternatively, you can replace half of the coconut flour in the Carrot Cake Applesauce Muffins with leftover wet pulp. The pulp can be stored in the freezer until you're ready to prepare the muffins.

Pour the milk into a glass jar for storage and store it in the refrigerator. Contents will settle; shake before serving.

Batch Cooking and Leftovers: This recipe can be easily doubled, but you may have to work in batches since the size of your blender will be a limiting factor.

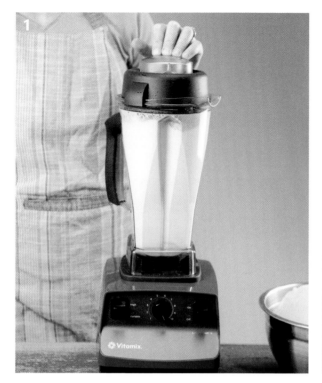

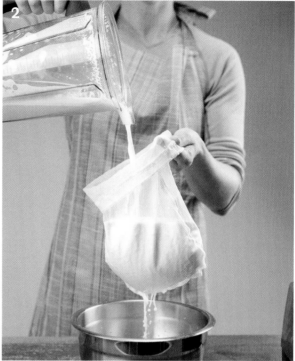

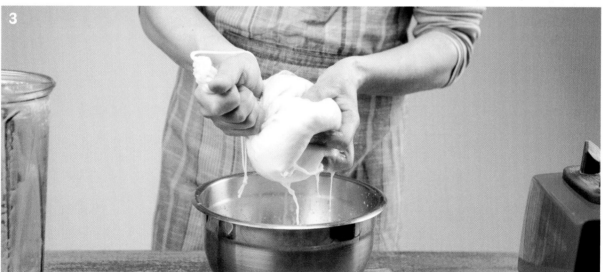

Step 1. Blend the unsweetened shredded coconut with warm water for about a minute or until the coconut becomes a fine meal. **Step 2.** Pour the milk through a nut milk bag over a large mixing bowl. **Step 3.** Squeeze the milk from the bag using two hands.

date-sweetened hot chocolate

active minutes   total time   servings

Store-bought hot chocolate mixes are often made with high-fructose corn syrup and hydrogenated oils. Why would you ever prepare such a thing when you can instead enjoy an amazing cup of guiltless, date-sweetened hot chocolate? I can't think of a more perfect hot beverage to enjoy as a special treat with the kids on a cold day. You can make this into a sweetened coffee beverage as a substitute for sugar-laden coffee drinks. To do so, simply reduce the amount of milk by half and sub in 1 cup (235 ml) of coffee or espresso. Sweetened coffee beverages are a source of unnecessary calories and sugar, and this substitute may help slowly wean you from your morning sugar bomb. Gradually reduce the amount of dates that you add until you can eventually skip the sweetness altogether.

2 cups (475 ml) Homemade Almond Milk

3 tablespoons cacao powder

3 dates, pitted

¼ teaspoon vanilla extract

Combine all the ingredients in a high-powered blender, and blend on high until the beverage reaches your desired temperature. If your blender does not heat foods, you can instead blend the ingredients together and then heat the hot chocolate in the microwave for about 1 minute or in a small saucepan on the stovetop.

Batch Cooking and Leftovers: You can certainly prepare a double batch, but it settles after about 20 minutes, so it's a beverage that you'll want to drink immediately.

sweet-tooth-zapping banana milkshake

active minutes   total time   servings   day   month

Don't underestimate the simplicity of this recipe—it's a quick, sweet, creamy, and perfectly balanced treat for yourself or your kids when you want to satisfy your sweet tooth in a healthy way—a guilty pleasure without the side of guilt! I like to keep a bag of prefrozen banana slices tucked away in the freezer for this milkshake or for quick snacks throughout the week. I'll often buy large bunches of bananas when they're on sale and nearing the end of their life. Not only is this treat easy and delicious, but it's also economical!

2 bananas, sliced and frozen
½ teaspoon cinnamon
½ teaspoon vanilla extract
1½ cups (175 ml) Homemade
  Almond Milk

Combine all the ingredients in a blender. Blend until smooth and creamy. Enjoy immediately.

Batch Cooking and Leftovers: I recommend preparing only the amount that you plan to consume immediately (or follow the instructions in *Freezing Smoothies*, page 222), but you can easily do a double batch.

Be sure to plan ahead for this recipe by freezing peeled and sliced bananas ahead of time.

Make It a Meal: Serve this as an after-school snack along with sugar-free beef jerky made with grass-fed beef.

Freezing Smoothies

Smoothies don't take an exorbitant amount of prep time, but the process can be streamlined by batch prepping and freezing. Start by preparing a double batch of whichever smoothie you prefer (your blender won't likely hold more). Pour the contents into freezer-safe Mason jars. Look on the side of the jar and you'll see a line that states, "for freezing." Only fill the jar to this line, allowing headspace for expansion. Overfilling will cause the jars to break. You can stop after just one batch or continue prepping consecutive batches since the blender is already dirty. Smoothies can be stored in the freezer for up to one month, so prep as many smoothies in one session as you'd like, keeping in mind that freezer space will likely be limited.

Transfer the smoothie to the refrigerator 12 to 24 hours before you want to drink it. It may still be slightly frozen, but it should be ready for drinking after about an hour of sitting at room temperature. If you drink smoothies for breakfast, this would mean transferring the smoothie to the countertop immediately upon waking and drinking it after you've gotten ready for the day. Give it a good shake before drinking. The smoothie will be slightly more watery than before it was frozen, but the flavor still will be excellent and the convenience may be worth the trade-off. You could also try freezing smoothies in kid-sized portions using reusable baby food pouches to send in packed lunches, but you'll have to experiment to see if the smoothie thaws by lunchtime. It can even act as the ice pack to keep foods cool, but the quality of your insulated lunch bag will influence the rate at which the smoothie thaws.

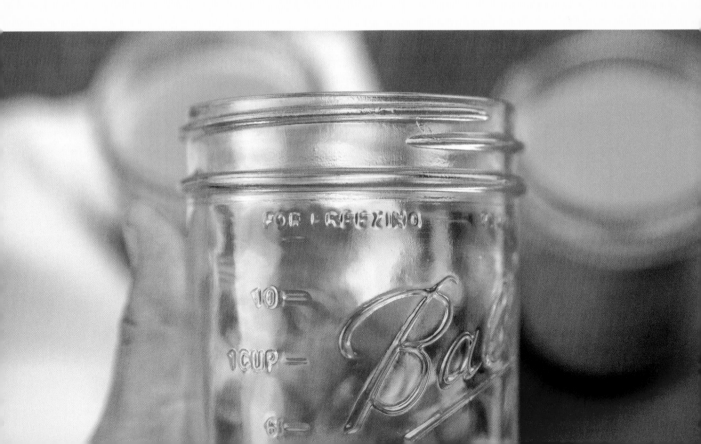

apple cinnamon smoothie

active minutes	total time	servings	day	month
5	5m	2	1	1

I love serving this smoothie when fresh apples become available at the end of the summer. When it's not quite cool enough to turn on the oven, this smoothie does a fabulous job at capturing the essence of fall flavors without the heat from warm foods. This Apple Cinnamon Smoothie can be served warm or chilled. For extra chill, slightly reduce the amount of almond milk and add in a few ice cubes. For a warm smoothie, allow the smoothie to blend in the blender until warm, or briefly heat the smoothie before serving.

2 large handfuls spinach

2 apples, core removed

½ cup (60 g) pecans

2 cups (470 ml) Homemade Almond Milk

1 teaspoon cinnamon

Combine all the ingredients in a blender and blend until completely smooth. Enjoy immediately.

Batch Cooking and Leftovers: Best if consumed immediately (or follow the instructions in *Freezing Smoothies*, page 222).

If preparing in advance, dice and freeze the apples on a parchment paper–lined baking sheet and then transfer the apples to a freezer-safe bag for long-term storage. The apples can then be used to prepare a frozen version of the smoothie. (A good option when apples are in season and you're looking for a preservation method that requires little effort.)

peanut butter and banana smoothie

active minutes   *total time*   *servings*   *day*   *month*

This simple smoothie is a great entry-level green drink for kids. The strong, familiar flavors of banana and peanut butter easily mask the flavor of spinach, making it nearly undetectable. Be sure to take a look at the recipe for the Sweet-Tooth-Zapping Banana Milkshake for some great ideas on prepping ahead.

2 large handfuls spinach
2 bananas, sliced and frozen
4 tablespoons peanut butter
1½ cups (355 ml) Homemade Almond Milk

Combine all the ingredients in a blender and blend until completely smooth. Enjoy immediately.

Batch Cooking and Leftovers: Best consumed immediately (or follow the instructions in *Freezing Smoothies,* page 222).

Be sure to dice and freeze the bananas in advance. (I always have frozen bananas on hand.)

my favorite mango smoothie

| 5 active minutes | 5m total time | 2 servings | 1 day | 1 month |

I absolutely love the flavor of mango combined with just the right amount of sweetness from banana. While I enjoy all of the smoothie recipes in this book, this recipe is by far my favorite. I have even prepared it for a group of preschoolers whose parents were shocked that their child would ever drink such a thing! It's a truly delicious green smoothie.

2 large handfuls spinach
2 cups (240 g) frozen
  diced mango
1 banana
6 tablespoons hemp hearts
2 cups (470 ml) Homemade
  Almond Milk

Place all the ingredients in a blender and blend until completely smooth. Enjoy immediately.

Batch Cooking and Leftovers: Best if consumed immediately (or follow the instructions in *Freezing Smoothies*, page 222).

I most often buy frozen diced mangoes, but you can freeze your own by spreading the diced mango on a parchment paper–lined baking sheet and freezing. See Avocado-Mango Salsa for instructions on how to cut a mango.

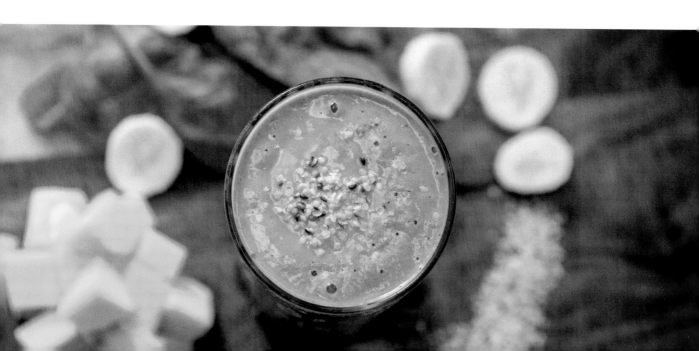

tropical paradise smoothie

  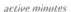

5 active minutes   **5m** total time   **2** servings   **1** day   **1** month

This is a perfectly beautiful green smoothie that captures the bright flavors of a tropical island. Sweet tropical fruits are nicely complemented with tart limes and creamy bananas. Enjoy this smoothie on a hot day when a large, hot meal just doesn't feel appetizing or when you want something cool and refreshing to curb your appetite.

2 small handfuls spinach

4 kale leaves

1 cup (120 g) frozen diced mango

1 cup (170 g) frozen diced
    pineapple

1 banana

2 cups (475 ml) coconut water

2 tablespoons lime juice

Combine all the ingredients in a blender and blend until completely smooth. Enjoy within 2 hours.

Batch Cooking and Leftovers: Best if consumed immediately (or follow the instructions in *Freezing Smoothies*, page 222).

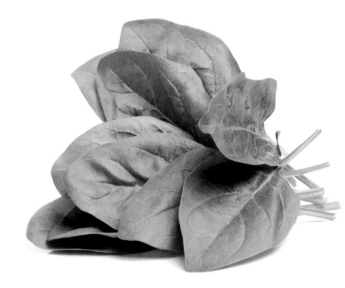

truly green smoothie

active minutes | total time | servings | day | month

You could call this smoothie a "salad in a blender." I absolutely adore the creamy, green goodness of this smoothie. Not only do I love its refreshing savory flavor, but I also instantly feel like I've done something good for my body. Try serving the smoothie with a couple of Hard-Boiled Eggs for a quick, easy, and nutrient-dense meal on a hot summer day. Some people might find the high fiber load in this smoothie to be challenging to digest. If this is the case, omit the water and avocado, blend all of the ingredients (you'll have to keep pushing them down into the blades, but they'll eventually start to blend), and strain the mixture through a nut milk bag or cheesecloth to extract the juice. This technique can be used to juice any of your favorite fruits and vegetables without the use of a juicer. Juices should not be frozen and should be consumed within 24 hours. They'll start to settle, but you just need to give them a good shake before consuming.

2 large handfuls spinach

8 outer romaine leaves, roughly torn into pieces

2 celery stalks, roughly chopped

1 green apple, cored

½ large cucumber, roughly chopped

½ lemon, peeled and seeds removed

½ avocado

1 small piece of white onion (about 2 tablespoons chopped)

Pinch of salt

2 cups (475 ml) water

8 ice cubes

Combine all the ingredients in a blender and blend until completely smooth. Enjoy within 2 hours.

Batch Cooking and Leftovers: Best if consumed immediately (or follow the instructions in *Freezing Smoothies*, page 222).

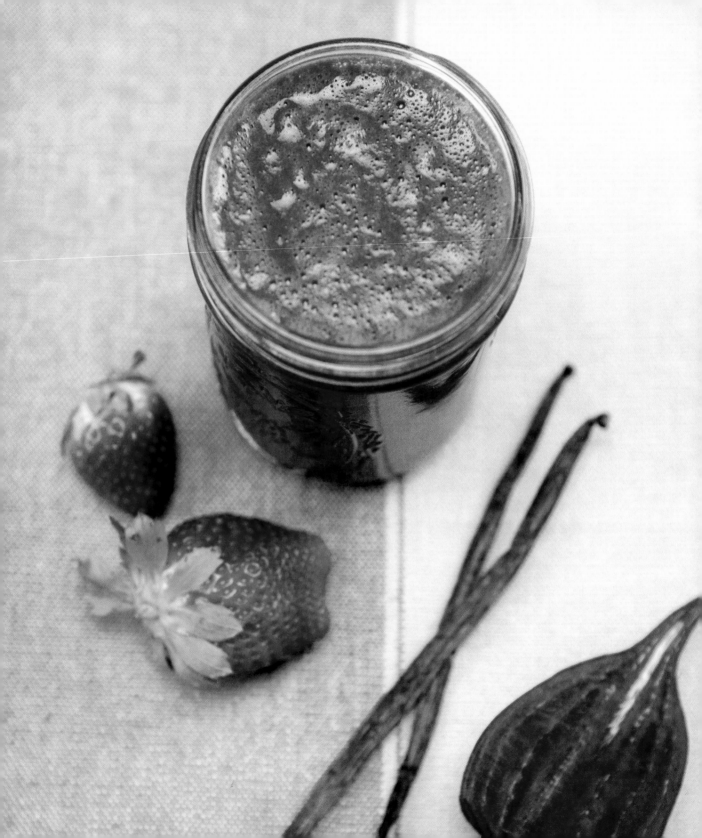

vanilla strawberry beet smoothie

| 5 | 5m | 2 | 1 | 1 |
| active minutes | total time | servings | day | month |

"Beets and strawberries?" you say. Don't knock it until you've tried it! The powerful liver-detoxifying properties of raw beets are subtly paired with refreshing strawberries and hints of vanilla. The high antioxidant content of this deep red smoothie will get a big thank-you from your body's detoxifying mechanisms. It's one of my favorites, given its rich color and powerful health benefits. Try subbing the strawberries with frozen dark sweet cherries and blueberries for a sweeter, darker smoothie.

2 large handfuls spinach

2 small beets, peeled and roughly chopped

2 cups (130 g) frozen strawberries

2 tablespoons hemp hearts

½ teaspoon vanilla extract

Dash of cinnamon

2 cups (475 ml) water

Combine all the ingredients in a blender and blend until completely smooth. Enjoy within 2 hours.

Batch Cooking and Leftovers: Best if consumed immediately (or follow the instructions in *Freezing Smoothies*, page 222).

winter immunity tea

active minutes   *total time*   *cups of tea*

My family frequently drinks this tea going into cold and flu season in the fall and throughout the winter. The mild flavors help to support your immune system in the fight against bacterial and viral infections. As with all herbal remedies, consistency is necessary in order to yield results.

4 tablespoons dried echinacea (best if a mix of roots, stems, and flowers)
3 tablespoons dried rose hips
3 tablespoons dried nettle

Combine all the ingredients in a small jar with a lid and shake until evenly mixed.

Use a tea ball to steep 1 tablespoon of tea mixture in 1 cup (235 ml) of hot water and enjoy. You can use a French press to make a larger quantity of tea at one time. Enjoy daily during cold and flu season or drink up to 3 cups per day when sick.

Batch Cooking and Leftovers: Loose tea can be stored out of direct sunlight for up to a year.

Winter Immunity Tea shown with Tummy Ache Tea and Bedtime Tea.

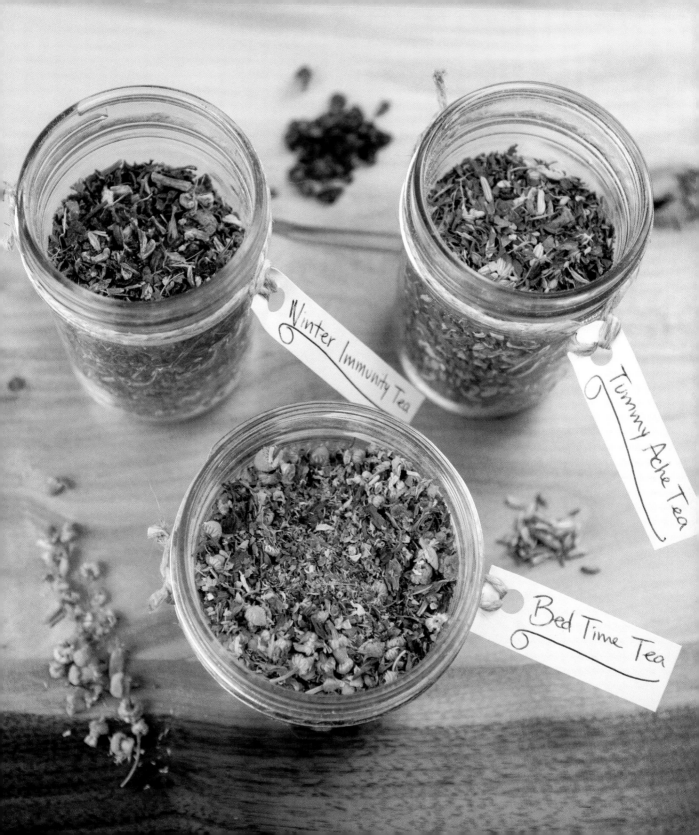

tummy ache tea

5 active minutes   **10m** total time   **11** cups of tea

You don't necessarily have to have a tummy ache to enjoy the soothing benefits of this calming tea. My kids love this tea's glowing warmth when they're not feeling well, but they also like it as an after-dinner drink that helps settle a full stomach before bed. Add a couple of drops of stevia for a lightly sweetened tea.

5 tablespoons dried peppermint
3 tablespoons dried ginger
3 tablespoons fennel seeds

Combine all the ingredients in a small jar with a lid and shake until evenly mixed.

Use a tea ball to steep 1 tablespoon of tea mixture in 1 cup (235 ml) of hot water and enjoy. You can use a French press to make a larger quantity of tea at one time. Enjoy daily or drink up to 3 cups per day when sick.

Batch Cooking and Leftovers: Loose tea can be stored out of direct sunlight for up to a year.

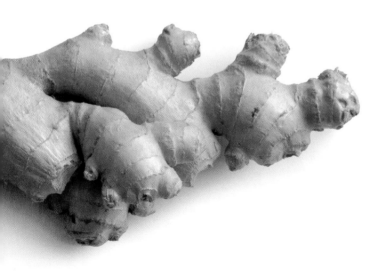

bedtime tea

active minutes
5

total time
10m

cups of tea
11

Having a tea on hand specifically for bedtime can help set the tone for a smooth transition to the bedroom and a good night's rest. The only caveat is that you shouldn't allow your child to drink too much immediately before going to sleep or they might wet the bed! We often enjoy this calming tea about an hour before bedtime. Its fragrant and relaxing essence is the perfect way to close the day. Note that people with ragweed allergies may have a mild allergic response to chamomile.

5 tablespoons dried chamomile

3 tablespoons dried catnip

3 tablespoons dried lemon balm

Combine all the ingredients in a small jar with a lid and shake until evenly mixed.

Use a tea ball to steep 1 tablespoon of tea mixture in 1 cup (235 ml) of hot water and enjoy. You can use a French press to make a larger quantity of tea at one time.

Batch Cooking and Leftovers: Loose tea can be stored out of direct sunlight for up to a year.

hibiscus zinger iced tea

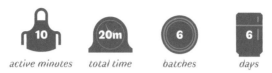

active minutes 10 · total time 20m · batches 6 · days 6

I love the tart, refreshing flavor of zinger teas, but it's nearly impossible to find a store-bought version that doesn't contain added flavoring. Luckily, you can easily make your own! You can drink this as a hot tea, but I prefer to make large batches to enjoy as an ice-cold beverage on a hot day. Shown on page 213.

2 cups (100 g) dried
  hibiscus petals
1¼ cups (95 g) dried orange peel
1 cup (26 g) dried spearmint
1 cup (30 g) dried lemongrass
1 cup (75 g) dried rose hips
Water
Ice

Combine the dried herbs in a ½-gallon-sized (or 2-liter) jar that allows for some headspace at the top. You won't be able to shake your herbs for mixing if they're too tightly packed. Cover the jar with a lid and shake in varying directions until the herbs are evenly distributed throughout. If you don't have a jar large enough, mix the ingredient together in a large bowl and pack the tea into smaller jars (this is also a great idea for holidays gifts).

To make one batch of iced tea (approximately 1 gallon), bring 6 cups (1.5 liters) water to just under a boil.

Place 1 cup (50 g) of dried tea into a ½-gallon-sized jar or bowl and pour the hot water on top. Allow the tea to steep for 10–15 minutes, stirring occasionally.

Fill a gallon-sized (3.8-liter) pitcher or pourable jar two-thirds full of ice. Place a metal fine-mesh strainer over the top of your pitcher or jar and carefully pour the hot tea through the strainer over the ice. Fill the pitcher or jar to the top with cold water or more ice to yield a gallon of iced tea.

Stir the iced tea and serve immediately or store in the refrigerator.

Batch Cooking and Leftovers: Loose tea can be stored out of direct sunlight for up to a year. Once the tea is prepared, it should then be stored for 6 days in the refrigerator as a cold beverage.

If doubling the recipe be sure to use adequately sized containers.

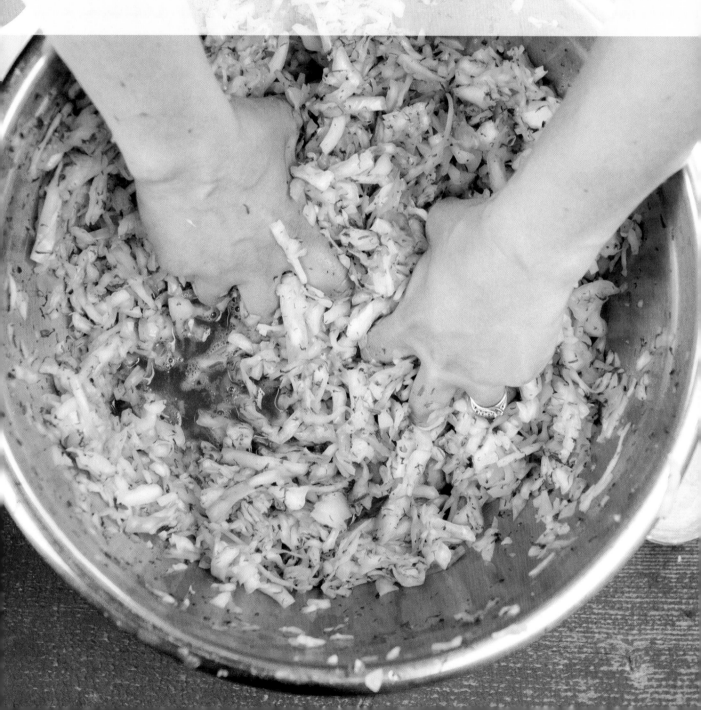

ferments

basic brine

active minutes *total time* *quart (945 ml)* *months*

You can ferment most any vegetable (such as broccoli, cauliflower, peppers, etc.) using brine. I've included recipes for some of my favorites here. Leafy greens like kale, collards, spinach, and cabbage can be fermented using the dry salt method—the method demonstrated in Dill Pickle Kraut (page 242). The process is straightforward: You add salt and massage the greens to release their juices. In other words, leafy greens will create their own brine. But vegetables like carrots, green beans, and cauliflower cannot be massaged in this way and instead require the addition of brine. The key to successfully fermenting any vegetable is making sure the vegetable stays submerged in the brine during fermentation. This prevents the growth of undesirable molds and bacteria, and guarantees proliferation of *Lactobacillus* and other beneficial bacteria and yeasts. I have included a few techniques for mold prevention in these recipes, but using a fermenting weight along with a pickle pipe or air lock is by far the most successful and effective method. You can start fermenting using these recipes, but you can also experiment with your own creations using this simple brine. It's best to avoid using chlorinated water for brines since it may prevent the growth of beneficial bacteria. However, it'll still work if this is all you have. Brine recipes generally call for 1–3 tablespoons of salt per quart (945 ml) of water. I've found that 2 tablespoons of salt creates my preferred saltiness and texture. Adding too little salt results in a mushy vegetable, but adding too much can make your vegetables too salty. Experiment to find your own perfect ratio of salt to water.

2 tablespoons salt
1 quart (945 ml) water

Dissolve the salt in the water and pour the brine over your desired vegetables.

Batch Cooking and Leftovers: Only prepare the amount of brine that you'll need to ferment your desired vegetables.

The recipe can be easily doubled or tripled if preparing large batches of ferments.

fermented salsa fresca

15 *active minutes* **2–3d** *total time* **8–10** *servings* **2** *months*

This salsa is one of the easiest ferments to incorporate into your diet on a regular basis. It's versatile, refreshing, and brings a uniquely delicious and nutritious flavor to your favorite dishes. I most often enjoy this salsa with Garlicky Greens, topped with two or even three fried eggs and some diced avocado for a quick and nutritious breakfast meal. Use this fermented salsa to replace store-bought salsa for any occasion.

3 cups (510 g) diced tomatoes
½ cup (55 g) finely diced onions
¾ cup (85 g) finely diced
  green pepper
2 cloves garlic, minced
Juice from 1 lime
2 teaspoons salt
2 tablespoons minced cilantro

Mix all the ingredients together in a medium-sized bowl. Allow the mixture to sit for about 5 minutes while the tomatoes release some of their juices, creating a brine.

Spoon the vegetables into a quart-sized jar, leaving about 2 inches (5 cm) of headspace at the top of the jar. Leave behind as much liquid as possible since there will be excess. Pack the salsa into the jar and pour in just enough liquid to completely submerge the salsa.

Place a fermenting weight on top of the salsa, if available. Alternatively, you can partially fill a small Ziploc bag with water and use this as a weight instead.

Place a clean towel or cheesecloth around the top of the jar and secure the cloth with a rubber band. You can also use an air lock or pickle pipe if you have one. Lastly, you can use a jar lid, but you will need to "burp" the jar (simply unscrew the lid just enough to release the gases and tighten it when done) every day.

Allow the salsa to sit at room temperature for 2–3 days. Place a tight lid on the salsa when fermentation is complete and transfer it to the refrigerator.

Batch Cooking and Leftovers: Preparing an extremely large batch is a great idea since this salsa is so versatile and seems to easily make its way into many dishes. Increase the amount of garlic to three cloves if doubling the recipe, four cloves if tripling, or five cloves if quadrupling.

Make It a Meal: Serve over Mexican Shredded Beef, shredded romaine lettuce, Garlicky Guacamole, Pico de Gallo, and grilled corn on the cob for a filling and colorful taco salad bowl.

basily carrots

active minutes   total time   servings   months

Basily carrots are the perfect ferment recipe for the novice! These carrots are bright and crunchy, and they have the added benefits of being partially digested by microbes. Carrots are a great snack for kids, so why not increase the nutritional value by fermenting before serving? Your kids will love the unique flavors and their tummies will thank you for the probiotic-rich foods! Be sure to see my note regarding mold (see the Dilly Beans recipe, page 240). I like to use tall, 24-ounce (0.7-liter) jars, because my kids seem to enjoy eating the longer carrots. But you can use any jar you'd like; just cut the carrots to the appropriate size. The great thing about fermenting is that you can even use an old salsa or marinara sauce jar if that's all you have. Try other fresh herbs in the place of basil such as rosemary, tarragon, sage, or any other herb that your family enjoys.

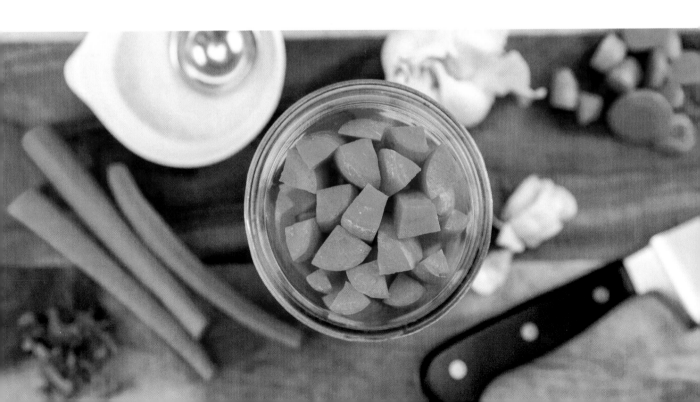

¾–1 pound (340–455 g) carrots,
    washed
5 fresh basil leaves, thinly sliced
1 clove garlic, smashed and peeled
½ recipe for Basic Brine

Cut the carrots into long, thinly sliced or french fry–shaped sticks. Trim the carrot length so that when standing upright in a wide-mouth 24-ounce jar (or whatever sized jar), there is approximately 1½ inches (3.8 cm) of space between the end of the carrot and the top of the jar.

Place the basil and garlic into the bottom of the jar and pack the carrots upright into the jar as tightly as you can. The tighter the carrots, the less likely they'll be able to float when the brine is added.

Pour the brine over top of the carrots, making sure that the carrots are completely submerged.

Place a fermenting weight on top of the carrots, if available. Alternatively, you can partially fill a small Ziploc bag with water and use this as a weight instead. However, the weight isn't necessary as long as your carrots are *very* tightly packed.

Place a clean towel or cheesecloth around the top of the jar and secure the cloth with a rubber band. You can also use an air lock or pickle pipe if you have one. Or you can secure a lid onto the jar, but you will need to "burp" the jar (simply unscrew the lid just enough to release the gases and tighten it when done) every day.

Allow the carrots to sit at room temperature, completely submerged in brine, for 3–5 days. After 3 days, check the flavor of your carrots to decide if you'd like to ferment them any longer. Once your desired flavor has been achieved, remove the cloth, lid, and weight, and store the carrots (with a lid) in the refrigerator.

Batch Cooking and Leftovers: Do not freeze ferments, since freezing will destroy the living yeasts and bacteria responsible for the fermentation process. You can easily double, triple, or even quadruple the recipe to save time in the future and have ferments on hand. Consider mixing and matching your vegetables for a variety of ferments.

Make It a Meal: Put into a lunch box along with Sage and Rosemary Sausage Patties, sliced cucumbers and red peppers, Roasted and Salted Walnuts, and a Chocolate Banana Cupcake.

dilly beans

10 active minutes   5d total time   10 servings   3 months

I used to prepare dilly beans by canning, but I haven't canned a thing (except for applesauce) since discovering ferments! These perfectly crunchy little beans are tangy, garlicky, and have just the right amount of dill. The added nutritional benefits of fermenting compared with canning make it my first choice when storing excess foods from the garden. A small amount of mold can grow on the brine surface at times. Simply scrape the mold from the surface and enjoy your dilly beans. Discoloration of the beans or mold growing on the beans themselves is a sign that something has gone wrong. Mold shouldn't grow if the beans stay submerged in the brine, but if it does happen, toss the beans and start again. See Dill Pickle Kraut (page 242) for information about where you can learn more regarding fermentation safety and troubleshooting.

1 pound (455 g) green beans, washed and trimmed
3 large dill leaves or 1 dill flower head
2 cloves garlic, smashed and peeled
½ teaspoon whole mustard seed
½ recipe for Basic Brine

Trim the green bean length so that when standing upright in a wide-mouth quart-sized jar, there is approximately 1½ inches (3.8 cm) of space between the end of the bean and the top of the jar.

Place the dill, garlic, and mustard into the bottom of the jar and pack the green beans upright into the jar as tightly as you can. The tighter the beans the less likely they'll be able to float when the brine is added.

Pour the brine over the top of the green beans, making sure that the beans are completely submerged. Place a fermenting weight on top of the beans, if available. Alternatively, you can partially fill a small Ziploc bag with water and use this as a weight instead. However, the weight isn't necessary as long as your beans are *very* tightly packed.

Place a clean towel or cheesecloth around the top of the jar and secure the cloth with a rubber band. You can also use an air lock or pickle pipe if you have one. Lastly, you can secure a lid onto the jar, but you will need to "burp" the jar (simply unscrew the lid just enough to release the gases and tighten it when done) every day.

Allow the green beans to sit at room temperature, completely submerged in brine, for 5 days. After 5 days, remove the cloth, lids, and weights, and transfer the beans (with a lid) to the refrigerator.

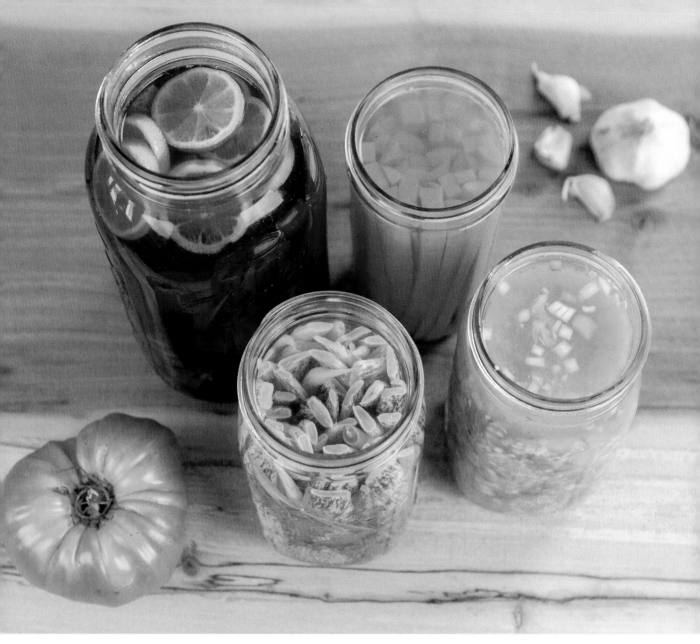

From top left and moving clockwise: Beet Kvass with Lemon, Basily Carrots, Fermented Salsa Fresca, and Dilly Beans.

Make It a Meal: Dilly beans can be eaten whole as a side or snack, or they can be finely chopped and added to salads including an Everyday Salad, The Tuna Salad Upgrade, and Grilled Chicken Salad with Fresh Vegetables.

Serve with Basily Carrots and a handful of Roasted and Salted Walnuts or Deviled Eggs for a great after-school snack.

dill pickle kraut

active minutes   total time   quarts (1.7 kg)   months

There's a reason that flavored krauts have suddenly become popular—they're amazing! I've tried a few different kraut flavors, but dill pickle–flavored kraut is by far my favorite. This versatile condiment elevates the flavor profile of any dish and also provides gut-enhancing microbiota. The microbial population changes over time as the kraut ferments; you can have all of it if you start to eat the kraut as early as 10 days after fermentation begins and continue to let it ferment as you slowly eat away at your creation. To do so, simply remove a large enough portion of the kraut to last for about a week, replace the cabbage leaves, weights, and lid, and allow the fermentation to continue while you enjoy the small sample batch. Some people let krauts ferment for months on end. This is possible with many ferments as long as the vegetable remains submerged in the brine. Exposure to air will cause it to go bad. You can find fermentation troubleshooting information on the North Carolina State Cooperative Extension Home Food Preservation resource page. Look under the Pickles and Fermented Foods section. You can easily find this resource with a Google search.

3½ pounds (1.6 kg) whole cabbage (do not buy preshredded cabbage for ferments)

1–1½ tablespoons salt

4 tablespoons packed, minced dill

1 clove garlic, minced

¾ teaspoon whole mustard seed

You'll need to work with a bowl much larger than you think because you'll be massaging the cabbage, which tends to make a mess. Your equipment needs to be clean, but not sterile.

Remove two large outer leaves from the cabbage, trying to keep them intact, and set them aside (do not shred these leaves). Shred the remaining cabbage using a knife or food processor. Sprinkle salt over the cabbage as you add it to the bowl. Adding salt as you chop allows the salt to start breaking down the cabbage cells and extracting the water to create a brine.

Add the remaining ingredients, mix, taste, adjust the salt if necessary, and allow the cabbage to sit for about 5 minutes to let the salt start removing the juices.

Using clean hands, massage the cabbage with as much force as possible until you've created enough brine to completely cover the cabbage when packed into jars. This process can take up to 10 or 15 minutes depending

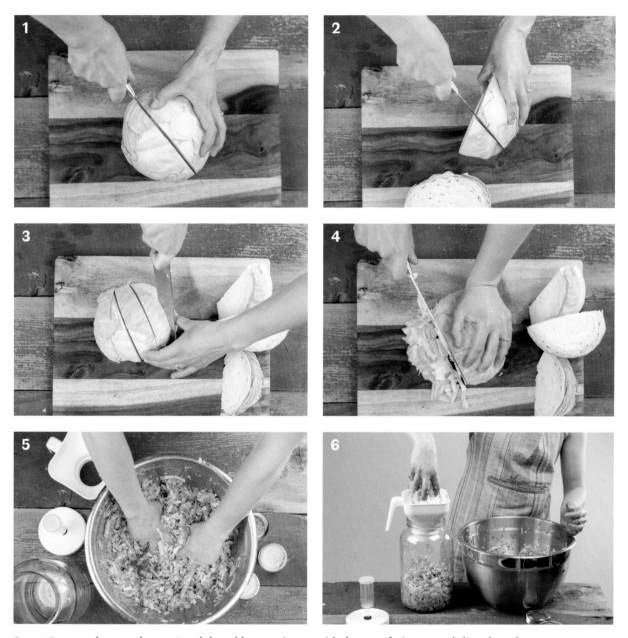

Step 1. Reserve the outer leaves. Stand the cabbage on its top with the stem facing up, and slice along the core to remove about half of the cabbage. **Step 2.** Continue to slice along the core, removing the final wedges. **Step 3.** Cut the cabbage half and wedges into smaller sections before shredding. **Step 4.** Shred the cabbage half and wedges. Salt the shredded cabbage as you add it to the bowl. **Step 5.** Use your hands to massage the juices from the salted cabbage. **Step 6.** Place the cabbage into a large glass jar (I've doubled the recipe and am using a gallon-sized jar in the photo). Use a funnel if available.

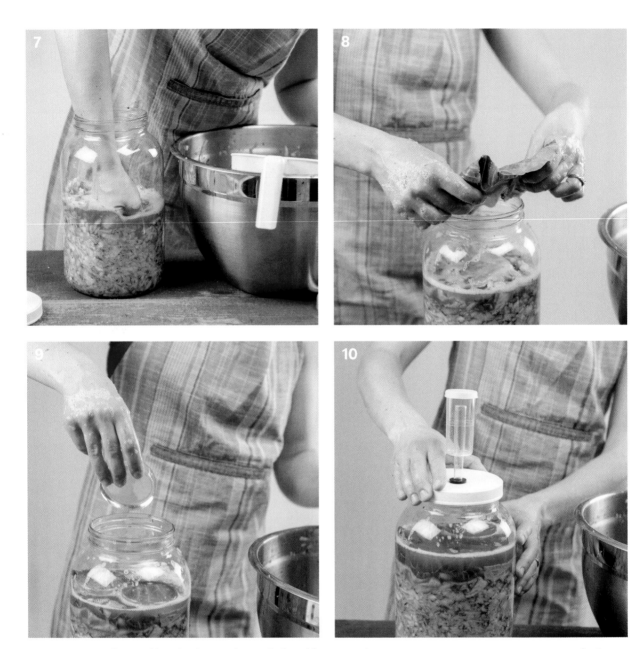

Step 7. Use your fist or a blunt kitchen tool to pack the cabbage into the jar as you go. You want to remove as much air as possible. **Step 8.** Fit the reserved outer cabbage leaves into the jar and place them on top of the shredded cabbage to form a barrier. **Step 9.** Place fermentation weights or a Ziploc bag filled with water on top of the large cabbage leaves to keep everything submerged. **Step 10.** Place an air lock lid on the jar, or secure a clean towel over the top of the jar using a rubber band.

on your efficiency, your technique, and the water content of the cabbage. I find it easiest to place the bowl on the floor and sit above it, allowing me to use my body weight to massage the cabbage.

Using one ½-gallon-sized or two quart-sized jars, tightly pack the cabbage into the jar(s), pressing firmly to remove any air bubbles. Pour the remaining brine over the top of the cabbage so that it's completely submerged.

Neatly fold the reserved cabbage leaves to create a barrier that will prevent the cabbage from floating above the brine. The shape and size of your folded leaf should fit tightly inside the jar, right on top of the kraut.

Place a fermenting weight or small Ziploc bag filled with water directly onto the large cabbage leaf to keep everything weighted down. Be sure to remove any small pieces of cabbage that are stuck to the inside of the jar and exposed to air. Cabbage exposed to air will often mold.

Place an air lock (preferred method) or cheesecloth secured with a rubber band on top of your jar(s). Allow the kraut to sit at room temperature for a minimum of 10 days, but 3 weeks or longer is ideal in order to achieve greater microbial diversity.

If white mold begins to grow on the brine surface, simply remove it as best you can. The kraut is still safe to eat. Remove the whole cabbage leaves, weights, and air lock or cheesecloth, place a lid on the jar, and transfer it to the refrigerator for storage.

Batch Cooking and Leftovers: Once you get comfortable with the kraut-making process, I recommend buying a gallon-sized fermenting jar and doubling this recipe to save time.

Make It a Meal: I use kraut to top most breakfast meals.

Dice a bowl of fresh tomatoes, top it with two fried eggs, Garlicky Guacamole, and Dill Pickle Kraut. Serve the dish with a Carrot Cake Applesauce Muffin or a piece of fruit for a brightly colored, fresh breakfast.

beet kvass with lemon

active minutes

total time

cup (60–120 ml)

months

There's nothing quite like beet kvass to bring out the rich color, powerful liver-supporting antioxidants, and earthy flavor of beets. The flavor of this highly nutritious beverage is perfected with a twist of citrus or the addition of a few slices of fresh ginger before fermenting. You can use whey, sauerkraut juice, or kvass for a starter culture. I initially used juice from Dill Pickle Kraut (which provided a less-than-desirable flavor), but now I reserve the last ¼ cup (60 ml) of kvass for use in the next batch. Kvass will occasionally turn out thick and viscous, a texture created by excess sugars in the beets. The texture will improve slightly after 2–3 weeks of refrigeration but can be avoided by using fewer beets in future batches.

2 teaspoons salt

1½ quarts (1.4 l) water

½ lemon, thinly sliced

¾ pound (340 g) beets,
  tops removed

¼ cup (60 ml) starter liquid
  (see note above)

Dissolve the salt in the water and set aside.

Place the lemon slices at the bottom of a ½-gallon-sized Mason jar.

Dice the beets into ¾- to 1-inch (1.9–2.5 cm) cubes, enough to fill the jar one-third full. Place the beets on top of the lemons and pour the brine over the beets. A few beets will float, but they'll mostly stay on the bottom of the jar.

Cover the kvass with an air lock, or a cheesecloth or towel secured with a rubber band, and allow the kvass to ferment on the countertop for about 3 days. If a film starts to grow, remove it as best you can and allow the kvass to continue fermenting.

Once fermentation is complete, strain the kvass into a large bowl, discard the beets, and pour the kvass into glass jars with plastic lids for refrigeration (metal lids will corrode).

Batch Cooking and Leftovers: Some people recommend that you let kvass age for a couple of weeks before drinking it (I only do this when it has a viscous texture).

Make It a Meal: Serve as an after-dinner drink to aid in digestion, or use it to replace the water in the Truly Green Smoothie.

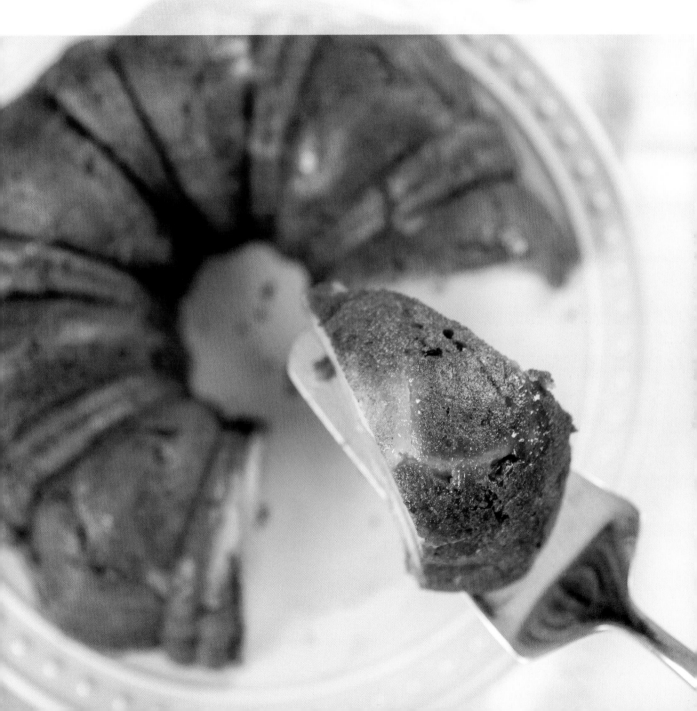

sweet treats

coconut whipped cream

active minutes   total time   servings   weeks

This rich, creamy, fluffy, and just-sweet-enough topping is a wonderful substitute for dairy-based whipped cream. In fact, the additional flavors of vanilla and coconut make it even more delicious! Use this whipped cream as a topping for any of the cakes or pies in this book, or over fruit for a light and nutritious after-dinner dessert.

1 can (13.5 ounces [398 ml]) coconut cream
4 drops stevia extract
½ teaspoon vanilla extract

Place the can of coconut cream into the refrigerator and allow it to chill for at least 8 hours.

Place a glass bowl in the freezer for about 10 minutes before making your whipped cream.

Turn the can of coconut cream upside down and open it from the bottom. Pour out the liquid and reserve this for using in smoothies or cooking. Use a spoon to remove the remaining cream and place it into your chilled bowl.

Use a hand mixer to whip the cream for about 7 minutes, until it appears fluffy and peaks form. You don't have to be as cautious about over-whipping as you do with dairy-based whipping cream. You really can't mess it up unless you don't whip it long enough.

Add the stevia and vanilla, and whip the coconut cream for another 2 minutes. Serve immediately.

Batch Cooking and Leftovers: If stored in the refrigerator, whip the coconut cream for a minute or two before serving. This recipe can be easily doubled.

chocolate icing

active minutes

total time

cups (650 g)

week

months

Unlike other attempts at dairy-free icing, this recipe holds up at room temperature. You may get a bit of melting if temperatures exceed 80°F (27°C), but overall it performs incredibly well. I served it at my son's fifth birthday party on Chocolate Banana Cupcakes and everyone agreed that the rich chocolate and coconut undertones made it the best chocolate icing they'd ever had! You can create beautiful icing toppings using an icing pipe, which you can purchase at most grocery stores. This extra decorative step will give your grain-free desserts a professional and enticing look. You can also use this icing to top Chocolate Walnut Brownies.

1 cup (200 g) coconut oil
1 cup (280 g) pitted Medjool
   dates, packed
1 teaspoon vanilla
⅔ cup (160 ml) almond milk
Pinch salt
⅔ cup (110 g) cacao powder

Combine the coconut oil, dates, vanilla, and almond milk in a high-powered blender. Blend the mixture till it's creamy and very few date pieces remain.

Add the salt and cacao powder and blend the icing again for about 10 seconds or till well combined.

The icing is slightly warm when it comes out of the blender but can be used immediately or stored at room temperature for up to 1 day.

Batch Prepping and Leftovers: Makes enough to ice 24 cupcakes. If pulling from the freezer or fridge, allow the icing to return to room temperature and stir before trying to spread or pipe it onto cupcakes.

chocolate walnut freezer fudge

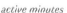

active minutes *total time* *pieces* *months*

10 active minutes · 1h 10m total time · 24 pieces · 3 months

You will *love* everything about this creamy, chocolaty, and perfectly sweet freezer fudge! Walnuts provide a distinct and delicious crunch to a thick and decadent dessert that satisfies the craving of the chocoholic. The fudge becomes too soft at room temperature, so you'll need to serve it with a plate positioned over an ice pack or ice if you're serving it at a party and want to leave it out for guests. Or you can simply walk around with a tray to treat your guests. Either way, I guarantee it won't last long! This recipe is similar to the Chocolate Icing recipe, but the elimination of almond milk and the addition of avocado makes it creamier. Freezer fudge is a good treat to send to school as a replacement food for your child when the other kids in the class are eating processed treats. Speak to the teacher about the possibility of storing the fudge in a freezer and about providing your child with one or two pieces of fudge when the rest of the class is eating a food you'd prefer your child not eat. Your child still gets to enjoy a sweet treat, but it will be in a form that you can feel good about. Don't forget to omit the walnuts if your child's classroom is nut-free. You can instead add sunflower seeds or shredded coconut flakes.

½ cup (100 g) coconut oil, solid (not melted)
½ avocado
½ cup (140 g) pitted Medjool dates, packed
½ teaspoon vanilla
¼ cup (22 g) cacao powder
½ cup (55 g) chopped walnuts

Combine the coconut oil, avocado, dates, and vanilla in a high-powered blender. Blend the mixture until it's creamy and very few date pieces remain. Try not to overblend, as this creates heat and will cause the coconut oil to separate from the rest of the fudge. You can't avoid it entirely, but try to keep blending to a minimum.

Add the cacao powder and blend the fudge again for about 10 seconds or until well combined.

Stir in the walnuts by hand and spread the entire mixture into an inch-thick (2.5 cm) slab on a parchment paper–lined baking sheet. Freeze the fudge for about 1 hour, remove it from the freezer, and slice it into 24 equal-sized pieces.

Serve immediately or return the fudge to the freezer for storage.

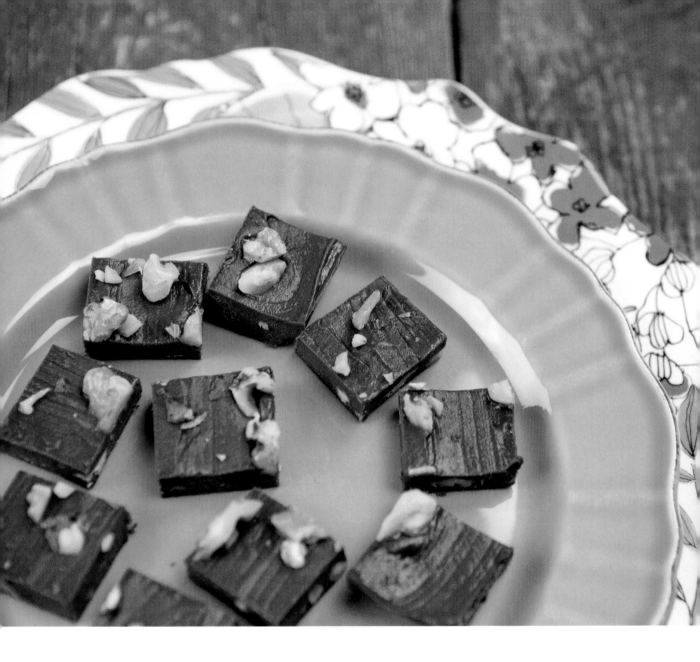

Batch Cooking and Freezing: You can easily double the recipe for a premade treat on special occasions. However, I'm wary of leaving treats around since they're often too tempting. I prefer to prepare this recipe only when there's a special occasion!

chocolate avocado mousse

5	5m	4	3	
active minutes	total time	servings	days	

I've tried varying recipes for chocolate avocado mousse and this recipe is by far the most delicious—it's creamy, sweet, chocolaty, rich, and absolutely decadent. Best of all, it's made from ingredients you can feel good about eating!

½ cup (120 ml) almond milk
7 pitted Medjool dates
¼ teaspoon vanilla extract
2 ripe avocados
2 tablespoons almond butter
  (or SunButter)
⅓ cup (28 g) cacao powder
Pinch of salt

Blend the almond milk, dates, and vanilla extract in a blender or food processor until the dates are blended into the almond milk.

Add in the remaining ingredients and blend till a completely smooth mousse is formed.

Best if chilled for an hour before serving but can be served immediately.

Batch Cooking and Leftovers: You can double this recipe, but work in batches if you're wanting to triple or quadruple it.

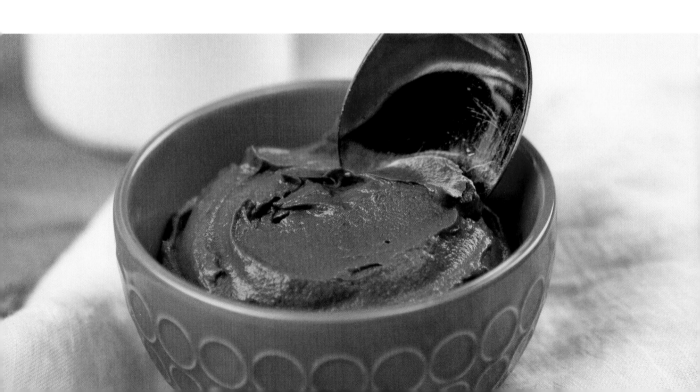

vegan vanilla milkshake

active minutes   *total time*   *servings*

This vanilla milkshake is creamy and sweet enough to convince any nonbeliever that healthier sweet treats can be both nutritious and delicious! Serve this milkshake in a decorative glass with a fun straw and your children won't likely blink an eye at this dairy-free substitute. Dates pack a lot of sugar, but their digestion is slowed by the presence of fiber, making dates an excellent way to sweeten a healthy treat.

¼ cup (36 g) almonds
3 pitted Medjool dates
1 tablespoon unsweetened
  shredded coconut
½ tablespoon chia seeds
1⅓ cups (155 g) ice
⅓ cup (80 ml) almond milk
  or water
¼ teaspoon vanilla extract

Blend all the ingredients together in a high-powered blender until a smooth milkshake is formed. Serve immediately.

Batch Cooking and Leftovers: Work in batches if you want to double the recipe, since this milkshake is challenging to blend.

mango lime ice cream

active minutes   total time   servings

This oh-so-simple dessert is absolutely marvelous! I've prepared it for my kids when they have friends over on hot days and everyone seems to love it. Creamy mangoes and avocado with just a hint of lime is oh so good! I prefer it topped with chopped pecans, but this is an optional addition. Preparing these frozen desserts in a blender feels intimidating once you see the workload required of your machine, but your concerns can be alleviated by first reading the blender's owner's manual for guidance. Dishes like this really put a blender to the test, which is why I suggest you buy good equipment (see *Kitchen Equipment Essentials*, page 45, for more information).

3 cups (360 g) frozen
  diced mangoes

½ ripe avocado

¼ cup (60 ml) almond milk

10 drops stevia

Juice from ½ lime

¼ teaspoon vanilla extract

Pinch of salt

¼ cup (30 g) pecans, chopped
  (optional)

Combine all the ingredients except the pecans in a high-powered blender or food processor until a well-blended frozen dessert forms. Top the ice cream with pecans and serve immediately. Does not store well.

Batch Cooking and Leftovers: Doubling the recipe will overload your blender, so you'll have to work in batches.

creamy fruit pops

active minutes · total time · popcicles · months

This recipe is similar to Mango Lime Ice Cream, yet the use of whole mangoes rather than frozen mangoes, and the resulting consistency, prevents the two from being interchangeable. I've searched high and low for Popsicles that I'd be okay with serving to my kids as a special treat on hot days, and I'm sorry to say that it's much like trying to find a needle in a haystack. Luckily, Popsicle molds aren't very expensive and making your own takes minimal time and effort. Your kids (and their friends) will love that you're serving up delicious and nutritious summer-time treats! Try replacing the dates with 10 drops of stevia to reduce the amount of sugar and carbs.

2 ripe mangoes, peeled and diced

½ ripe avocado

2 pitted Medjool dates (soaked for a minimum of an hour if you don't have a good blender or food processor)

Juice from 1 lime

Pinch of salt

Combine all the ingredients in a blender or food processor and blend until completely smooth and creamy.

Spoon the mixture into six BPA-free Popsicle molds, tapping each mold on the counter to remove any air bubbles. Freeze the Popsicles for a minimum of 2 hours.

Run each Popsicle mold under warm water for 30–45 seconds before trying to pull the frozen Popsicle from the mold. This will prevent you from pulling too hard and accidentally removing the Popsicle stick, leaving the Popsicle stuck in the mold.

Batch Cooking and Leftovers: The recipe can be easily doubled, but you'll need more than just six molds.

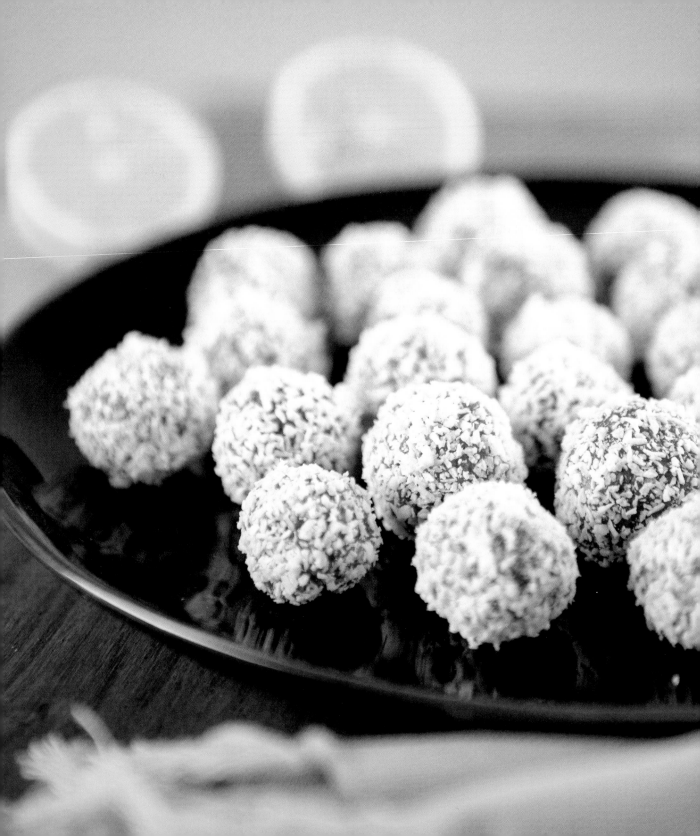

lemon coconut date balls

20	**20m**	**30**	**2**	**3**
active minutes	*total time*	*1-inch* balls*	*weeks*	*months*

These delightful, citrusy little morsels are one of my favorite sweets to serve at Christmastime. If you like lemon bars then you will love this healthy alternative! I also enjoy that this recipe summons participation from even the youngest of kids—almost anyone can roll a paste into a ball and dip it in coconut! Like the Chocolate Walnut Freezer Fudge, this is another great recipe to store at school. Be sure to read my notes in the freezer fudge recipe for more information. Some people like using this recipe as energy bites during exercise to replace bars. You can increase the protein content by adding a few tablespoons of protein powder, and you can form the balls into a different shape, like small bars or squares. Be sure to do some research before purchasing a protein powder since there's a wide range of quality when it comes to sports supplements. Lastly, adding more salt to the recipe can help to replace electrolytes during exercise.

1½ cups (190 g) walnuts

1⅓ cups (375 g) pitted Medjool
   dates, packed

Juice and zest from 1 lemon

⅔ cup (75 g) shredded
   unsweetened coconut, divided

Pinch of salt

* 2.5 cm

Process the walnuts and dates in a food processor until small pieces form. Add in the lemon juice and zest, ⅓ cup (38 g) of the shredded coconut, and the salt, and continue to process until a paste forms and all ingredients are well chopped and combined.

Fill a small dish with water to use to occasionally wet the palms of your hands. Keeping your hands moist while forming the coconut date balls will keep the mixture from sticking to your hands. Roll the mixture into approximately 30, 1-inch-sized (2.5 cm) balls.

Once you've formed all the balls, pour the remaining shredded coconut into a bowl and roll each ball in coconut until it's completely covered.

Chill the coconut date balls for about 1 hour before serving.

Batch Cooking and Leftovers: The recipe can be doubled, but you'll have to work in batches.

nut-free chocolate superfood bites

20 active minutes **20m** total time **30** bites **2** weeks **3** months

My son was allergic to a number of tree nuts when he was a toddler, which proved to be a challenge when trying to find healthy, gluten-free desserts. I decided to instead make my own toddler-friendly dessert by modifying a recipe that originally called for walnuts, dates, and cacao. The walnuts were easy to replace, but I realized that the recipe could be taken a step further by enhancing the antioxidant benefits through added superfoods. Goji berries are an excellent source of vitamin C and are a unique berry in that they contain all eight essential amino acids. In other words, they're a complete protein. Mulberries are a good source of iron and one of my favorite dried berries for their superior taste and texture. Raw cacao is one of nature's best sources of antioxidants, and is an excellent source of iron, magnesium, and even calcium. Maca powder is made from the root of a cruciferous plant and boasts benefits including improved energy and reduced blood pressure; it can also help the body adapt to stress (an adaptogenic herb). As you can see, these bites aren't just designed to taste sweet and chocolaty, they're designed to pack a substantial nutritional punch!

1 cup (280 g) pitted Medjool dates, packed
¼ cup (28 g) dried goji berries
¼ cup (28 g) dried mulberries
½ cup (75 g) sunflower seeds
½ cup (75 g) pumpkin seeds
3 tablespoons raw cacao
1–2 tablespoons water
1 heaping tablespoon maca powder
2 teaspoons vanilla
Pinch of salt
½ cup (55 g) shredded coconut (optional)

Process all the ingredients except the shredded coconut in a food processor until the seeds are in small bits and the dates and dried berries have made a paste.

Fill a small dish with water to occasionally wet the palms of your hands. Keeping your hands slightly moist while forming the bites will keep the mixture from sticking to your hands. Roll the mixture into approximately 30, 1-inch-sized (2.5 cm) balls.

Once you've formed all the balls, pour the shredded coconut into a bowl and roll each ball in coconut until it's completely covered.

Chill the bites for about 1 hour before serving.

Batch Cooking and Leftovers: The recipe can be doubled, but you'll have to work in batches.

chocolate ice cream

active minutes	*total time*	*small portions*	*months*
15	2h 15m	6	2

It's hard to believe that something so simple can be so delicious and visually appealing. While my kids certainly enjoy this ice cream recipe, it's my husband and I who devour it. This ice cream is sweet enough for kids, sophisticated enough for adults, and easy enough for anyone to prepare.

2 cans (5.4 ounces [160 ml] each) coconut cream
4 pitted Medjool dates
½ teaspoon vanilla extract
1 pound (455 g) frozen dark sweet cherries
¼ cup cacao powder
½ cup (60 g) chopped walnuts (optional)

Place the coconut cream, dates, and vanilla extract into a blender or food processor and blend until creamy and well combined. Add in the cherries and cacao powder and blend until you reach a smooth, creamy consistency.

Pour the mixture into a bread pan, smooth it flat, and allow the ice cream to freeze for about 2 hours or until it can be scooped. Serve the ice cream immediately topped with chopped walnuts, if using.

Batch Cooking and Leftovers: If the ice cream is frozen solid, allow it to soften in the refrigerator for about 1½ hours before serving to improve texture.

This recipe can be doubled, but larger amounts need to be prepared in batches and you'll need to increase the amount of time the ice cream is chilled and thawed.

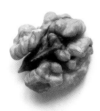
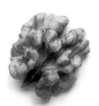
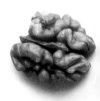

chocolate walnut brownies

active minutes   *total time*   *small brownies*   *week*   *month*

These brownies take very little time to prepare, but you *must* be patient in waiting for them to cool. If you can overcome the urge to prematurely dig into these mouthwatering morsels, you will not be disappointed! The brownies need adequate time to cool so they bind together, creating a moist and flavorful Chocolate Walnut Brownie. Try topping them with Chocolate Icing, but halve that recipe since you won't need the entire amount. The sweetness of the brownies seems to improve over time, so advance preparation is an advantage. Don't forget to invite the kids to help you prepare this easy dessert!

½ cup (100 g) coconut oil, melted, plus more for greasing

3 eggs

½ cup (140 g) pitted Medjool dates, packed

2 teaspoons vanilla

⅓ cup (30 g) coconut flour

½ cup (43 g) cacao powder

¼ teaspoon baking powder

¼ teaspoon salt

⅔ cup (75 g) chopped walnuts, divided

Preheat the oven to 350°F (177°C).

Place the oil, eggs, dates, and vanilla into a blender and blend till a smooth batter forms. Add all the other ingredients except the walnuts, and blend again to form a smooth batter.

Set aside 2 tablespoons of walnuts and mix the remaining walnuts into the batter using a mixing spoon.

Pour the batter into a greased 7 × 11-inch (18 × 28 cm) or 9 × 9-inch (23 × 23 cm) baking pan. Evenly sprinkle the remaining walnuts on top and bake the brownies for 18 minutes.

Allow the brownies to completely cool for 2 hours. Brownies are best served chilled.

Batch Cooking and Leftovers: If preparing a double batch, double the ingredients. Blend the first four ingredients as instructed, but then transfer the batter to a bowl to mix in the remaining ingredients by hand. The larger amount of batter will be too much for your blender. Continue with the remainder of the recipe as instructed.

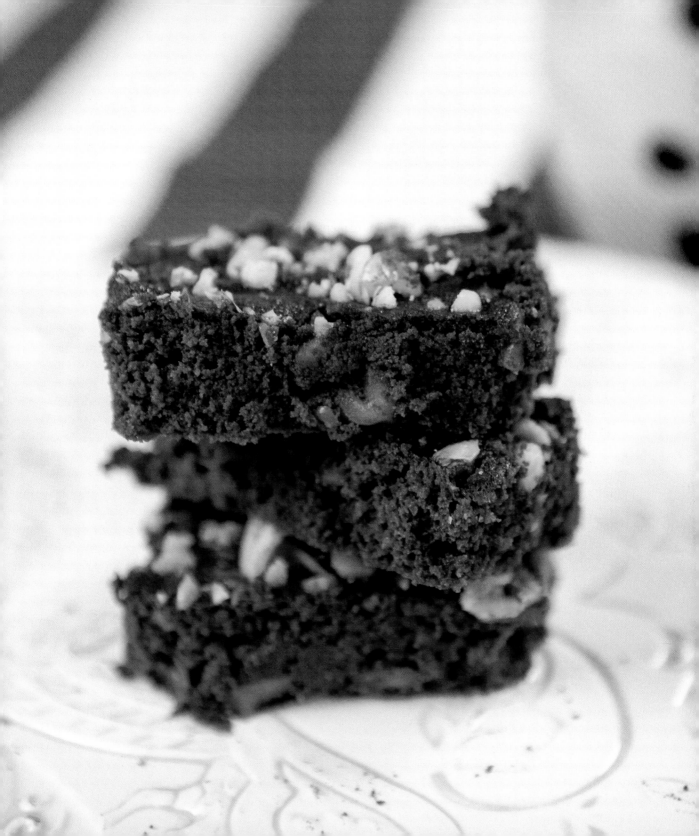

chocolate banana cupcakes

active minutes   *total time*   *cupcakes**   *week*   *month*

These chocolaty cupcakes withstood the ultimate taste test—my five-year-old's birthday party! They're beautifully rich, mildly sweet, and form the perfect base for Chocolate Icing. With sweetness provided only by overripe bananas, these are a treat that can be served (without icing) on a regular basis. Your child will love opening their lunch box to find a delicious chocolate treat! The bananas should be yellow and covered in brown spots, but not black.

7 slightly overripe bananas

4 eggs

½ cup (100 g) coconut oil

½ cup (70 g) cassava flour

½ cup (47 g) almond flour

⅔ cup (60 g) cacao powder

2 teaspoons vanilla

1 teaspoon baking powder

1 teaspoon baking soda

½ teaspoon salt

* the exact amount will depend on the size of the bananas

Preheat the oven to 350°F (177°C).

Peel and roughly chop the bananas into 2-inch (5 cm) pieces. Place the bananas in a blender or food processor with all the other ingredients and blend until a smooth batter is formed.

Divide the batter into approximately 24 silicon muffin molds or muffin paper–lined muffin cups, filling each cup about three-quarters full. These cupcakes will rise, but not quite as well as a traditional cupcake. They'll also shrink a bit as they cool.

Bake the cupcakes for 20 minutes. Allow the cupcakes to completely cool before icing.

Batch Cooking and Leftovers: You'll have to work in batches if doubling the recipe, but leftovers can be easily frozen, and can be quickly assembled as a dessert for a special occasion.

apple spice bundt cake

| 25 active minutes | 1h 15m total time | 16 servings | 1 week | 1 month |

My mother made the most delicious apple cake when I was a kid, but it was a tradition I could no longer enjoy once we discovered my son's allergy to wheat. I wanted to include a recipe that brought me back to my childhood memories of a warm kitchen filled with the delightful fragrance of apples and cinnamon. Not only does this date-sweetened cake fill my heart with warm memories, but it also quickly became a new family tradition for special occasions. With a texture and flavor profile that very closely mimic a cake made with traditional flour, you simply cannot go wrong! Shown on page 247.

5 cups (565 g) peeled and
  sliced apples, about 4–5
  medium apples
⅔ cup (185 g) pitted Medjool
  dates, packed
½ cup (120 ml) avocado oil
4 eggs
½ cup (120 ml) water
2 teaspoons vanilla
4 ripe plantains,
  peeled and chopped
⅔ cup (95 g) cassava flour
1 teaspoon baking soda
1 teaspoon baking powder
2 teaspoons cinnamon
¼ teaspoon ginger powder
¼ teaspoon nutmeg
½ teaspoon salt
2 tablespoons coconut oil,
  for greasing

Preheat the oven to 350°F (177°C).

Peel and thinly slice the apples and set aside.

Using a high-powered blender or food processor, blend the dates, avocado oil, eggs, water, and vanilla till the dates are completely puréed, about 30 seconds.

Add all the other ingredients except the apples and coconut oil into the blender or food processor and blend until a batter has formed, about 1 minute. Mix the apples into the batter using a mixing spoon, and evenly pour the batter into a greased 10-inch (25 cm) Bundt pan. Be sure to evenly distribute the apples throughout.

Bake the cake for 45–50 minutes or until an inserted knife comes out clean.

Allow the cake to cool for about 10 minutes and remove it from the pan by turning the pan upside down onto a cooling rack. Allow the cake to cool for 2 hours before serving.

Batch Cooking and Leftovers: Cut into individual slices before freezing so that you can portion out individual pieces every now and then.

Work in batches if doubling the cake.

pumpkin pie with hazelnut crust

active minutes	total time	servings	week	month
20	1h 10m	8	1	1

Although this pie isn't an exact replica of the condensed milk–sweetened version that most of us are accustomed to, its deliciously unique flavors and perfectly sweet creaminess are enough to impress any guest. The toasted flavor of the hazelnut crust gives this pie a unique twist on the holiday classic. Serve each slice topped with a dollop or two of homemade Coconut Whipped Cream. For a pecan crust, use 2 cups (220 g) of pecans in the place of the hazelnuts.

CRUST

1½ cups (215 g) whole hazelnuts
2 tablespoons (25 g) coconut oil, more for greasing
1 egg white, reserve yolk for filling
Pinch of salt

FILLING

1 can (15 ounces [425 g]) pumpkin purée
1 can (5.4 ounces [160 ml]) unsweetened coconut cream
2 eggs
1 egg yolk
½ cup (140 g) pitted Medjool dates, packed
1 teaspoon vanilla extract
2 teaspoons pumpkin pie spice
Pinch of salt

CRUST INSTRUCTIONS

Preheat the oven to 350°F (177°C).

Grind the hazelnuts into a coarse flour using a blender or food processor. Mix in the remaining ingredients by hand until well combined.

Place the crust mixture into a greased pie pan and use fingers to evenly press the mixture into the pan, taking the time to form an even crust. Use a fork to poke holes along the bottom of the crust.

Bake the crust for 7 minutes while preparing the filling.

FILLING INSTRUCTIONS

Combine all the filling ingredients in a blender or food processor and gently blend until the batter is smooth.

Pour the mixture into the warm piecrust and bake the pie for 45 minutes or until set.

Allow the pie to completely cool before serving.

Batch Cooking and Leftovers: This recipe can be easily doubled as long as you have two pie pans.

acknowledgments

The first thanks goes to my editor, Makenna, who had the vision, faith, and patience to help me write a book that I never dreamed possible. Thanks to Mom and Dad who taught me how to be strong in the face of adversity. I wouldn't be fighting for solutions without that strength. Thanks to the many family members, especially D.D., Pops, Gramps, and Grandma Barbara, who offered emotional and financial help throughout this process. I couldn't have done it without such good helpers. Thanks to Nancy whose generosity is a model for serving others less fortunate than ourselves. I give my word to pay her generosity forward, hopefully 10 times over. Thanks to all of the friends who encouraged, inspired, provided a shoulder to cry on, and watched my children while I wrote. Most of all, thanks to my husband (and photographer), who will forever be my biggest fan and source of support. I couldn't imagine a better partner in life. This book took a village and I'm thankful for each member who played a role.

Appendix A

Menus

In this section I have included four weeks of menus to get you started on developing a meal plan for your family. Note that the menus operate as a four-week set. You'll be preparing large batches of certain recipes, eating a portion immediately, and freezing leftovers for later weeks. This approach will save you time in the long run. Each menu includes breakfast, lunch, and dinner. However, please note that the menus do *not* incorporate snack foods. Snacks greatly vary depending on your needs, preferences, and budget, so I leave this up to you to decide for yourself. Look over the *Quick and Easy Snacks* sidebar (page 170) and add your snack choices to your shopping list. Be mindful that you may be able to use ingredients for snacks that are already on your main shopping list. If, for example, you see that you'll have excess celery one week (maybe a recipe calls for five stalks, but you must purchase an entire bunch), you can incorporate the extras into your weekly snack plan. Extra ingredients can also be used creatively on days when you've scheduled leftover meals.

Salad toppings such as olives, nuts, seeds, or avocados aren't listed in these menus, either. The vegetable ingredients for each week's Everyday Salad are listed, but salad toppings are such an individual thing. For example, I'm of the opinion that a salad is incomplete without green or kalamata olives, but my husband essentially says the same about walnuts or sunflower seeds. We start with the same "base" salad, but we

finish it to our own preference. Be sure to add any necessary items (snacks and salad toppings) to your shopping list to prevent multiple trips to the store.

The menus assume that leftovers from dinner will be served for lunches, including packed lunches for the kids. (See *Packed Lunches for Kids*, page 280, for more information.) The only exception is the menu for Week 4, which incorporates an additional meal to serve for lunch. Friday's are a "free night." Use this night to eat whatever you would like whether eating at a restaurant or preparing an acceptable packaged meal. I have found that a free night is a welcomed break at the end of a long week.

Every family has different caloric needs based on age, sex, activity level, and individual metabolism, so it's up to you to determine how the meal plans can meet all your family's needs. You may need to buy a few extra items, or double a few more recipes. Unfortunately, I can't paint an exact portrait of *your* specific needs. However, be cautious in thinking that the menus will produce *too much food*, unless you don't plan to serve leftovers for lunches. Yes, the menus yield large quantities of food, but remember that they are designed to fill the stomachs of an average of four individuals for an entire week. Leftovers can always be frozen or repurposed for subsequent snacks or meals. Also keep in mind that you don't want to be preparing separate meals for your children. Dinner is dinner. Lunch is lunch. Establish some boundaries around mealtimes and stick to your decision. (For readers who crave more detailed descriptions of recommended prep sequences that walk you through each step, you can download a PDF at deeprootedwellness.com/grainfree.)

As you may recall from part 1, suitable fats for cooking include coconut oil, olive oil, lard, and a handful of others (see *A Word on the Recipes and Menus*, page 66, for details regarding cooking fats and oils). Each recipe specifies the type of fat that is best for that particular dish, but fats are often interchangeable. Choose whichever fats you prefer to use for cooking, but know that substitutions can't always be made, such as the case of avocado oil—it is virtually tasteless, making it the best oil to use when you want to avoid adding a flavorful oil. Coconut oil often adds a sweet flavor to foods, making it a good choice for recipes like Plantain Muffins. Lard has a high smoke point, making it the best option for frying. Avocado oil is another good option for frying, but it's not nearly as economical as using lard or reserved animal fats.

You Want Me to Do *What* on Saturdays?

Head on over to Instagram and you'll see that #meal-prepsaturdays and #mealprepsundays are a real thing among food prep gurus! A typical busy workweek starts on Monday, which means you won't have time to get the majority of your food prep done at the beginning of the week. I therefore suggest starting your meal prep week on Saturday since this is the start of your weekend, thus you are available to get busy in the kitchen. The food that you prep on Saturday will create the beginning of a meal plan that you start to follow on Sunday. Your brain may be resistant to this idea, but I give you my word that it's the best way to accomplish a *lot* of work in the kitchen in as little time as possible.

A Note about Ingredients Lists

The ingredients lists reflect every ingredient you'll need to prepare each meal plan. (As I already mentioned, these lists do not include snacks, salad toppings, or additional ingredients you may want for lunches.) The ingredients lists are as exact as possible in order to set you up for complete success in the kitchen. You'll see that I've calculated total needs for items like salt, olive oil, and spices for each week. While an exact list may seem like overkill to take with you shopping, this actually provides you with the opportunity to check these pantry items to guarantee you have enough before heading to the store. Many of the pantry items and frozen meats might already be available in your home. If so, the shopping trip should be primarily limited to fresh ingredients and those ingredients that need to be restocked.

week one menu

Recipes and Quantities Needed

Prepare the recipes with the indicated quantities to make this week's plan work. Please note that one breakfast prepared this week will be served on Saturday of Week 2 (see *Week Two Menu*, page 271).

BREAKFAST RECIPES

Pecan Bread: Prepare two batches of the Pecan Bread Variation for a total of four loaves of bread. Store two loaves in the refrigerator and freeze the other two for use in Week 3.

Probiotic Pork and Vegetables: Double the recipe and store half in the refrigerator and half in the freezer for use in Week 3.

Vegetable Egg Scramble with Avocado and Salsa: You'll be preparing this recipe on four separate occasions, but the chopped vegetables will be prepared in advance to reduce your cooking time throughout the week.

Fermented Salsa Fresca: This will serve as the condiment for the Vegetable Egg Scramble with Avocado and Salsa.

Apple Walnut Crisp Cereal: This recipe yields 16 servings but will only be served once per week. You'll therefore reserve a fourth of the recipe in the refrigerator to eat during Week 1, and the other 12 servings will be frozen into three evenly sized portions for Weeks 2, 3, and the very end of Week 4.

Homemade Coconut Milk: The milk to accompany the Apple Walnut Crisp Cereal.

LUNCH AND DINNER RECIPES

Everyday Salad: This week's salad incorporates two large heads of romaine lettuce, one pint of cherry tomatoes, one large cucumber, two large carrots, one 14-ounce (396 g) can of artichoke hearts, one red pepper, and six ounces (170 g) of alfalfa sprouts.

Red Wine Lemon Vinaigrette: Double the recipe and refrigerate any leftover dressing for use in Week 4.

Not Quite Your Mama's Chili: Double the recipe and freeze half to be used in Week 3.

Beef Stock: To be used in Not Quite Your Mama's Chili.

Simple Whole Roasted Chicken: Prepare two whole chickens. Store one in the refrigerator and the other in the freezer for a future meal (there will be a handful of items left over in the freezer after completing the four weeks' worth of meal plans; this is one of such items).

Grain-Free Gravy: Freeze any leftovers for future use.

Roasted Non-Starchy Vegetables: Prepare this recipe using green beans.

Red and Yellow Rosemary Potatoes

Cottage Pie: Double the stuffing recipe, use half of the recipe to assemble the pie as instructed, and freeze the other half for use in Week 2.

Greek-style "Pasta" Bowls: This dish will be assembled using the following four recipes:

> **Simple Spaghetti Squash:** Prepare two.
> **Grilled Chicken Breasts with Basil and Thyme:** Use half for this week and freeze the other half for use in Week 3.
> **Sun-Dried Tomato Tapenade:** While not indicated, this recipe could be doubled and frozen.
> **Simple Vegan Pesto:** While not indicated, this recipe could be doubled and frozen.

Shrimp Scampi with Tomatoes and Zoodles: Serve this dish over leftover Simple Spaghetti Squash.

week one menu

	Breakfast	Lunch	Dinner
Saturday	Leftovers; Prepare for Future Meals	Leftovers; Prepare for Future Meals	Leftovers; Prepare for Future Meals
Sunday	Probiotic Pork and Vegetables + Pecan Bread	Leftovers; Prepare for Future Meals	Not Quite Your Mama's Chili + grain-free tortilla chips + Everyday Salad + Vinaigrette
Monday	Probiotic Pork and Vegetables + Pecan Bread	Not Quite Your Mama's Chili + grain-free tortilla chips	Simple Whole Roasted Chicken + Grain-Free Gravy + Roasted Green Beans + Red and Yellow Rosemary Potatoes
Tuesday	Apple Walnut Crisp Cereal + Homemade Coconut Milk	Simple Whole Roasted Chicken + Grain-Free Gravy + Roasted Green Beans + Red and Yellow Rosemary Potatoes	Cottage Pie + Everyday Salad + Vinaigrette
Wednesday	Vegetable Egg Scramble with Avocado and Salsa (use Fermented Salsa Fresca) + Pecan Bread	Cottage Pie + Everyday Salad + Vinaigrette	Greek-style "Pasta" Bowls with Grilled Chicken Breasts + Sun-Dried Tomato Tapenade + Simple Vegan Pesto + Everyday Salad + Vinaigrette
Thursday	Vegetable Egg Scramble with Avocado and Salsa (use Fermented Salsa Fresca) + Pecan Bread	Greek-style "Pasta" Bowls with Grilled Chicken Breasts + Sun-Dried Tomato Tapenade + Simple Vegan Pesto + Everyday Salad + Vinaigrette	Shrimp Scampi with Tomatoes and Zoodles over leftover Simple Spaghetti Squash
Friday	Vegetable Egg Scramble with Avocado and Salsa (use Fermented Salsa Fresca) + Pecan Bread	Cottage Pie + Everyday Salad +Vinaigrette	FREE NIGHT

ingredients list for week one

Meat, Seafood, Eggs, and Bones

- [ ] beef bones, 3 lbs. (1.4 kg)
- [ ] chicken breasts, 5 lbs. (2.3 kg)
- [ ] eggs, 16
- [ ] ground beef, 8 lbs. (3.6 kg)
- [ ] ground pork, 4 lbs. (1.8 kg)
- [ ] shrimp, peeled and deveined, 1 lb. (455 g)
- [ ] whole chickens, 2 (4 lbs. [910 g] each)

Vegetables and Fresh Herbs

- [ ] alfalfa sprouts, 1 package
- [ ] cabbages, 2 small (2 lbs. [910 g] each)
- [ ] carrots, 16
- [ ] celery, 3 bunches
- [ ] cherry tomatoes, 1 pint
- [ ] cucumber, 1
- [ ] fresh basil, 1 bunch
- [ ] fresh cilantro, 1 small bunch
- [ ] fresh parsley, 1 bunch
- [ ] garlic, 5 heads
- [ ] green beans, 2 lbs. (910 g)
- [ ] green peppers, 3
- [ ] kale, 4 bunches
- [ ] red onions, 2
- [ ] red peppers, 3
- [ ] red potatoes, 2 lbs. (910 g)
- [ ] Roma tomatoes, 1.6 lbs. (735 g)
- [ ] romaine lettuce, 2 large heads
- [ ] spaghetti squash, 2 (3–4 lbs. [1.4–1.8 kg] each)
- [ ] spinach, 1 lb. (455 g)
- [ ] sweet potatoes, 4 lbs. (1.8 kg)
- [ ] yellow onions, 12
- [ ] yellow potatoes, 2 lbs. (910 g)
- [ ] zucchinis, 8 medium

Fruit

- [ ] apples, 4 lbs. (1.8 kg)
- [ ] avocados, 6
- [ ] plantains, 8 ripe
- [ ] lemon, 1 (zest + juice)
- [ ] lime, 1

Other

- [ ] coarse-ground mustard, 2 Tbsp.
- [ ] frozen organic corn, 2 lbs. (910 g)
- [ ] frozen peas, 2 lbs. (910 g)
- [ ] grain-free tortilla or plantain chips, 8 servings
- [ ] raw sauerkraut, 2 cups (340 g)
- [ ] white wine (dry), ½ cup (120 ml)

Pantry Items

- [ ] artichoke hearts, 14 oz. (396 g) can
- [ ] baking powder, 4 tsp.
- [ ] baking soda, 2 tsp.
- [ ] capers, 2 Tbsp.
- [ ] diced tomatoes, 2 cans (14.5 oz. [410 g] each)
- [ ] dried black beans, 1 lb. (455 g)
- [ ] green olives, ½ cup (65 g)
- [ ] kalamata olives, 12.1 oz. (343 g) jar + ¾ cup (100 g)
- [ ] pecans, chopped, 3 cups (140 g)
- [ ] pine nuts, ¼ cup (32 g)
- [ ] sunflower seeds, raw, 2 cups (290 g)
- [ ] sun-dried tomato halves, 9
- [ ] tomato paste, 2 cans (6 oz. [170 g] each)
- [ ] unsweetened shredded coconut, 2 cups (225 g)
- [ ] vanilla extract, 1½ tsp.
- [ ] walnuts, raw, 1½ lbs. (680 g)

Fats, Oils, and Vinegars

- [ ] cooking fat, 10 Tbsp.
- [ ] cooking oil, 1 cup (235 ml) + 2 Tbsp.
- [ ] coconut oil, 1½ cups (300 g)
- [ ] olive oil, 1¾ cup (415 ml)
- [ ] raw apple cider vinegar, 4 Tbsp.
- [ ] red wine vinegar, ½ cup (120 ml)
- [ ] vinegar, 1 Tbsp.

Dried Herbs and Spices

- [ ] bay leaves, 3
- [ ] chili powder, 2 Tbsp.
- [ ] cinnamon, 4 Tbsp.
- [ ] cumin powder, 1 Tbsp.
- [ ] dried basil, 8 tsp.
- [ ] dried oregano, 2 tsp.
- [ ] dried parsley, 2 Tbsp.
- [ ] dried rosemary, 1 Tbsp.
- [ ] dried sage, 3 Tbsp.
- [ ] dried tarragon, 2 Tbsp.
- [ ] dried thyme, 1 Tbsp.
- [ ] garlic powder, 3 Tbsp.
- [ ] onion powder, 1 Tbsp. + 1 tsp.
- [ ] pepper, to taste
- [ ] red pepper flakes, pinch
- [ ] sea salt, 10 Tbsp.
- [ ] smoked paprika, 1½ tsp.

week two menu

Recipes and Quantities Needed

BREAKFAST RECIPES

Carrot Cake Applesauce Muffins: Prepare a single batch to yield 24 muffins.

Cauliflower-Sausage Breakfast Casserole: Double the sausage-and-onion mix, use half to assemble the casserole, and freeze the other half to make the casserole again in Week 4.

Spaghetti Squash Porridge

Apple Walnut Crisp Cereal: Remove one of the three bags frozen during Week 1.

Homemade Coconut Milk: Prepare a single recipe to serve with Apple Walnut Crisp Cereal on Friday.

LUNCH AND DINNER RECIPES

Everyday Salad: This week's salad incorporates one pound (455 g) of mixed greens, a small red cabbage, a half pound (225 g) of raw beets, two medium carrots, half of a small red onion, and one half cup (70 g) sunflower seeds.

Fresh Basil and Garlic Balsamic Vinaigrette: Double the recipe and refrigerate any leftover dressing for use in Weeks 3 and 4.

Italian-style "Pasta" Bowls: Assemble this dish by preparing:

Simple Spaghetti Squash: Prepare two squashes, one for the porridge and one for the "Pasta" Bowls.

Hearty Meat Bolognese: Prepare a single recipe as instructed, reserve half for use this week, and freeze the other half for use in Week 4.

Pecan Parmesan "Cheese": Double the recipe, reserve half for use this week, and freeze the other half for use in Week 4.

Pulled Mojo Chicken: Prepare a single recipe as instructed, use half this week, and freeze the other half for use in Week 4.

Plantain Tortillas

Chimichurri Sauce: Double the recipe, use half for a taco topping this week, and freeze the other half for use in Week 4.

Pico de Gallo

Garlicky Guacamole

Cottage Pie: Use the frozen stuffing prepared during Week 1 and complete the recipe as instructed.

Turmeric-Ginger Baked Chicken

Coconut Lime Cauliflower Rice

Chicken Stock: About three quarts will be used to make White Bean, Fennel, and Sausage Stew, and the remaining quart will be used in Week 3 for Creamy Cauliflower Soup.

White Bean, Fennel, and Sausage Stew

Additional needs: One head of shredded romaine to serve with the Plantain Tortillas and Pulled Mojo Chicken on Monday and Tuesday.

week two menu

	Breakfast	Lunch	Dinner
Saturday	Vegetable Egg Scramble with Avocado and Salsa (use Fermented Salsa Fresca) + Pecan Bread (left over from Week 1)	Leftovers	Leftovers
Sunday	Cauliflower-Sausage Breakfast Casserole + Carrot Cake Applesauce Muffins	Leftovers	Italian-style "Pasta" Bowls with Hearty Meat Bolognese + Pecan Parmesan "Cheese" + Everyday Salad + Vinaigrette
Monday	Spaghetti Squash Porridge	Italian-style "Pasta" Bowls with Hearty Meat Bolognese + Pecan Parmesan "Cheese" + Everyday Salad + Vinaigrette	Pulled Mojo Chicken + Plantain Tortillas + Chimichurri + Pico de Gallo + Garlicky Guacamole + shredded lettuce
Tuesday	Cauliflower-Sausage Breakfast Casserole + Carrot Cake Applesauce Muffins	Everyday Salad + Pulled Mojo Chicken + Chimichurri + Pico de Gallo + Garlicky Guacamole	Cottage Pie + Everyday Salad + Vinaigrette
Wednesday	Spaghetti Squash Porridge	Cottage Pie + Everyday Salad + Vinaigrette	Turmeric-Ginger Baked Chicken + Coconut Lime Cauliflower Rice + Everyday Salad + Vinaigrette
Thursday	Cauliflower-Sausage Breakfast Casserole + Carrot Cake Applesauce Muffins	Turmeric-Ginger Baked Chicken + Coconut Lime Cauliflower Rice + Everyday Salad + Vinaigrette	White Bean, Fennel, and Sausage Stew
Friday	Apple Walnut Crisp Cereal + Homemade Coconut Milk	Turmeric-Ginger Baked Chicken + Everyday Salad + Vinaigrette	FREE NIGHT

ingredients list for week two

Meat, Seafood, Eggs, and Bones

- ☐ chicken breasts, 2½–3 lbs. (1.1–1.4 kg)
- ☐ chicken thighs, 7 lbs. (3.2 kg)
- ☐ ground breakfast sausage, 4 lbs. (1.8 kg)
- ☐ ground beef, 3 lbs. (1.4 kg)
- ☐ sausage links, 2 lbs. (910 g)
- ☐ eggs, 31
- ☐ chicken bones, 2 lbs. (910 g)

Vegetables and Fresh Herbs

- ☐ basil, 1 bunch
- ☐ beets, ½ lb. (225 g)
- ☐ carrots, 13
- ☐ cauliflower, 2 large heads
- ☐ celery, 2 bunches
- ☐ cilantro, 3 bunches
- ☐ fennel bulb, 1
- ☐ garlic, 3 heads
- ☐ grape tomatoes, 1 pint
- ☐ green pepper, 1
- ☐ jalapeño pepper, 1
- ☐ mixed greens, 1 lb. (455 g)
- ☐ mushrooms, 1 lb. (455 g)
- ☐ onions, 6
- ☐ parsley, 3 bunches
- ☐ red cabbage, 1 small
- ☐ red onions, 2
- ☐ red pepper, 3
- ☐ Roma tomatoes, 2
- ☐ tomato, 1
- ☐ romaine, 1 head

- ☐ spaghetti squash, 2 (3–4 lbs. [1.4–1.8 kg] each)
- ☐ sweet potatoes, 4 lbs. (1.8 kg)
- ☐ zucchinis, 2

Fruit

- ☐ avocados, 2
- ☐ lemons, 3
- ☐ limes, 4
- ☐ orange, 1
- ☐ plantains, green/yellow, 2

Other

- ☐ nutritional yeast, 2 Tbsp.
- ☐ white wine (dry), 1 cup (235 ml)

Pantry Items

- ☐ baking powder, 2 tsp.
- ☐ baking soda, ½ tsp.
- ☐ coconut milk, 2 cans (13.5 oz. [398 ml] each)
- ☐ coconut cream, 5.4 oz. (160 ml) can
- ☐ coconut flour, 1 cup (130 g)
- ☐ crushed tomatoes, 2 cans (28 oz. [793 g] each)
- ☐ diced fire-roasted tomatoes, 2 cans (14.5 oz. [411 g] each)
- ☐ dried white beans, 1 lb. (910 g)
- ☐ fire-roasted crushed tomatoes, 2 cans (28 oz. [793 g] each)
- ☐ pecans, 1 cup (120 g)
- ☐ raisins, 1¼ cups (215 g)
- ☐ sunflower seeds, ½ cup (70 g)

- ☐ unsweetened shredded coconut, 2 cups (225 g)
- ☐ unsweetened applesauce, 2 cups (490 g)
- ☐ vanilla extract, 1 Tbsp.
- ☐ walnuts, 1½ cups (170 g)

Fats, Oils, and Vinegars

- ☐ avocado oil, ¼ cup (60 ml)
- ☐ balsamic vinegar, 1 cup (235 ml)
- ☐ coconut oil, ½ cup (100 g)
- ☐ cooking fat, 4 Tbsp.
- ☐ olive oil, 2 cups (475 ml)
- ☐ raw apple cider vinegar (or red wine vinegar if preferred for the Chimichurri Sauce), ¼ cup (60 ml)
- ☐ vinegar, 1 Tbsp. + 1 tsp.

Dried Herbs and Spices

- ☐ bay leaves, 2
- ☐ cinnamon, 4 Tbsp. + 1 tsp.
- ☐ cumin powder, 2 tsp.
- ☐ dried basil, 1½ Tbsp.
- ☐ dried oregano, 2½ Tbsp. + 2½ tsp.
- ☐ dried parsley, 2 Tbsp.
- ☐ dried rosemary, 1½ Tbsp.
- ☐ dried thyme, ½ Tbsp.
- ☐ garlic powder, 1 Tbsp.
- ☐ ginger powder, 1 tsp.
- ☐ onion powder, 1 Tbsp.
- ☐ sea salt, 5 Tbsp. + 2¼ tsp.
- ☐ smoked paprika, 1 tsp.
- ☐ turmeric powder, 1 tsp.

week three menu

Recipes and Quantities Needed

BREAKFAST RECIPES

Eat Your Greens Frittata

Pecan Bread: Use the two loaves frozen during Week 1 from the freezer.

My Favorite Mango Smoothie: You'll prepare a double batch twice during the week (Tuesday and Friday), enough to serve four individuals on two different days.

Hard-Boiled Eggs: Use 24 eggs in total: 16 eggs are to accompany the smoothie for breakfasts (2 per person, serving four people on two mornings), 4 are for the Massaged Kale Salad with Lentils, and the remainders can be used for snacks.

Probiotic Pork and Vegetables: Use the leftovers frozen during Week 1.

Apple Walnut Crisp Cereal: Use one of the remaining two bags that were frozen from Week 1.

Homemade Coconut Milk: Prepare a single recipe to serve with Apple Walnut Crisp Cereal on Thursday.

LUNCH AND DINNER RECIPES

Everyday Salad: This week's salad incorporates one head of napa cabbage, one half small red onion, one medium cucumber, one pint of grape tomatoes, and a small bunch of radishes.

Italian Dressing: Double the recipe and refrigerate leftovers for use in Week 4.

OMGrain-Free Chicken Tenders

Roasted Non-Starchy Vegetables: Prepare this recipe using broccoli.

Crispy Sweet Potato Fries

Herbed Beef Burgers

Red and Yellow Rosemary Potatoes

Summer Cucumber and Tomato Salad

Not Quite Your Mama's Chili: Use the frozen leftovers from Week 1.

Grilled Chicken Salad with Fresh Vegetables: Prepare this dish using frozen Grilled Chicken Breasts with Basil and Thyme from Week 1.

Homemade Mayonnaise: Prepare this for use in the chicken salad.

Roasted Roots: Prepare this recipe using two pounds (910 g) of carrots and two pounds (910 g) of beets.

Creamy Cauliflower Soup: Prepare a double batch using leftover Chicken Stock from Week 2 along with a fresh batch made this week.

Chicken Stock: Prepare a double batch and reserve leftovers for Week 4.

Perfectly Baked Bacon: Prepare two pounds (910 g) and crumble or chop it into bacon pieces to be served with the Creamy Cauliflower Soup.

Massaged Kale Salad with Lentils

Dill Pickle Kraut: The kraut won't be ready for a minimum of 10 days, making it available as a condiment by the end of Week 4. Moving forward, sauerkraut should be prepared at least once every three weeks.

Additional needs: Grain-free tortilla chips or plantain chips to serve with Not Quite Your Mama's Chili.

week three menu

	Breakfast	Lunch	Dinner
Saturday	Cauliflower-Sausage Breakfast Casserole + Carrot Cake Applesauce Muffins (left over from Week 2)	Leftovers	Leftovers
Sunday	Eat Your Greens Frittata + Pecan Bread	Leftovers	OMGrain-Free Chicken Tenders + Roasted Non-Starchy Vegetables (broccoli) + Crispy Sweet Potato Fries
Monday	Eat Your Greens Frittata + Pecan Bread	Creamy Cauliflower Soup with bacon + OMGrain-Free Chicken Tenders (and/or Hard-Boiled Eggs) + Everyday Salad + Italian Dressing	Herbed Beef Burgers + Red and Yellow Rosemary Potatoes + Summer Cucumber and Tomato Salad
Tuesday	My Favorite Mango Smoothie + Hard-Boiled Eggs	Herbed Beef Burgers + Red and Yellow Rosemary Potatoes + Summer Cucumber and Tomato Salad	Not Quite Your Mama's Chili + grain-free tortilla chips + Everyday Salad + Italian Dressing
Wednesday	Probiotic Pork and Vegetables + Pecan Bread	Not Quite Your Mama's Chili + grain-free tortilla chips + Everyday Salad + Italian Dressing	Grilled Chicken Salad with Fresh Vegetables + Roasted Roots + Everyday Salad + Italian Dressing
Thursday	Apple Walnut Crisp Cereal + Homemade Coconut Milk	Grilled Chicken Salad with Fresh Vegetables + Roasted Roots + Everyday Salad + Italian Dressing	Creamy Cauliflower Soup with bacon + Massaged Kale Salad with Lentils
Friday	My Favorite Mango Smoothie + Hard-Boiled Eggs	Creamy Cauliflower Soup with bacon + Massaged Kale Salad with Lentils	FREE NIGHT

ingredients list for week three

Meat, Seafood, Eggs, and Bones

- [ ] bacon, thinly sliced, 2 lbs. (910 g)
- [ ] chicken tenders, 2 lbs. (910 g)
- [ ] chicken bones, 2 lbs. (910 g)
- [ ] eggs, 36
- [ ] ground beef, 3 lbs. (1.4 kg)

Vegetables and Fresh Herbs

- [ ] basil, 1 bunch
- [ ] beets, 2 lbs. (910 g)
- [ ] broccoli, 2 lbs. (910 g)
- [ ] cabbage, 3½ lbs. (1.6 kg)
- [ ] carrots, 7 individual + 2 lbs. (910 g)
- [ ] cauliflower, 2 heads
- [ ] celery, 1 bunch
- [ ] cucumbers, 2 lbs. (910 g)
- [ ] dill, 1 small bunch
- [ ] garlic, 3 heads
- [ ] grape tomatoes, 2 pints
- [ ] heirloom tomatoes, 1 lb. (455 g)
- [ ] kale, 3 bunches
- [ ] parsley, 1 bunch
- [ ] napa cabbage, 1 head
- [ ] radishes, 1 small bunch
- [ ] red onion, 1
- [ ] red pepper, 1
- [ ] red potatoes, 2 lbs. (910 g)
- [ ] spinach, 1 lb. (455 g)
- [ ] sweet potatoes, 2 lbs. (910 g)
- [ ] tomato, 1 large or 2 Roma
- [ ] yellow potatoes, 2 lbs. (910 g)
- [ ] yellow onions, 8

Fruit

- [ ] avocados, 3
- [ ] bananas, 4
- [ ] lemons, 2

Other

- [ ] Dijon mustard, 2 Tbsp. + 2½ tsp.
- [ ] frozen diced mangoes, 8 cups (960 g)
- [ ] grain-free tortilla chips, 2 bags (5 oz. [142 g] each)
- [ ] raw sauerkraut, 2 cups (340 g)

Pantry Items

- [ ] coconut cream, 2 cans (5.4 oz. [160 ml] each)
- [ ] French lentils, 1 cup (210 g)
- [ ] hearts of palm, 14-oz. (396 g) can
- [ ] hemp hearts, 24 Tbsp.
- [ ] unsweetened shredded coconut, 3½ cups (395 g)
- [ ] raw almonds, 4 cups (570 g)

Fats, Oils, and Vinegars

- [ ] avocado oil (or olive oil if preferred for the Homemade Mayonnaise), ¾ cup (175 ml)
- [ ] cooking fat, 6 Tbsp.
- [ ] cooking oil, ½ cup (120 ml)
- [ ] lard (or grease from bacon), 1 cup (220 g)
- [ ] olive oil, 1 cup (235 ml) + 2½ Tbsp.
- [ ] raw apple cider vinegar, 5 Tbsp.
- [ ] red wine vinegar, 3 Tbsp.
- [ ] vinegar, 1 Tbsp.
- [ ] white vinegar, ½ cup (120 ml)

Dried Herbs and Spices

- [ ] bay leaves, 2
- [ ] crushed red pepper flakes, ⅛ tsp.
- [ ] cumin powder, ¼ tsp.
- [ ] dried basil, 1½ tsp.
- [ ] dried oregano, 1 Tbsp. + 1⅛ tsp.
- [ ] dried parsley, 2 tsps.
- [ ] dried rosemary, 1 Tbsp. + 2 tsps.
- [ ] garlic powder, 2 Tbsp. + 1 tsp.
- [ ] mustard seed, ¾ tsp.
- [ ] onion powder, 2 Tbsp. + 1 tsp.
- [ ] pepper, to taste
- [ ] salt, ½ cup (130 g)

week four menu

Recipes and Quantities Needed

BREAKFAST RECIPES

Banana Nut Bread: Double the recipe, use half this week, and freeze the other two loaves for use in the future (beyond the meal plans covered in this book).

Cauliflower-Sausage Breakfast Casserole: Use the pork-and-onion mixture frozen from Week 2.

Spaghetti Squash Porridge

Apple Walnut Crisp Cereal: Use the final bag of frozen cereal made in Week 1 (to be used early next week, beyond the meal plans in his book).

Homemade Coconut Milk: Used for the Apple Walnut Crisp Cereal.

LUNCH AND DINNER RECIPES

Everyday Salad: This week's salad incorporates one pound (455 g) of spinach, a 14-ounce (396 g) can of artichoke hearts, one red pepper, one bunch of green onions, and one cup (115 g) of chopped walnuts.

Dressings: Pull all leftover dressing from Weeks 1, 2, and 3 from the refrigerator.

Pulled Mojo Chicken: Use the frozen chicken prepared in Week 2.

Plantain Tortillas

Avocado-Mango Salsa: Double the recipe, using half for tacos and the other half for the baked salmon.

Chimichurri Sauce: Use the frozen sauce from Week 2.

Baked Salmon with Avocado-Mango Salsa

Grain-Free Tabbouleh

Coconut and Cinnamon Sweet Potato Mash: Double the recipe to use as a side for multiple meals.

Italian-style "Pasta" Bowls: Assemble this dish using the following recipes:

> **Hearty Meat Bolognese:** Use the frozen Bolognese from Week 2.
>
> **Pecan Parmesan "Cheese":** Use the frozen Parmesan from Week 2.

40-Minute Beef Stew

Beef Stock: Prepare Beef Stock to be used in the 40-Minute Beef Stew.

Shrimp and Mixed Vegetable Green Curry

Coconut Lime Cauliflower Rice

Turkey Cucumber Rolls

Creamy Carrot Ginger Soup: Use the leftover Chicken Stock from Week 3 to prepare this soup.

Additional needs: Shredded romaine lettuce for use with grain-free tacos.

week four menu

	Breakfast	Lunch	Dinner
Saturday	Probiotic Pork and Vegetables + Pecan Bread (left over from Week 3)	Leftovers	Leftovers
Sunday	Cauliflower-Sausage Breakfast Casserole + Banana Nut Bread	Leftovers	Pulled Mojo Chicken + Plantain Tortillas + Avocado-Mango Salsa + Chimichurri Sauce + shredded romaine lettuce
Monday	Cauliflower-Sausage Breakfast Casserole + Banana Nut Bread	Everyday Salad + Pulled Mojo Chicken + Chimichurri Sauce	Baked Salmon with Avocado-Mango Salsa + Grain-Free Tabbouleh + Coconut and Cinnamon Sweet Potato Mash
Tuesday	Spaghetti Squash Porridge	Pulled Mojo Chicken + Grain-Free Tabbouleh + Coconut and Cinnamon Sweet Potato Mash	Italian-style "Pasta" Bowls + Hearty Meat Bolognese + Pecan Parmesan "Cheese" + Everyday Salad + leftover dressing
Wednesday	Cauliflower-Sausage Breakfast Casserole + Banana Nut Bread	Italian-style "Pasta" Bowls + Hearty Meat Bolognese + Pecan Parmesan "Cheese" + Everyday Salad + leftover dressing	40-Minute Beef Stew + Everyday Salad + leftover dressing
Thursday	Spaghetti Squash Porridge	40-Minute Beef Stew + Everyday Salad + leftover dressing	Shrimp and Vegetable Mixed Green Curry + Coconut Lime Cauliflower Rice
Friday	Cauliflower-Sausage Breakfast Casserole + Banana Nut Bread	Creamy Carrot Ginger Soup + Turkey Cucumber Rolls + Everyday Salad + leftover dressing	FREE NIGHT

ingredients list for week four

Meat, Seafood, Eggs, and Bones

- [ ] eggs, 28
- [ ] salmon, 1½ lbs. (680 g)
- [ ] shrimp, peeled and deveined, 1 lb. (455 g)
- [ ] turkey breast, sliced, 16 slices, about 14 oz. (395 g)
- [ ] stew beef, 2 lbs. (910 g)
- [ ] beef bones, 3 lbs. (1.4 kg)

Vegetables and Fresh Herbs

- [ ] basil, 1 small bunch (minced 2 Tbsp.)
- [ ] carrots, 11 individual + 2 lbs. (910 g)
- [ ] cauliflower, 3 heads
- [ ] celery, 2 bunches
- [ ] cilantro, 1 bunch
- [ ] English cucumbers, 5
- [ ] garlic, 4 heads
- [ ] ginger, 1-inch (2.5 cm) piece
- [ ] green beans, 1 lb. (450 g)
- [ ] green onions, 1 bunch
- [ ] kale, 1 bunch
- [ ] onions, 6
- [ ] parsley, 1 bunch
- [ ] red pepper, 2
- [ ] red onion, 1
- [ ] romaine, 1 head
- [ ] spaghetti squash, 2 (3–4 lbs. [1.4–1.8 kg] each)
- [ ] spinach, 1 lb. (455 g)
- [ ] sweet potatoes, 6 lbs. (1.4 kg)
- [ ] tomato, 1 large
- [ ] yellow potatoes, 2 lbs. (910 g)

Fruit

- [ ] avocados, 2
- [ ] bananas, 12 overripe
- [ ] lemon, 1
- [ ] lime, 2
- [ ] mangoes, 2
- [ ] plantains, 2

Other

- [ ] coarse-ground mustard, 2 Tbsp.
- [ ] green curry paste, 2 Tbsp.
- [ ] hummus, 16 oz. (455 g)

Pantry Items

- [ ] almond flour, 3 cups (290 g)
- [ ] artichoke hearts, 14 oz. (396 g) can
- [ ] baking powder, 4 tsp.
- [ ] baking soda, 2½ tsp.
- [ ] coconut cream, 5.4 oz. (160 ml) can
- [ ] coconut milk, 3 cans (13.5 oz. [398 ml] each)
- [ ] raisins, ½ cup (85 g)
- [ ] unsweetened shredded coconut, 2 cups (225 g)
- [ ] vanilla extract, 2 Tbsp. + 1 tsp.
- [ ] walnuts, chopped, 3¾ cups (430 g)

Fats, Oils, and Vinegars

- [ ] avocado oil, ¼ cup (60 ml)
- [ ] coconut oil, 1½ cups (300 g) + 2 Tbsp.
- [ ] cooking oil, 1½ Tbsp.
- [ ] olive oil, ¼ cup (60 ml)
- [ ] vinegar, 1 Tbsp. + 1 tsp.

Dried Herbs and Spices

- [ ] bay leaves, 5
- [ ] cinnamon, 2 Tbsp. + 1½ tsp.
- [ ] dried tarragon, 1 tsp.
- [ ] nutmeg, 2 tsp.
- [ ] pepper, to taste
- [ ] salt, 4 Tbsp. + 1¼ tsp.

Appendix B

Packed Lunches for Kids

The majority of your kids' lunches should be comprised of leftovers. Although many of the meals described in this book pack well, not all of them do. It's very important to buy a leak-proof lunch box, which will guarantee flexibility and freedom when it comes to what you pack. Refer to the sidebar *Lunch Boxes for Whole-Food Meals* on page 40 for lunch box recommendations.

I spent quite a bit of time researching packed lunch ideas for kids and I was disappointed by the lack of protein options and the excess of carbohydrates. Kids need balanced lunches. Try to refrain from loading their lunch box with fruit, muffins, crackers, pastas, and breads, even if those are their favorite foods. If they have the option to eat something, chances are they'll at least try it. If you find they're avoiding a certain food day after day, take a break from it for a few days, but don't give up hope that they won't develop a taste for it later! Lunches (and snacks, for that matter) that are heavily loaded with carbohydrates won't provide your child with the energy, stamina, and brainpower to successfully and gracefully make it through the school day. Try to shift your focus to healthy fats and proteins, and then fill in the gaps with those beloved carbs, in healthier forms.

The meal plans assume that dinner leftovers will be served for lunch, but there are the rare instances when

serving a leftover may be challenging. For example, you may not be able to easily pack the White Bean, Fennel, and Sausage Stew prepared during the second week's plan unless you have a thermos for keeping the soup warm. Save the soup for the weekend when it's easier to reheat. Instead, pack a meal for the kids using a different leftover dinner.

Another strategy for packing a lunch in a pinch, or when leftovers won't suffice, is to keep a few easy lunch options on hand. Try store-bought wraps made from coconut meat (coconut wraps) with natural deli meats, organic chips, and raw vegetables. Other quick options include tuna salad, sardines, and Hard-Boiled Eggs. Foods like the Plantain Muffins, Carrot Cake Applesauce Muffins, Plantain Blender Pancakes, Grilled Chicken Breasts with Basil and Thyme, Mexican Shredded Beef, and Perfectly Baked Bacon are examples of recipes that can be easily frozen. See *Recipes That Freeze Well*, page 285. Simply create lunch-sized portions of these foods and store them in the freezer for times when you need a few extra items to pack for the kids. Transfer those items to the refrigerator the night before and they'll be ready to serve by lunchtime the following day.

Green smoothies are another quick option when you need to fill a lunch box with a nutritious food. You can buy refillable baby food pouches or squeeze

Foods That Pack Well for School Lunches

PROTEINS	SIDES	BREADS/MUFFINS
Hard-Boiled Eggs	Summer Cucumber and Tomato Salad	Hearty Almond Flour Bread
"Pasta" Bowls	Everyday Salad with choice of dressing	Plantain Sandwich Bread
Simple Egg Salad	Grilled Zucchini and Yellow Squash	Carrot Cake Applesauce
The Tuna Salad Upgrade	Roasted Non-Starchy Vegetables	Muffins
Simple Whole Roasted Chicken	Grain-Free Tabbouleh	Plantain Muffins (with Pecan
Pulled Mojo Chicken	Roasted Brussels Sprouts with Bacon	Bread Variation)
Grilled Chicken Breasts with	Coconut Lime Cauliflower Rice	Plantain Blender Pancakes
Basil and Thyme	Coconut and Cinnamon Sweet Potato Mash	Banana Nut Bread
Grilled Chicken Salad with	Roasted Roots	
Fresh Vegetables	Dilly Sweet Potato Salad	**DIPS AND FILLERS**
OMGrain-Free Chicken Tenders	Kobocha Casserole with Pecans	Garlicky Guacamole
Herbed Beef Burgers	Cold-Pack Dill Pickles	Avocado-Mango Salsa
Mexican Shredded Beef	Basily Carrots	Fiesta Sunflower Seed Hummus
Cottage Pie	Dilly Beans	Apple Walnut Crisp Cereal
Perfectly Baked Bacon	Apple Cinnamon Smoothie	Superfoods Trail Mix
Deviled Eggs	Peanut Butter and Banana Smoothie	Coconut Cream Goji Bites
Turkey Cucumber Rolls	My Favorite Mango Smoothie	Roasted and Salted Walnuts

pouches that hold anywhere from four to eight ounces of food. Prepare the green smoothie recipe as instructed, divide it among however many pouches you have, and freeze them as quick additions to lunch boxes. Be sure to show your children how to mash and shake the pouches a bit to ensure that the ingredients get mixed together (a small amount of separation can occur after freezing). Alternatively, you can purchase insulated, spill-proof water bottles with larger straws that will easily hold a green smoothie.

The following lunch suggestions are built using many of the recipes in this book, but some incorporate easy, quick, and healthy components that can be thrown together when leftovers aren't available. You'll have to plan ahead for some of these components, being sure to add the ingredients to your meal

plan, while other components can be thrown together with items that should already be stocked in your pantry and freezer. If you're trying to maximize your time efficiency in the kitchen, then it's also a good idea to plan dinners around foods you know will pack well. These strategies will all feel more natural the longer you cook from this book, and as you develop an intuitive meal plan catered to your schedule and preference.

LUNCH 1

Sliced Grilled Chicken Breasts with
  Basil and Thyme
Small Everyday Salad with dressing of choice
Carrot Cake Applesauce Muffins
Olives or nuts and seeds

LUNCH 2

Turkey Cucumber Rolls
Sliced raw vegetables with Fiesta
    Sunflower Seed Hummus
Plantain Muffins
Olives or nuts and seeds
Grape tomatoes

LUNCH 3

Hard-Boiled Eggs or Deviled Eggs
Small Everyday Salad with
    dressing of choice
Apple slices
Nut or seed butter

LUNCH 4

Turkey sandwich made from
    Plantain Sandwich Bread,
organic deli meats, lettuce,
    Homemade Mayonnaise,
    and mustard
Sliced raw vegetables with Fiesta
    Sunflower Seed Hummus
Applesauce or fruit

LUNCH 5

The Tuna Salad Upgrade
Dilly Sweet Potato Salad
Coconut Cream Goji Bites
Sliced raw vegetables

LUNCH 6

Grilled Chicken Salad with
    Fresh Vegetables
Red and Yellow Rosemary
    Potatoes

Small Everyday Salad with
    choice of dressing
Coconut Cream Goji Bites

LUNCH 7

Pulled Mojo Chicken
Garlicky Guacamole
Pico de Gallo
Grain-free chips or
    Plantain Tortillas
Shredded romaine lettuce

LUNCH 8

Simple Egg Salad
Roasted Roots
Roasted Non-Starchy Vegetables
    (green beans or broccoli)
Superfoods Trail Mix

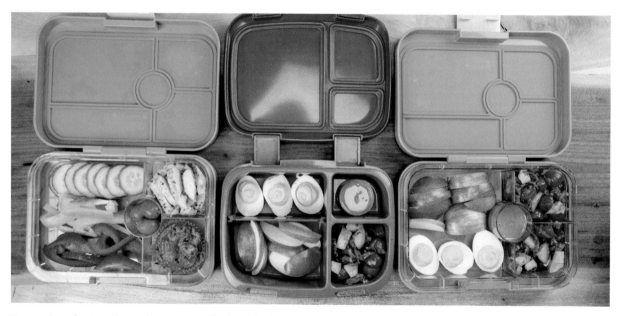

Suggestions for Lunch 1 and Lunch 3 are both packed in the Yumbox Tapas lunch box, and Lunch 2 is also packed in the Bentgo Fresh for comparison's sake. The two lunches pack similarly, but the dipper container in the Yumbox Tapas offers a space for the peanut butter while the Bentgo Fresh required the use of an additional container.

Appendix C

Holiday Meals and Healthy Celebrations

Holidays are not an excuse to throw a healthy diet to the wayside and fall deep into the junk food trap. Holidays are supposed to be a time when we get a break from the day-to-day so that we can rejuvenate and feel refreshed. I don't know about you, but "refreshed" is not how I feel after eating a boatload of unhealthy meals. So that I can use holidays as a time to truly recharge, I select a number of healthy foods for my family and friends to enjoy.

I provide two different meal plans to serve to your family and guests during most any celebration, whether that be a birthday, Christmas, Hanukkah, New Year's, Thanksgiving, or Easter. I've included a few holiday-specific foods in the section *Snacks and Smaller Meals* (page 169), such as the Apple Slice Monsters and the Strawberry Santas. Every family has their own traditions, so hopefully these plans can be catered to meet your own needs. For example, my family has established the tradition of celebrating Christmas Day with a smorgasbord of finger and snack foods. I select one or two healthy desserts that we'll also enjoy, and we spend the day munching away. Thanksgiving is a bit more traditional in that we celebrate with a large, sit-down meal. Both of these plans take quite a bit of prep work, so I like to start preparing a day or two in advance, which is not uncommon for large holiday meals.

Snacks and Appetizers

Every food in this plan is a finger food, which makes for a fun and easy afternoon of celebration interjected with frequent snacking. This seems to work particularly well for young kids who are often too busy to eat a full meal. Be sure to give yourself plenty of prep time for the fermented vegetables (Basily Carrots and Dilly Beans) and the Cold-Pack Dill Pickles. These need to be started at least a week in advance.

FINGER FOODS

Deviled Eggs
Bacon-Bundled Green Beans
Turkey Cucumber Rolls
Large tray of sliced mixed vegetables for dipping
Roasted and Salted Walnuts
Cold-Pack Dill Pickles
Basily Carrots
Dilly Beans
Organic sweet potato chips

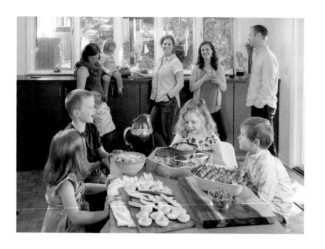

Traditional Sit-Down Dinner

I haven't included a recipe for a Thanksgiving turkey in this book, but you can easily find one online if you prefer turkey over chicken. If you use a turkey, you'll want to double the amount of vegetables used to prepare the Grain-Free Gravy since a turkey is so much larger than a whole chicken.

THE FEAST

Simple Whole Roasted Chicken (2 total; or 1 turkey)
Grain-Free Gravy
Everyday Salad: spinach, red onion, shaved fennel, and walnuts
Fresh Basil and Garlic Balsamic Vinaigrette
Roasted Brussels Sprouts with Bacon
Kobocha Casserole with Pecans
Red and Yellow Rosemary Potatoes

DESSERT

Apple Spice Bundt Cake
Pumpkin Pie with Hazelnut Crust
Coconut Whipped Cream

BEVERAGES

Hibiscus Zinger Iced Tea
Hot tea of your choice

DIP SELECTION

Garlicky Guacamole
Sun-Dried Tomato Tapenade
Fiesta Sunflower Seed Hummus
    (or another store-bought variety)

SWEET TREATS

Lemon Coconut Date Balls
Chocolate Walnut Brownies

BEVERAGES

Infused Water
Hot tea of your choice

Appendix D

Recipes That Freeze Well

EVERYDAY BASICS

Beef Stock

Chicken Stock

Homemade Lard or Tallow

Pecan Parmesan "Cheese"

Saving Excess Fat from Cooked Meats

Simple Spaghetti Squash

BREAKFASTS AND "BREADS"

Apple Walnut Crisp Cereal

Asparagus and Mushroom Quiche with
    Almond Flour Crust

Banana Nut Bread

Carrot Cake Applesauce Muffins

Cauliflower-Sausage Breakfast Casserole
    (prepared dish or cooked sausage only)

Eat Your Greens Frittata

Hearty Almond Flour Bread

Perfectly Baked Bacon

Plantain Blender Pancakes

Plantain Muffins with
    Pecan Bread Variation

Probiotic Pork and Vegetables

Sage and Rosemary Sausage Patties
    (best frozen raw)

Spaghetti Squash Porridge

MAIN COURSES

Cottage Pie (stuffing or whole pie)

Garlic and Cumin Slow Roast with Napa Cabbage

Grilled Chicken Breasts with Basil and Thyme

Flavorful Turkey Burgers (freeze raw)

Herb-Encrusted Drumsticks

Herbed Beef Burgers (freeze raw)

Mexican Shredded Beef

OMGrain-Free Chicken Tenders

Pulled Mojo Chicken

Simple Whole Roasted Chicken

Turmeric-Ginger Baked Chicken

VEGETABLE SIDES AND SALADS

Coconut and Cinnamon Sweet Potato Mash

Garlicky Greens

Kobocha Casserole with Pecans
    (prepared dish or cooked squash only)

Red and Yellow Rosemary Potatoes
    (reheat in the oven)

Roasted Roots (reheat in the oven)

SOUPS AND STEWS

40-Minute Beef Stew

Apple Butternut Soup

Black Bean and Vegetable Soup

Chicken and Vegetable Coconut Curry Soup
Chicken Noodle Soup (without the noodles)
Creamy Carrot Ginger Soup
Creamy Cauliflower Soup
Not Quite Your Mama's Chili
White Bean, Fennel, and Sausage Stew

SNACKS AND SMALLER MEALS
Bacon Liver Pâté
Coconut Cream Goji Bites
"Pasta" Bowls
Roasted and Salted Walnuts
Superfoods Trail Mix

SAUCES, DIPS, AND DRESSINGS
Chimichurri Sauce
Fresh Basil and Garlic Balsamic Vinaigrette
Grain-Free Gravy
Hearty Meat Bolognese
Italian Dressing
Red Wine Lemon Vinaigrette
Simple Vegan Pesto
Sun-Dried Tomato Tapenade
Thai Peanut Sauce

SMOOTHIES AND OTHER DRINKS
Apple Cinnamon Smoothie
Bedtime Tea
Homemade Almond Milk
My Favorite Mango Smoothie
Peanut Butter and Banana Smoothie
Sweet-Tooth-Zapping Banana Milkshake
Tropical Paradise Smoothie
Truly Green Smoothie
Tummy Ache Tea
Vanilla Strawberry Beet Smoothie
Winter Immunity Tea

SWEET TREATS
Apple Spice Bundt Cake
Chocolate Banana Cupcakes
Chocolate Ice Cream
Chocolate Icing
Chocolate Walnut Brownies
Chocolate Walnut Freezer Fudge
Creamy Fruit Pops
Lemon Coconut Date Balls
Nut-Free Chocolate Superfood Bites
Pumpkin Pie with Hazelnut Crust

resources

WEBSITES

Chris Kresser: www.chriskresser.com

Chris Masterjohn, PhD: www.chrismasterjohnphd.com

Dr. Mark Hyman: www.drhyman.com

Environmental Working Group: www.ewg.org

Institute for Responsible Technology:
www.responsibletechnology.org

Mother Earth News: www.motherearthnews.com

Paleo Leap: www.paleoleap.com

The Paleo Mom, Sarah Ballantyne, PhD:
www.thepaleomom.com

The Weston A. Price Foundation: www.westonaprice.org

BOOKS

Campbell-McBride, Natasha. *Gut and Psychology Syndrome: Natural Treatment for Autism, Dyspraxia, A.D.D., Dyslexia, A.D.H.D., Depression, Schizophrenia.* York, PA: Medinform Publishing, 2015.

Davis, William. *Wheat Belly.* New York: Rodale, Inc., 2011.

Fallon Morell, Sally, and Thomas Cowan. *The Nourishing Traditions Book of Baby & Child Care.* Washington, DC: New Trends Publishing, Inc., 2013.

Fallon, Sally, and Mary Enig. *Nourishing Traditions: The Cookbook That Challenges Politically Correct Nutrition and the Diet Dictocrats.* Washington, DC: New Trends Publishing, Inc., 2001.

Fraker, Cheri, et al. *Food Chaining: The Proven 6-Step Plan to Stop Picky Eating, Solve Feeding Problems, and Expand Your Child's Diet.* Cambridge, MA: Da Capo Lifelong Books, 2007.

Katz, Sandor. *The Art of Fermentation.* White River Junction, VT: Chelsea Green Publishing, 2012.

Katz, Sandor. *Wild Fermentation.* White River Junction, VT: Chelsea Green Publishing, 2016.

Know, Lee. *Michochondria and the Future of Medicine.* White River Junction, VT: Chelsea Green Publishing, 2017.

Morstein, Mona. *Mastering Your Diabetes.* White River Junction, VT: Chelsea Green Publishing, 2017.

Perlmutter, David. *Grain Brain: The Surprising Truth about Wheat, Carbs, and Sugar—Your Brain's Silent Killers.* New York: Little, Brown and Company, 2013.

Perro, Michelle, and Vincanne Adams. *What's Making Our Children Sick?* White River Junction, VT: Chelsea Green Publishing, 2017.

Pitchford, Paul. *Healing with Whole Foods: Asian Traditions and Modern Nutrition*, 3rd ed. Berkeley, CA: North Atlantic Books, 2002.

Pollan, Michael. *In Defense of Food: An Eater's Manifesto.* New York: The Penguin Press, 2008.

notes

CHAPTER 1:
THE RESTRICTIVE DIET FOR OPTIMAL HEALTH

1. University of California Los Angeles Newsroom, "This Is Your Brain on Sugar."
2. K. Yaffe et al., "Diabetes, Glucose Control, and 9-Year Cognitive Decline among Older Adults without Dementia."
3. M. Lenoir et al., "Intense Sweetness Surpasses Cocaine Reward."
4. Anthony Samsel and Stephanie Seneff, "Glyphosate, Pathways to Modern Diseases II."
5. Pavel Grasgruber et al., "Food Consumption and the Actual Statistics of Cardiovascular Diseases."
6. Pavel Grasgruber et al., "Food Consumption and the Actual Statistics of Cardiovascular Diseases."
7. R. De Sousa et al., "Intake of Saturated Trans Unsaturated Fatty Acids and Risk of All Cause Mortality, Cardiovascular Disease, and Type 2 Diabetes."
8. Sarah Ballantyne, "Why Grains Are Bad: Part 3, Nutrient Density and Acidity."
9. David S. Ludwig and Walter C. Willett, "Three Daily Servings of Reduced-Fat Milk: An Evidence-Based Recommendation?"
10. Lenard I. Lesser et al., "Relationship between Funding Source and Conclusion among Nutrition-Related Scientific Articles."
11. R. J. Scharf et al., "Longitudinal Evaluation of Milk Type Consumed and Weight Status in Preschoolers."
12. C. S. Berkey et al., "Milk, Dairy Fat, Dietary Calcium, and Weight Gain."
13. K. Dahl-Jorgensen, "Relationship between Cows' Milk Consumption and Incidence of IDDM in Childhood."
14. Duff Wilson, "Harvard Medical School in Ethics Quandary."

bibliography

Ahmed, S. H., K. Guillem, and Y. Vandaele. "Sugar Addiction: Pushing the Drug-Sugar Analogy to the Limit." *Current Opinion in Clinical Nutrition and Metabolic Care* 16, no. 4 (July 2013): 434–439.

Allbritton, Jen. "Wheaty Indiscretions: What Happens to Wheat, from Seed to Storage." Accessed May 22, 2017. www.westonaprice.org/health-topics/modern-foods /wheaty-indiscretions-what-happens-to-wheat-from -seed-to-storage.

Ballantyne, Sarah. "Are All Lectins Bad? (And What Are Lectins, Anyway?)" Accessed May 2, 2017. www .thepaleomom.com/lectins-bad.

Ballantyne, Sarah. "Olive Oil Redemption: Yes, It's a Great Cooking Oil!" Accessed Feb. 22, 2018. www.thepaleomom .com/olive-oil-redemption-yes-its-a-great-cooking-oil.

Ballantyne, Sarah. "The Great Dairy Debate." Accessed April 22, 2017. www.thepaleomom.com/the-great-dairy-debate.

Ballantyne, Sarah. "Why Grains Are Bad—Part 1: Lectins and the Gut." Accessed May 2, 2017. www.thepaleomom .com/why-grains-are-bad.

Ballantyne, Sarah. "Why Grains Are Bad—Part 2: Omega 3 vs. 6 Fats." Accessed May 2, 2017. www.thepaleomom .com/why-grains-are-bad-for-you-part-2.

Ballantyne, Sarah. "Why Grains Are Bad—Part 3: Nutrient Density and Acidity." Accessed May 2, 2017. www .thepaleomom.com/how-do-grains-legumes-and -dairy-cause.

Berkey, C. S., H. R. Rockett, W. C. Willett, and G. A. Colditz. "Milk, Dairy Fat, Dietary Calcium, and Weight Gain: A Longitudinal Study of Adolescents." *Archives of Pediatric and Adolescent Medicine* 159, no. 6 (June 2005): 543–550.

Bethene Ervin, R., Brian K. Kit, Margaret D. Carroll, and Cynthia L. Ogden. "Consumption of Added Sugar Among U.S. Children and Adolescents, 2005–2008." *National Center for Health Statistics Data Brief* no. 87 (2012). Accessed May 2. www.cdc.gov/nchs/data /databriefs/db87.pdf.

Bock, Kenneth, and Cameron Stauth. *Healing the New Childhood Epidemics: Autism, ADHD, Asthma, and Allergies*. New York: Random House Publishers, 2008.

Campbell-McBride, Natasha. *Gut and Psychology Syndrome: Natural Treatment for Autism, Dyspraxia, A.D.D., Dyslexia, A.D.H.D., Depression, Schizophrenia*. York, PA: Medinform Publishing, 2015.

Campbell, T. Colin, and Thomas M. Campbell II. *The China Study: The Most Comprehensive Study of Nutrition Ever Conducted and the Startling Implications for Diet, Weight Loss and Long-Term Health*. Dallas: BenBella Books, Inc., 2006.

Center for the Science in the Public Interest. "43% of Products Marketed to Kids Are Artificially Dyed, Study Finds." Accessed Feb. 20, 2017. https://cspinet.org/new /201606131.html.

Centers for Disease Control and Prevention. "Adult Obesity Facts." Accessed May 3, 2017. www.cdc.gov /obesity/data/adult.html.

Centers for Disease Control and Prevention. "Diabetes Report Card 2014." Accessed May 2, 2017. www .cdc.gov/diabetes/pdfs/library/diabetesreportcard 2014.pdf.

Centers for Disease Control and Prevention. "Leading Causes of Death." Accessed May 15, 2017. www.cdc.gov /nchs/fastats/leading-causes-of-death.htm.

Colbin, Annemarie. *The Whole-Food Guide to Strong Bones: A Holistic Approach.* Oakland, CA: New Harbinger Publications, Inc., 2009.

Cornell University Extension Toxicology Network. "Pesticide Information Profile: Pyrethrins." Accessed Jan. 10, 2018. http://pmep.cce.cornell.edu/profiles/extoxnet/pyrethrins-ziram/pyrethrins-ext.html.

Cornell University Extension Toxicology Network. "Pesticide Information Profile: Rotenone." Accessed Jan. 10, 2018. http://pmep.cce.cornell.edu/profiles/extoxnet/pyrethrins-ziram/rotenone-ext.html.

D'Adamo, E. and Sonia Caprio. "Type 2 Diabetes in Youth: Epidemiology and Pathophysiology." *Diabetes Care* 34, suppl. 2 (May 2011): S161–S165.

Dahl-Jorgensen, K., G. Joner, and K. F. Hanssen. "Relationship between Cows' Milk Consumption and Incidence of IDDM in Childhood." *Diabetes Care* 14, no. 11 (Nov. 1991): 1081–1083.

Davis, William. *Wheat Belly.* New York: Rodale, Inc., 2011.

De Sousa, R., A. Mente, A. Maroleanu, A. Cozma, V. Ha, T. Kishibe, E. Uleryk, P. Budylowski, H. Schunemann, J. Beyene, and S. Anand. "Intake of Saturated Trans Unsaturated Fatty Acids and Risk of All Cause Mortality, Cardiovascular Disease, and Type 2 Diabetes: Systematic Review and Meta-Analysis of Observational Studies." *The BMJ* 351 (Feb. 2015): h3978.

Deming, D. M., K. C. Reidy, M. K. Fox, R. R. Briefel, E. Jacquier, and A. L. Eldridge. "Cross-Sectional Analysis of Eating Patterns and Snacking in the US Feeding Infants and Toddlers Study 2008." *Public Health Nutrition* 20 (March 2017): 1–9.

Ebbeling, Cara B., Janis F. Swain, Henry A. Feldman, William W. Wong, David L. Hachey, Erica Garcia-Lago, and David S. Ludwig. "Effects of Dietary Composition on Energy Expenditure during Weight-Loss Maintenance." *Journal of the American Medical Association* 307, no. 24 (June 2012): 2627–2634.

Egli, I., L. Davidsson, M. A. Juillerat, D. Barclay, and R. F. Hurrell. "The Influence of Soaking and Germination on the Phytase Activity and Phytic Acid Content of Grains and Seeds Potentially Useful for Complementary Feeding." *Journal of Food Science* 67, no. 9 (Nov. 2002): 3484–3488.

Emory Health Sciences. "High-Fructose Diet in Adolescence May Exacerbate Depressive-Like Behavior." *Science Daily* (Nov. 18, 2014). www.sciencedaily.com/releases/2014/11/141118141852.htm.

Environmental Working Group. "EWG's 2017 Shopper's Guide to Pesticides in Produce™: Clean Fifteen." Accessed Jan. 12, 2018. www.ewg.org/foodnews/clean-fifteen.php.

Environmental Working Group. "EWG's 2017 Shopper's Guide to Pesticides in Produce™: Dirty Dozen." Accessed Jan. 12, 2018. www.ewg.org/foodnews/dirty-dozen.php.

Fallon Morell, Sally, and Thomas Cowan. *The Nourishing Traditions Book of Baby & Child Care.* Washington, DC: New Trends Publishing, Inc., 2013.

Food and Agriculture Organization of the United Nations. "Part 3: Feeding the World." Accessed on May 12, 2017. www.fao.org/docrep/018/i3107e/i3107e03.pdf.

Fraker, Cheri, et al. *Food Chaining: The Proven 6-Step Plan to Stop Picky Eating, Solve Feeding Problems, and Expand Your Child's Diet.* Cambridge, MA: Da Capo Lifelong Books, 2007.

Grasgruber, Pavel, Martin Seberea, Eduard Hrazdira, Sylva Hrebickova, and Jan Cacek. "Food Consumption and the Actual Statistics of Cardiovascular Diseases: An Epidemiological Comparison of 42 European Countries." *Food and Nutrition Research* 60 (Sept. 2016): 10.3402/fnr.v60.31694. Accessed Feb. 18, 2018. www.ncbi.nlm.nih.gov/pmc/articles/PMC5040825.

Harvard Health Publishing, Harvard Medical School. "The Truth about Fats: The Good, the Bad, and the In-Between." Accessed Feb. 22, 2018. www.health.harvard.edu/staying-healthy/the-truth-about-fats-bad-and-good.

Ho, M. H., W. H. Wong, and C. Chang. "Clinical Spectrum of Food Allergies: A Comprehensive Review." *Clinical Reviews in Allergy and Immunology* 46, no. 3 (June 2014): 225–240.

Hyman, Mark. "Got Proof? Lack of Evidence for Milk's Benefits." Accessed April 25, 2017. http://drhyman.com /blog/2013/07/05/got-proof-lack-of-evidence-for -milks-benefits.

Hyman, Mark. "Milk Is Dangerous for Your Health." Accessed April 23, 2017. http://drhyman.com/blog /2013/10/28/milk-dangerous-health.

Institute for Responsible Technology. "Appendix 2: Glyphosate Bans and Restrictions across the Globe." Accessed April 26, 2017. http://responsibletechnology .org/irtnew/wp-content/uploads/2016/01/2-Glyphosate -Bans-and-Restrictions-Across-the-Globe.pdf.

Institute for Responsible Technology. "State-of-the-Science on the Health Risks of GM Foods." Accessed Jan. 11, 2018. https://responsibletechnology.org/irtne w/docs/state_science_gmo.pdf.

Jimenez, P., P. Garcia, A. Bustamante, A. Barriga, and P. Robert. "Thermal Stability of Oils Added with Avocado (*Persea americana* cv. Hass) or Olive (*Olea europaea* cv. Arbequina) Leaf Extracts during the French Potatoes Frying." *Food Chemistry* 221 (April 2017): 123–129.

Ji, Sayer. "Opening Pandora's Bread Box: The Critical Role of Wheat Lectin in Human Disease." Accessed June 1, 2017. www.greenmedinfo.com/page/opening-pandoras -bread-box-critical-role-wheat-lectin-human-disease.

Kresser, Chris. "Why Your Genes Aren't Your Destiny." Accessed June 2, 2017. https://chriskresser.com /why-your-genes-arent-your-destiny.

Landreth, G. E., L. K. Williams, and C. McCutchen. "Wheat Germ Agglutinin Blocks the Biological Effects of Nerve Growth Factor." *Journal of Cell Biology* 101 (Nov. 1985): 1690–1694.

Lenoir, M., Fuschia Serre, Lauriane Cantin, and Serge H. Ahmed. "Intense Sweetness Surpasses Cocaine Reward." *PLoS ONE* 8 (August 2007): e698.

Lesser, Lenard I., Cara B. Ebbeling, Merrill Goozner, David Wypij, and David S. Ludwig. "Relationship between Funding Source and Conclusion among Nutrition-Related Scientific Articles." *PLoS Medicine* 4, no. 1 (Jan. 2007): 41–46.

Ludwig, David S., and Walter C. Willett. "Three Daily Servings of Reduced-Fat Milk: An Evidence-Based Recommendation?" *JAMA Pediatrics* 167, no. 9 (Sept. 2013): 788–789.

Mayo Clinic. "Children's Nutrition: 10 Tips for Picky Eaters." Accessed on Feb. 16, 2018. www.mayoclinic. org/healthy-lifestyle/childrens-health/in-depth /childrens-health/art-20044948.

Monsanto. "Monsanto Receives Key Import Approval to Enable 2018 Launch of Vistive® Gold Soybean." Accessed Feb. 22, 2018. https://monsanto.com /spotlight/articles/monsanto-receives-key-import -approval-enable-2018-launch-vistive-gold-soybean.

Myers, John, Michael Antoniou, Bruce Blumberg, et al. "Concerns Over Use of Glyphosate-Based Herbicides and Risks Associated with Exposures: A Consensus Statement." *Environmental Health* 15 (2016): 19.

Nagel, Ramiel. "Living with Phytic Acid." Accessed May 2, 2017. www.westonaprice.org/health-topics /vegetarianism-and-plant-foods/living-with -phytic-acid.

Nestle, Marion. "Did the Low-Fat Era Make Us Fat?" *PBS Frontline*. Accessed May 12, 2017. www.pbs.org/wgbh /pages/frontline/shows/diet/themes/lowfat.html.

Paleo Leap. "What Is Wrong with Grains?" Accessed May 2, 2017. https://paleoleap.com/what-is-wrong-with-grains.

Perlmutter, David. *Grain Brain: The Surprising Truth about Wheat, Carbs, and Sugar—Your Brain's Silent Killers*. New York: Little, Brown and Company, 2013.

Pitchford, Paul. *Healing with Whole Foods: Asian Traditions and Modern Nutrition*, 3rd ed. Berkeley, CA: North Atlantic Books, 2002.

Pollan, Michael. *In Defense of Food: An Eater's Manifesto*. New York: The Penguin Press, 2008.

Rothamsted Research Archives. "Broadbalk Winter Wheat Experiment." Accessed April 22, 2017. www.era.rothamsted.ac.uk/index.php?area=home&page=index&dataset=4.

Roundup. *Preharvest Staging Guide*. Accessed April 28, 2017. https://usrtk.org/wp-content/uploads/2016/09/Monsanto-application-guide-for-preharvest.pdf.

Samsel, Anthony, and Stephanie Seneff. "Glyphosate, Pathways to Modern Diseases II: Celiac Sprue and Gluten Intolerance." *Interdisciplinary Toxicology* 6, no. 4 (2013): 159–184.

Samsel, Anthony, and Stephanie Seneff. "Glyphosate's Suppression of Cytochrome P450 Enzymes and Amino Acid Biosynthesis by the Gut Microbiome: Pathways to Modern Diseases." *Entropy* 15, no. 4 (2013): 1416–1463.

Scharf, R. J., R. T. Demmer, and M. D. DeBoer. "Longitudinal Evaluation of Milk Type Consumed and Weight Status in Preschoolers." *Archives of Disease in Childhood* 98 (2013): 335–340.

Taubes, Gary. *Why We Get Fat and What to Do about It*. New York: Anchor Books, 2010.

United States Department of Agriculture and United States Department of Health and Human Services. "Dietary Guidelines for Americans 2010." Accessed May 5, 2017. https://health.gov/dietaryguidelines/dga2010/DietaryGuidelines2010.pdf.

United States Department of Agriculture Economic Research Service. "Sugar Sweeteners Yearbook Tables." Accessed May 4, 2017. www.ers.usda.gov/data-products/sugar-and-sweeteners-yearbook-tables/sugar-and-sweeteners-yearbook-tables.

United States Department of Agriculture. "Wheat's Role in the U.S. Diet." Accessed May 2, 2017. www.ers.usda.gov/topics/crops/wheat/wheats-role-in-the-us-diet.

United States Food and Drug Administration. "Final Determination Regarding Partially Hydrogenated Oils (Removing Trans Fat)." Accessed on Feb. 22, 2018. www.fda.gov/Food/IngredientsPackagingLabeling/FoodAdditivesIngredients/ucm449162.htm.

University of California Los Angeles Newsroom. "This Is Your Brain on Sugar: UCLA Study Shows High-Fructose Diet Sabotages Learning, Memory." Accessed May 2, 2017. http://newsroom.ucla.edu/releases/this-is-your-brain-on-sugar-ucla-233992.

University of California San Francisco—Sugar Science. "Hidden in Plain Sight: Added Sugar Is Hiding in 74% of Packaged Foods." Accessed May 3, 2017. http://sugarscience.ucsf.edu/hidden-in-plain-sight/#.WoGLs5PwbBJ.

Vasconcelos, I. M., and J. T. Oliveira. "Antinutritional Properties of Plant Lectins." *Toxicon* 15, no. 44 (Sept. 2004): 385–403.

Wilson, Duff. "Harvard Medical School in Ethics Quandary." *New York Times* (March 2, 2009). Accessed May 3, 2017. https://archive.nytimes.com/www.nytimes.com/2009/03/03/business/03medschool.html.

World Health Organization. "Guideline: Sugars Intake for Adults and Children." Accessed May 8, 2017. http://apps.who.int/iris/bitstream/10665/149782/1/9789241549028_eng.pdf?ua=1.

Yaffe, K., C. Falvey, N. Hamilton, et al. "Diabetes, Glucose Control, and 9-Year Cognitive Decline among Older Adults without Dementia." *Archives of Neurology* 69, no. 9 (Sept. 2012): 1170–1175.

Ziegler, E. E. "Adverse Effects of Cow's Milk in Infants." *Nestlé Nutrition Workshop Series: Pediatric Program* 60 (2007): 185–196.

Zielger, P., R. Briefel, M. Ponza, T. Novak, and K. Hendricks. "Nutrient Intakes and Food Patterns of Toddlers' Lunches and Snacks: Influence of Location." *Journal of American Dietetic Association* 106, suppl. 1 (Jan. 2006): S124–S134.

recipe index

index

birthday celebrations, 39–40.
See also celebration and
holiday foods
black beans
in chili, 160–61
in vegetable soup, 158–59
blackberry-sage water, 215
blenders
children using, 37
cost of, 46
high-powered, 45–46, 47
for tube-fed meal
preparation, 46
Blendtec blender, 46
blood loss, occult intestinal, 23
blueberries, 26
in apple slice monsters, 178
body mass index
in cystic fibrosis, 31
and low-fat milk in diet, 23
bok choy and red peppers with
Thai peanut sauce, 133
Bolognese sauce with meat, 210
bone health
dairy products in, 20,
21–22, 27
minerals in, 8–9
pH affecting, 8–9
phytic acid affecting, 12
bone stock and broth, 22, 54
brain
fat in, 18
sugar affecting, 2, 9, 10–12
bran, 12
milling affecting, 16
phytic acid in, 12, 13
breads, 87–96
almond flour, 88
banana nut, 69, 96
pecan, 92–93
phytic acid in, 13
plantain sandwich, 89
wheat in, 16
breakfast, 69–96
meal planning for, 58, 60–61
menu suggestions for,
268–79
potatoes with rosemary in, 137
sweet potatoes in, 136
breast-feeding, 23, 25

brine for ferments, 236, 238–41
basic recipe for, 236
Broadbalk Winter Wheat
Experiment, 16–17
broccoli, 22
fermented, 236
roasted, 126
brownies, chocolate walnut, 260
brussels sprouts, 22
roasted, with bacon, 130
buckwheat, 12
budget-friendly solutions, 53–54
bulk purchases in, 49, 51,
53–54
vegetable gardening in,
50–51, 54
bulk purchases, 51, 53–54
of spices, 54
stocking pantry and freezer
with, 49
bundt cake, apple spice, 247, 263
burgers
beef, 114
turkey, 113
butternut soup with apples,
156–57
buying foods. *See* shopping

C
cabbage
fermented, 236, 242–45
in krauts, 242–45
napa, slow roasted beef with
garlic, cumin, and, 116–17
preparation tips, 132, 243
roasted wedges with
tahini-miso sauce, 132
cake, apple spice, 247, 263
calcium
and bone health, 8, 21–22
phytic acid binding with, 12
sources of, 22
Campbell-McBride, Natasha, 32
cancer, glyphosate affecting risk
for, 17
candy, 30, 38, 39
canola oil, 19
carbohydrates, 3
and cardiovascular disease
risk, 18

in grains, 12
cardiovascular disease, 3, 18, 27
carrots
with basil, 238–39
fermented, 236, 238–39
in muffins with applesauce,
87
roasted, 126, 138–39
in soup with ginger, 153
casein, 24
cassava flour
in apple spice cake, 263
in chocolate banana
cupcakes, 262
cast iron pans, 47
catnip in bedtime tea, 233
cauliflower
fermented, 236
hash browns, 77
riced, 128, 131
and sausage in breakfast
casserole, 73
in soup, creamy, 150–51
in tabbouleh, grain-free, 128
celebration and holiday foods,
39–40, 67, 283–84
apple slice monsters, 178
apple spice bundt cake,
247, 263
banana snowmen, 177
chocolate banana cupcakes,
262
lemon coconut date balls, 257
outside of school and
home, 42
in schools, 38–39
strawberry santas, 175
Center for Science in the Public
Interest, 29
Centers for Disease Control
and Prevention, 9
CFTR protein in cystic
fibrosis, 6–7
chamomile in bedtime tea, 233
change to healthier diet, 43–54
taking small steps in, 43–44
time required for, 44–45
chicken, 102–12
baked, with turmeric and
ginger, 109

budget-friendly, 54
in coconut curry soup with
vegetables, 164–65
and gravy, 212
grilled breasts in salad with
fresh vegetables, 108
grilled breasts with basil and
thyme, 104–5, 108
herb-encrusted drumsticks,
112
leftover, uses of, 57
in pasta bowls, 187
pulled mojo, 103
tenders, grain-free, 110–11,
133
in turnip noodle soup,
166–67
whole roasted, 102, 212
chicken stock, 54, 102, 112,
152, 154
children, 29–42
cystic fibrosis in, 8, 31–32,
33, 34
dairy intake of, 22–23, 24–25
diabetes in, 10, 29, 32, 38
eating away from home,
38–42
eating new foods, 23, 33–36
food intolerances and
allergies in, 23
in food preparation, 35, 36–38
foods marketed to, 29–31
GAPS diet in, 32–33, 34
healthy eating habits in, 33–36
loving nourishment of, 31–32
obesity in, 9
phytic acid in diet of, 12
as picky eaters, 31–32, 33–36
sugar intake of, 3, 4, 9, 29, 30,
38–39
chili, 40, 54, 160–61
chimichurri sauce, 198
The China Study, 24, 25
chocolate
in brownies with walnuts, 260
in cupcakes with bananas, 262
in fudge with walnuts, 250–51
hot beverage, date-sweet-
ened, 220
ice cream, 259

about the author

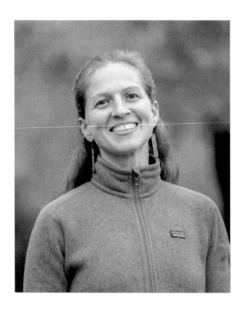

Leah M. Webb, MPH, CHC, obtained her health coach certification from the Institute for Integrative Nutrition after earning a bachelor of science degree in environmental biology from Appalachian State University and a master of public health degree in environmental health sciences from Georgia Southern University. She has worked in nutrition and gardening education since 2009 with a focus on engaging children in healthy eating habits through experiential learning and discovery. Leah started and runs the Deep Rooted Wellness blog, on which she posts stories and tips regarding nutrition, gardening, and healthy families. Leah lives in the mountains of North Carolina with her husband, T. C., and her two children, Owen and June. Owen has a life-threatening anaphylactic allergy to wheat, and June has cystic fibrosis, a genetic disease severely impacting the lungs and pancreas. Leah's commitment to a restrictive, nutrient-dense diet has played an important role in her children's integrative care. When not at work, you'll find Leah in her garden, tending to her chickens, volunteering in her children's schools, or engaging in a variety of forms of exercise that feel nourishing.